The authors wish to advise people of Aboriginal and Torres Strait Islander descent, that this book contains names and images of persons who are now deceased.

We wish to thank the following Warlpiri people whose photographs appear in the book. We have been unable to find all Warlpiri names listed at this stage.

Tilo Nangala, Rosie Nangala Fleming, Nell Nangala, Lydia Nangala Samson, Jimmy Jungarrayi Spencer, Jillie Nakamarra Spencer, Candy Napaljarri, Judy Nampijinpa Granites, Wikija Nampijinpa, Portia Napanangka, Nigel Japangardi, Renee Napangardi Marshall, Lynette Nampijinpa Daniels, Johnny Wayne Jungarrayi, Janey Napanangka Langdon, Gracey Napangardi, Michael Nelson Jakamarra, Jeannine Nungarrayi Egan, Anthony Jampijinpa Egan, Raelene Napurrurla Kennedy, Oscar Jungarrayi Wayne, Gavin Japaljarri Spencer, Alice Napanangka Granites, Chrissy Nampijinpa Fry, Bess Nungarrayi France, Clarrise Nampijinpa Fry, Violet Nampijinpa Brown, Harry Jakamarra Nelson, Jillie Nakamarra Spencer, Cindy Napaljarri, Wikija Nampijinpa, Renne Napangardi Marshall and Benjamin Japangadi.

If you are able to identify any of the un-identified people, please contact us at press@adelaide.edu.au

YUENDUMU
legacy of a longitudinal growth study in Central Australia

by
Tasman Brown
Grant C Townsend
Sandra K Pinkerton
James R Rogers

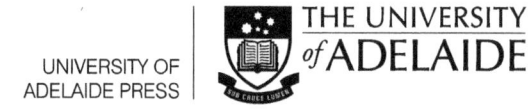

Published in Adelaide by

University of Adelaide Press
Barr Smith Library
The University of Adelaide
South Australia
5005
press@adelaide.edu.au
www.adelaide.edu.au/press

The University of Adelaide Press publishes externally refereed scholarly books by staff of the University of Adelaide. It aims to maximise the accessibility to its best research by publishing works through the internet as free downloads and as high quality printed volumes on demand.

Electronic Index: this book is available from the website as a down-loadable PDF with fully searchable text. Please use the electronic version to serve as the index.

© 2011 The Authors

This book is copyright. Apart from any fair dealing for the purposes of private study, research, criticism or review as permitted under the Copyright Act, no part may be reproduced, stored in a retrieval system, or transmitted, in any form or by any means, electronic, mechanical, photocopying, recording or otherwise without the prior written permission. Address all inquiries to the Director at the above address.

For the full Cataloguing-in-Publication data please contact National Library of Australia: cip@nla.gov.au

ISBN (electronic) 978-0-9870730-0-6
ISBN (paperback) 978-0-9807230-9-0

Book design: Céline Lawrence / John Emerson / Midland Typesetters
Cover design: Emma Spoehr. Photograph supplied by the authors.

Foreword

During my orthodontic training in the 1960s, like most orthodontists in that era, I was quite interested in Raymond Begg's presentation of the large dental arches and well-aligned teeth that are characteristic of Australian Aborigines. As it became possible to measure tongue and lip pressures against the teeth and relate them to the etiology of malocclusion, I thought it would be of considerable interest to evaluate intra-oral pressures in Australian Aboriginal people. That led to initial contact with Tas Brown and Murray Barrett at the University of Adelaide, and with their help I obtained a Fulbright fellowship to carry out such a study while on sabbatical leave from the University of Kentucky. With three children in tow, my wife and I travelled by ship to Sydney, and I cemented my reputation as an eccentric by continuing to Adelaide by train. When I got off the train wearing cowboy boots, I'm sure I was the strangest looking specimen of visiting professor the welcoming group had ever seen.

At that point the regular collection of growth data at Yuendumu was coming to an end, and a number of related studies already had been carried out there. With Murray Barrett as the expedition leader and David Parker and Leslie Reynolds to help, we sent my research equipment up to Alice Springs via train, flew up, rented a Land Rover, loaded it up and set out down the dirt track to Yuendumu. Sitting in what would have been the driver's seat in the US, I was asking myself how I had gotten into this mess long before we arrived. But it turned out very well. The fancy pressure recording equipment worked, Tom and Pat Fleming's hospitality was outstanding, the children at Yuendumu were very helpful (and appreciative of the Polaroid photos of themselves they got as a reward), and the data actually did shed some light on the equilibrium that determines tooth positions.

My experience was typical, not at all unique. As this book shows, a number of visitors with a research agenda were hosted at Yuendumu through the years, adding their contributions to the continuing effort of faculty at The University of Adelaide. This book is a valuable record of what was done there during the project. It pulls together the varied studies and puts them in perspective in a way that is likely to lead to further progress in understanding both the development of the dentition and facial/bodily development more generally. I'm pleased to have been a small part of the project, and delighted to have the opportunity to introduce the book.

William R. Proffit
Kenan Professor, Orthodontics
University of North Carolina School of Dentistry

Preface

This volume is about a special research project in Central Australia, the scientists from The University of Adelaide who were involved for many years and the Aboriginal children and adults who participated in the study. The project is unique for several reasons. Primarily, it concerned the dentitions and general growth of children from Yuendumu in the Northern Territory who researchers observed annually between 1951 and 1971. In contrast to a cross-sectional design, the value of longitudinal studies lies in a clearer insight into the range of variation in growth patterns between individuals and the extent of variations within the same individual over time. Although many longitudinal studies of modern European populations have been undertaken, there have been few opportunities for recording craniofacial and dental development in other groups. Moreover, such studies are extremely rare when the subjects are indigenous children growing up in an isolated community with limited but increasing contact with European society and customs. Although the field trips ceased in 1971, when Yuendumu was a vastly different community than it is today, ongoing data analysis continues to provide information of relevance, as it will in the future.

Records collected over the 20 years included measurements of the growing children, casts of their dentitions, radiographs and family data, all of which have provided an invaluable source of information about the Yuendumu population, their dental conditions and the growth patterns of the children. During this time 1717 sets of dental casts representing 446 subjects and serial records for 288 subjects were obtained. Many researchers have accessed this material - the principal investigators, postgraduate students and many scholars from overseas. To date, over 250 scientific publications have resulted from the Yuendumu project. In addition to observing dental development and craniofacial growth, the investigators were able to witness and record many of the customs and crafts of the Yuendumu people.

The first two chapters of this book are historical. They outline the foundations of the Yuendumu project with emphasis on the pioneer dental anthropologists who were active in South Australia during the early years of the 20th century. They also detail the events and personalities leading to the establishment of Yuendumu in 1946 and the beginning of the dental study in 1951. Chapters 3 and 4 deal with the field trips, the logistics entailed in prosecuting a long-term research project in the centre of Australia, and the methodology developed. Two further chapters summarise many of the outcomes of the project with emphasis on dental morphology, dental development, dental occlusion and craniofacial growth. A biographical chapter follows describing the team members, their relationship with the Warlbiri people and some of the visiting researchers who have worked at Yuendumu or in our Adelaide laboratory. Chapter 8 describes more recent initiatives in genetics, craniofacial imaging and tooth wear that developed from the methodology used in the Yuendumu studies. This chapter also considers the present health, both oral and general, of the Yuendumu Aboriginal people and looks at the benefits of the research as well as the future of human longitudinal growth studies in general.

Finally, a complete bibliography of publications and theses arising from the research is included, together with an Appendix that contains a list of overseas visitors in the Yuendumu study, new growth tables for Yuendumu children with known birthdates and a selection of photographs of Yuendumu and its people.

Tasman Brown
Grant C Townsend
Sandra K Pinkerton
James R Rogers

The University of Adelaide

Dedication

This book is dedicated to Thomas Draper Campbell and Murray James Barrett, and to the Warlpiri adults and children who participated in the Yuendumu Growth Study.

Photographic acknowledgments

All photographs in this book unless otherwise attributed are the property of

The Cranio-facial Biology Research Unit,
School of Dentistry,
The University of Adelaide

Acknowledgments

We gratefully acknowledge the substantial financial support from the United States Public Health Service Research Grant DE02034-07 from the National Institute of Dental Research, National Institute of Health, Bethesda, Maryland, which ensured the continuity of the longitudinal study, and grants from the Wenner-Gren Foundation for Anthropological Research, New York, the Australian Institute of Aboriginal Studies and Torres Strait Islanders, Canberra, and the University of Adelaide.

Approval for the study was granted by the Minister of Territories, the Administrator of the Northern Territory, the Director of Welfare and the Director of the Commonwealth Office of Education and Native Affairs prior to visiting Yuendumu.

We also acknowledge the support of the National Health and Medical Research Council and the University of Adelaide in the data analysis phase in the 1970s and 1980s.

Jolyon Fleming and Ted Egan, both of Alice Springs, permitted us to use tributes to Jolyon's father, the late Reverend Tom Fleming, in Chapter 7. Those were among the many forwarded to the late Pat Fleming after Tom's death in 1990.

The text and many illustrations in Chapters 5 and 6 are based on the English translation of Tasman Brown's chapter, 'Occlusal Development and Function in Australian Aboriginals' in *Ortopedia Funcional Dos Maxilares* by Dr Wilma A Simões of São Paulo, Brazil, and published by Livaria Santos Editoria. Our gratitude is extended to Dr Wilma Simões and Dr Rui M Santos for permission to use these extracts. Permission to use the aerial photograph of Yuendumu in Chapter 2 was given by the copyright owners OzOutback Internet Services.

We would also like to thank Dr Bruce Simmons, former General Manager of Central Australian Oral Health Services, for his very thoughtful comments that we have included in Chapter 8.

We would also like to thank Bess Nungarrayi Price and her husband Dave for reading and commenting on a draft of the book. Bess is chair of the Northern Territory Government's Indigenous Affairs Advisory Council and also a member of the Commonwealth Government's Advisory Group on Violence Against Women. Bess was one of the participants in the Yuendumu study.

The collaboration and administrative assistance by colleagues and staff, both present and past, of The University of Adelaide are gratefully acknowledged. We also thank Ms Karen Squires, Administrative Assistant, Craniofacial Biology and Dental Education Group, School of Dentistry for her secretarial assistance.

Tasman Brown
Grant C Townsend
Sandra K Pinkerton
James R Rogers

Contents

Foreword		v
Preface		vii
Dedication		ix
Photographic acknowledgments		ix
Acknowledgments		x
1	**The Yuendumu Project: Anthropological Foundations**	1
	Physical and Dental Anthropology	3
	Early expeditions 1923–1939	14
2	**Yuendumu and the Warlpiri: Early History**	23
	Location and meaning of the word Yuendumu	23
	Expansion and conflict associated with European settlement	24
	Conflict between European pastoral interests and Warlpiri needs	27
	Establishment of Yuendumu (Rock Hill Bore) Settlement in 1946	28
	Baptist ministry of the Reverend Tom and Pat Fleming	33
	Physical characteristics of the Warlpiri	34
3	**Yuendumu: The Longitudinal Project 1951–1960**	45
	Anthropology in Adelaide pre-Yuendumu	45
	Dental Anthropology at Yuendumu	47
	Expeditions and locations	52
	X-occlusion	54
	Organisation, equipment and supplies	59
	Impact of Barrett's visit to Scandinavia in 1960	65
4	**Yuendumu: The Longitudinal Project 1961–1971**	69
	Initial preparations	69
	The Warlpiri and their kinship system	71

	Life at the Settlement during the longitudinal study	73
	Water supplies	74
	Bore water content	76
	Changing food habits	77
	Aims of the project	78
	Studies in the early 1960s	79
	Age classification	81
	Dental genetics	82
	Annual trips	83
	The work schedule	86
	Subject identification	88
	Limitations of the study	89
	Transition to computers	91
	OSCAR	94
	Later development of computer systems	95
	The collection	95
5	**Occlusal Development and Function in the Warlpiri**	**101**
	Introduction	101
	Morphology of the dental arches	104
	Food habits and masticatory movements	107
	Development of occlusion	111
	Variations in tooth size	112
	Tooth size relationships	117
	Tooth size correlations	121
	Dental crown features	123
6	**Facial Growth Patterns in the Warlpiri**	**135**
	Mid-facial prognathism	136
	Lip and tongue pressures in relation to occlusion	147
	Tooth wear and continuously changing occlusion	151
	Occlusal function in the worn dentition	160
	Functions of tooth cusps	164
7	**People and Personalities Involved with the Project**	**171**
	International researchers	171
	Other interest from the USA	182
	The Adelaide researchers	184

	Other staff on the project	192
	At Yuendumu	194
	The Missionaries: Tom Fleming (1909–1990) and Pat Fleming (1914–1995)	195
	The Flemings and the dental teams	196
8	**The Past, the Present and the Future**	**207**
	The end of field trips to Yuendumu and the post-1970 years	207
	Research in the 1970s	213
	Oral health of Yuendumu Aboriginal people from the 1950s to the present day	225
	General health and oral health in Yuendumu Aboriginals at the present time	230
	Did the Aboriginal people at Yuendumu benefit from the research?	233
	The future of human longitudinal growth studies	236
9	**The Research Legacy: Publications, theses and films directly relating to the Yuendumu Study**	**249**
	Publications	249
	Theses	261
	Films	263
Appendices		**265**
	Appendix A	266
	Appendix B	267
	Appendix C	291

Tables and Figures

Figure 1.1	Team members about to depart on the first visit to Yuendumu in 1951. Murray Barrett, top right, is standing above Draper Campbell	2
Figure 1.2	William Ramsay Smith at work	5
Figure 1.3	Specimens from The Ramsay Smith Bequest	8
Figure 1.4	Thomas Draper Campbell	9
Figure 1.5	Campbell's first major publication in dental anthropology	11
Figure 1.6	Percy Raymond Begg in front of his portrait that is displayed on the fourth floor of the Adelaide Dental Hospital building	14
Table 1.1	Early expeditions by researchers from The University of Adelaide showing the trip prefix, year and location	15
Figure 1.7	Map showing the locations of field expeditions sponsored by The Board for Anthropological Research (redrawn after a map used by TD Campbell)	16
Figure 1.8	Early photograph of unidentified Aboriginal people by Campbell	17
Figure 1.9	Campbell and unidentified children – from the 1950s (courtesy of PG Dellow)	18
Figure 2.1	Aerial view of Yuendumu (courtesy of OzOutback Internet Services)	24
Figure 2.2	Yuendumu environs	29
Figure 2.3	Yuendumu environs – water and greenery in a good season	31
Figure 2.4	Camp dogs watching a kangaroo cooking	32
Figure 2.5	Unidentified Warlpiri children with a goanna	32
Figure 2.6	Professor Andrew A Abbie at Kalumburu, Western Australia, 1963	35
Table 2.1	Yuendumu subjects with recorded birthdates: distribution by sex and number of serial records	36
Table 2.2	Summary of selected variables measured in young adults from Yuendumu (recorded age = 20 years)	37

Table 2.3	Biological growth parameters derived by the Preece-Baines model 1 for Aboriginal children (PHV = peak height velocity)	39
Figure 2.7	Mean constant curves for height and height velocity in Warlpiri boys and girls	40
Figure 2.8	Unidentified Warlpiri man and woman showing distinctive facial characters	65
Figure 2.9	Unidentified Yuendumu schoolboys	41
Figure 3.1	Murray Barrett filming at Yuendumu	48
Figure 3.2	Murray Barrett examining Anthony Jampijinpa Egan with Jeannine Nungarrayi Egan watching	49
Figure 3.3	Murray Barrett obtaining dental impressions in the early 1950s	50
Figure 3.4	Children licking condensed milk from their fingers	51
Table 3.1	Expeditions to Yuendumu and other locations between the years 1951–1959	53
Figure 3.5	Dental casts of an adolescent Warlpiri male illustrating a normal, healthy and functional dentition	54
Figure 3.6	X–occlusion: dental models showing a) occlusion of the teeth on the right side only b) in the central position where there is no maximum posterior tooth contact on either side c) occlusion of teeth on the left side only	55
Figure 3.7	Murray Barrett taking a photograph of an unidentified girl's mouth with a helper retracting her lips	58
Figure 3.8	Murray Barrett preparing a movie camera to film the cooking of a kangaroo over a fire in the background	58
Figure 3.9	Murray Barrett recording an unidentified Warlpiri speaker	60
Figure 3.10	Murray Barrett examining an unidentified boy	61
Table 3.2	The list of supplies sent by rail and land transport to Yuendumu in 1953	62
Figure 4.1	A typical shelter on the outskirts of Yuendumu. A group of European-style houses, provided by the Welfare Branch, with verandahs and water tanks typical of the late 1960s, are in the background	71
Table 4.1	Spellings used for the Warlpiri kinship names	72
Figure 4.2	Inside a school room at Yuendumu during the 1950s	73
Figure 4.3	The Yuendumu water towers	75
Figure 4.4	An unidentified woman preparing damper and a child drinking from a bucket	76

Figure 4.5	Examples of dental fluorosis	77
Figure 4.6	Tom Fleming at the Yuendumu store	78
Figure 4.7	Instrument used for measuring arch breadth and depth on dental models during the 1960s	80
Table 4.2	Dental criteria for grouping subjects and dental code used for field sheets and computer input	81
Figure 4.8	Examples of anomalies of the anterior teeth showing missing and peg-shaped lateral incisors (A) and a supernumerary tooth (B)	82
Figure 4.9	Sandy Pinkerton and Murray Barrett	83
Table 4.3	Team members of the Yuendumu field trips 1961–1971	84
Figure 4.10	Pat Fleming with a class of pupils from Yuendumu School c1965	85
Figure 4.11	Murray Barrett obtaining a dental impression	87
Figure 4.12	Harry Jakamarra Nelson with his serial trip prefix and number	88
Figure 4.13	Senior dental student Harold Clarke producing dental models in the field at Yuendumu during the 1968 field expedition	90
Figure 4.14	Raelene Napurrula Kennedy, Oscar Jungarrayi Wayne, Gavin Japaljarri Spencer, Alice Napanangka Granites, Chrissy Nampijinpa Fry, Bess Nungarrayi France, Clarrise Nampijinpa Fry, Violet Nampijinpa Brown in line to participate	91
Figure 4.15	A typical punch card deck that was used for data processing by the only mainframe computer located on The University of Adelaide campus in the 1960s	93
Figure 4.16	OSCAR – the record reader, decimal converter and card punch used to output coordinate data. Manufactured by Computer Industries Inc., Van Nuys, California	94
Figure 4.17	Murray Barrett recording a group of Yuendumu school children	96
Figure 5.1	Unidentified juvenile and adult Warlpiri males showing characteristic facial morphology	104
Figure 5.2	Maxillary dental models of Aboriginal and European Australians showing the marked differences in size and shape of the dental arch	105
Table 5.1	Frequencies of malocclusion and tooth crowding in seven populations	106
Table 5.2	Frequencies of tooth crowding in Aboriginal Australians, and modern and medieval Danes	107
Figure 5.3	A typical chewing cycle in an Australian Aboriginal person. The path of tooth contact during empty grinding is shown at the top of the cycle (after Beyron, 1964)	109
Table 5.3	Determinants of occlusal development and function	112

Table 5.4	Weighted mean estimates of contributions to tooth size variability in Australian Aboriginal people	113
Table 5.5	Coefficients of variation in molar tooth size of Australian Aboriginal people	115
Table 5.6	Tooth size correlations in the permanent dentition of Australian Aboriginal people – mesiodistal diameters above the diagonal, buccolingual below	116
Table 5.7	Differences in mesiodistal diameters of corresponding deciduous and permanent teeth and tooth groups expressed in mm	118
Table 5.8	Comparison of leeway space expressed in mm in several populations	119
Figure 5.4	Occlusal development in an Aboriginal girl aged 6.7, 11.7 and 12.7 years	120
Figure 5.5	Occlusal development in an Aboriginal girl aged 8.6, 10.4 and 12.4 years	120
Table 5.9	Tooth size correlations between corresponding deciduous and permanent teeth of Australian Aboriginal people	122
Table 5.10	Tooth size correlations between corresponding maxillary and mandibular teeth and tooth groups in Australian Aboriginal people	123
Figure 5.6	Dental features including Cusp 6, Cusp 5, Carabelli trait and shovel-shaped incisors	124
Table 5.11	Average ages of exfoliation and emergence in Australian Aboriginal people: time interval calculated as the age of emergence of a permanent tooth less the age of exfoliation of the deciduous precursor	127
Table 5.12	Ages of emergence for specified numbers of permanent teeth determined by ranking the mean emergence times of left and right teeth	129
Table 5.13	Intervals in years between the first and second phases of permanent tooth emergence calculated as the difference between ages at which the last lateral incisor emerges and the first canine or premolar emerges	130
Figure 6.1	Max Jungarrayi and friend displaying mid-facial prognathism	136
Figure 6.2	General craniofacial growth pattern - boy aged 6.9 to 16.3 years	137
Figure 6.3	Mandibular remodelling and tooth emergence shown by superimposition of growth records on stable reference structures	138
Figure 6.4	Mandibular growth and dental arch development	139
Figure 6.5	Maxillary growth and dental arch development	140
Table 6.1	Dimensional changes in the dental arches of an Australian Aboriginal boy	141

Figure 6.6	Changes in dental arch breadths with times of tooth emergence indicated	142
Figure 6.7	Changes in dental arch depths with times of tooth emergence indicated	143
Figure 6.8	Occlusal development in an Aboriginal boy aged 5.5, 6.9 and 8.5 years	145
Figure 6.9	Occlusal development in an Aboriginal boy aged 10.3, 11.3 and 13.3 years	146
Figure 6.10	Occlusal development in an Aboriginal boy aged 14.3, 15.3 and 16.3 years	146
Figure 6.11	Labial and lingual tongue pressures during swallowing in Australian Aboriginal people	147
Figure 6.12	Comparison of tongue pressures during swallowing in Australian Aboriginal people and North American whites	148
Figure 6.13	Comparison of resting tongue pressures in Australian Aboriginal people and North American whites	149
Figure 6.14	Comparison of resting tongue pressures in Australian Aboriginal people and North American whites	150
Figure 6.15	Dental casts of Aboriginal adults from Yuendumu, Central Australia (left) and Kalumburu, Northwest Australia (right), showing different degrees of tooth wear	153
Figure 6.16	Unidentified Warlpiri boy, from the film 'So they did eat' (the ebook version will link to an extract from the film)	154
Figure 6.17	Stages in occlusal wear of deciduous molars (after Barrett, 1958)	155
Figure 6.18	Photograph of dental model showing presence of helicoidal plane associated with varying amounts and direction of wear on the lower molar teeth	156
Figure 6.19	Severe tooth wear in an Aboriginal male from Kalumburu, Northwest Australia, aged about 70 years, showing loss of adjacent tooth contacts, deposition of secondary dentine, helicoidal occlusal plane and alveolar development	158
Figure 6.20	Dental casts of a Warlpiri girl aged 12.9, 15.9 and 29.9 years showing changing incisor relationships	162
Figure 7.1	Henry Lennart Beyron	171
Figure 7.2	Arne Björk	173
Figure 7.3	Beni Solow	175

Figure 7.4	Sven Helm	176
Figure 7.5	Tadashi Ozaki	177
Figure 7.6	William R Proffit	179
Figure 7.7	Stephen Molnar	181
Figure 7.8	Edward McNulty (left) and R McClean with unidentified Warlpiri boys at Yuendumu, 1967	183
Figure 7.9	Murray James Barrett	185
Figure 7.10	Tasman Brown	188
Figure 7.11	Alec Cran examines an unidentified Warlpiri man, 1955 (courtesy of PG Dellow)	192
Figure 7.12	Left, Elizabeth Fanning with a group of school girls in 1962, and right, Grant Townsend and an unidentified Warlpiri man in 1970	193
Figure 7.13	Murray Barrett and Jimmy Jungarrayi Spencer	194
Figure 7.14	Tom and Pat Fleming (courtesy of Jolyon Fleming)	195
Figure 7.15	Pat Fleming serving team member Michael Nugent at the Yuendumu store, 1969	198
Figure 7.16	Benjamin Japangadi and friends at a movie evening at Yuendumu	198
Figure 7.17	The "new" church at Yuendumu	200
Table 8.1	The distribution of 288 participants with the full range of records by age at first examination and the number of sets of serial records	208
Figure 8.1	Recent evulsion of a central incisor	210
Figure 8.2	Serial dental models of a Warlpiri boy from 8.57–15.57 years	211
Figure 8.3	Professors Tadashi Ozaki and Tasman Brown	212
Figure 8.4	Intraoral photographs showing Aboriginal children in the 1950s with considerable staining, oral debris and dental plaque but little evidence of oral disease	213
Figure 8.5	The title page of the memorial volume of Murray Barrett's collected papers	214
Figure 8.6	Grant Townsend, Lassi Alvesalo and John Mayhall at the University of Turku, Finland, in 1986	216
Figure 8.7	James Rogers completed an honours degree based on the twin data housed in the M J Barrett Laboratory, and an increasing number of students began research projects during the 1990s leading to honours or doctorate degrees. One of the students was Sue Taji, shown here discussing with Jim Rogers some dental models of twins	217
Figure 8.8	Lindsay Richards and John Kaidonis with "Cannibal"	218

Figure 8.9	Images of the upper dental models of a pair of monozygotic twins generated by a 3D laser scanner and appropriate software available in the Murray Barrett Laboratory at the School of Dentistry, The University of Adelaide (images produced by PhD student, Atika Ashar). This technology now enables 'virtual models' to be stored and accurate measurements obtained for research purposes	219
Figure 8.10	Panoral radiographs of a pair of monozygotic (so-called identical) twins showing mirror imaging for congenital absence of a permanent lower second premolar. In Twin A, the arrow shows a missing tooth on the left side whereas the equivalent tooth is missing on the right side in Twin B. The arrows pointing at the lower right third molar region show differences in the stages of dental development between the co-twins, perhaps reflecting epigenetic influences	220
Figure 8.11	Professor Bhim Savara, Sandy Pinkerton and Dr Amanda Abbott	221
Figure 8.12	Stereo-photography and contour maps of twins	221
Figure 8.13	Average faces of young adults from the Yuendumu collection. (1a) The male average. (1b) The same male average as 1a, but with the texture information preserved. (2a) The female average. (2b) The same female average as 2a, but with the texture information preserved (courtesy of Dr Carl Stephan)	223
Figure 8.14	Evidence of dental fluorosis	226
Figure 8.15	Working in the Adelaide laboratory in the early 1990s. Standing are Grant Townsend, Tas Brown and Lindsay Richards with Samvit Kaul and Rob Corruccini seated	228
Table 8.2	Mean deciduous dmft scores of Yuendumu children aged 5–10 years	229
Figure 8.16	Two Jungarrayi, Jimmy and Murray	234

1
The Yuendumu Project: Anthropological Foundations

On 14 August 1951, 15 members of an anthropological research expedition left Adelaide on a Trans Australia Airlines flight for Alice Springs. The University of Adelaide group was travelling to Yuendumu, a remote Aboriginal Reserve established by the Native Affairs Branch of the Commonwealth Government in 1946 as a supply depot for Wailbri (Warlpiri) Aboriginal people[1] from neighbouring regions. Yuendumu was located around a bore on the Alice Springs to Mount Doreen stock route, about 290 kilometres north-west of Alice Springs in the Northern Territory of Australia. Yuendumu Reserve offered a unique opportunity for a multidisciplinary team to observe a group of Aboriginal people who were at an early stage of transition from a nomadic and hunter-gatherer way of life to living on a settlement. Sponsored by the Board for Anthropological Research of The University of Adelaide, the 1951 expedition was the first of many subsequent research visits to Yuendumu.

Several eminent Adelaide scientists were among the team members: T Draper Campbell, Charles P Mountford and Norman B Tindale, anthropologists; H K Fry, anthropologist and medical practitioner; Andrew A Abbie and W Ross Adey, anatomists; Cedric Stanton Hicks, Hugh LeMessurier and David Kerr, physiologists; J Burton

---

1   Wailbri is one spelling of the name that the Aboriginal people of Yuendumu call themselves. Campbell and Barrett and their successors always used this spelling in their publications. Other writers have used different spellings, for example Walbiri, Wailbiri and more recently Warlpiri, which is preferred by the Institute of Aboriginal and Torres Strait Islander Studies, Canberra. To avoid confusion, Warlpiri is used in the present text.

Cleland, naturalist and pathologist. Thomas Draper Campbell, a highly experienced anthropologist, who had led many pre-war expeditions to remote regions of South and Central Australia, was the leader of the Yuendumu team. At the time he was Director of Dental Studies at The University of Adelaide and in 1954 he became the university's first Professor of Dentistry.

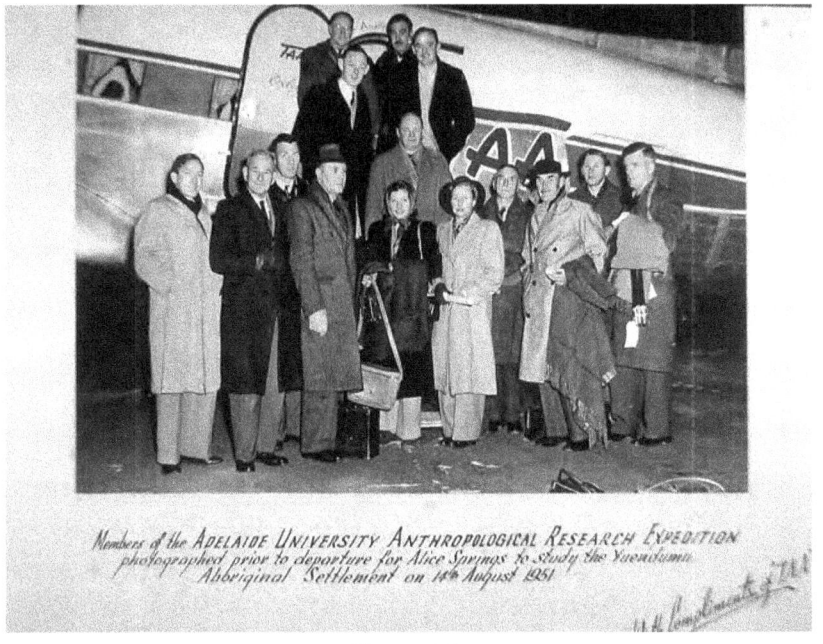

Figure 1.1
Team members about to depart on the first visit to Yuendumu in 1951.
Murray Barrett, top right, is standing above Draper Campbell

Murray James Barrett was a relatively junior member of the team. He was an ex-student of Draper Campbell and had recently been appointed to the staff of The University of Adelaide as Reader in Prosthetic Dentistry. He was particularly interested in dental morphology and masticatory function, and the observations he made during the initial visit to Yuendumu provided the stimulus for Barrett to plan an ongoing study of Warlpiri adults and children that would continue for a further 20 years of data gathering during annual trips to the Settlement. He immediately realised the wealth of material that would accrue from a well-planned and carefully executed longitudinal study. Even so, Barrett could hardly have visualised the results of his initiative. The ongoing study by Barrett and his colleagues resulted in a unique, extensive and irreplaceable collection of observations, recordings, photographs, genealogies and other records of an Aboriginal community. This material has attracted numerous local and overseas researchers and produced many theses and over 250 scientific papers (see Chapter 9). Research on these records continues in 2011, some 36 years after Barrett's death and 60 years after the first expedition to Yuendumu.

Physical and Dental Anthropology

For many years before the first Yuendumu expedition, an important research activity at The University of Adelaide involved the physical characteristics, lifestyle and customs of Australian Aboriginal people. Although there was no department of anthropology in the university, a long succession of scientists, mainly from other disciplines, particularly medicine and dentistry, had brought recognition that Adelaide was the major centre for research in physical anthropology in Australia. The South Australian Museum was also an active participant in these endeavours, particularly under the guidance of Edward Stirling during his term as Director. The history of the first Aboriginal contact with Europeans in South Australia and the subsequent development of physical anthropology and the sub-discipline of dental anthropology provided a focus for the later interest in Yuendumu and the success of the research that began in 1951. The following brief description of early contact with Aboriginal peoples in South Australia is important because it represented the foundations of physical anthropology in South Australia and would have been well known to Wood Jones and Draper Campbell.

Anthropological interest in South Australia was stimulated by the voyage of Matthew Flinders, the English navigator who charted the entire southern coast of Australia in 1802 in the *Investigator* (Flinders, 1814). The subsequent exploration by Charles Sturt, who used a whaleboat to chart the River Murray system in 1830, brought reports of good land for settling and descriptions of indigenous people he met along the river (Sturt, 1833). Sturt's explorations were instrumental in convincing a group of London businessmen to form the South Australian Association in 1833, with a view to establishing a viable colony in the south. Captain John Hindmarsh, the first Governor, proclaimed the British Province of South Australia on 28 December 1836 and soon afterwards Colonel William Light, the Surveyor General, laid out Adelaide to become the capital of the future state. At the time it was estimated that about 12,000 Aboriginal people inhabited the young colony (Dutton, 1978).

Settlers from Great Britain arrived in the new colony in rapidly increasing numbers, encouraged by reports of good grazing lands and property at relatively low prices. It appeared a wonderful opportunity for riches and a new life. Before long, colonisation had spread along the River Murray, along the coast to the south-eastern regions, and to the west. The early explorers of the middle to late 19th century ventured further to extend opportunities for profitable grazing. It was inevitable that friendly and hostile encounters would occur with Aboriginal people who resented the invasion of their lands by foreigners. The journals of well-known explorers of the inland included descriptions of the physical characteristics of Aboriginal people that were among the earliest anthropological accounts from South Australia. With the spread of colonisation, diseases that were often fatal were introduced to local indigenous people. This, together with the annexation of tribal lands, meant that there were few intact Aboriginal groups in South Australia by the end of the 19th century. For example, Graham Jenkin's *Conquest of the Ngarrindjeri* (1979) provides an important and detailed account of the contact history of European settlers and the Ngarrindjeri people of the lower River Murray lakes, including the work of George Taplin, who established the Point McLeay Mission in 1859.

Scientists enthusiastically pursued the study of "exotic" people from newly explored lands after the publication of Charles Darwin's *Origin of Species* (Darwin, 1859). Physical and social anthropology gained many new practitioners and increased status as scientific disciplines. The Aboriginal groups in South Australia attracted great interest and several texts of anthropological significance soon followed (Taplin, 1879; Curr, 1886-7; Stirling, 1896; Spencer and Gillen, 1899). The South Australian Museum was established by an Act of Parliament in 1856 and later played an important role in the development of anthropology, particularly under the guidance of Edward Stirling, who was Director of the Museum from 1889 until his death in 1919. Among his many scientific publications was an account of the Aboriginal burials at Swanport near the town of Murray Bridge on the River Murray (Stirling, 1911). By 1900, physical and social anthropology were well established in South Australia and interest in dental anthropology followed shortly.

Kirk (1985) has published a detailed account of early physical anthropology in Australia. His history refers to the 18th and 19th century explorers and anthropologists with their descriptions of Aboriginal people. Kirk also extended his survey to 20th century medical and anthropological investigators, with particular reference to the Board for Anthropological Research and the Board's sponsorship of field research in the 1920s-30s.

William Ramsay Smith 1859–1937

William Ramsay Smith was probably the first scientist in South Australia to take an interest in dental morphology and dental anthropology, fields in which he published articles and presented papers to scientific meetings. Ramsay Smith was a source of inspiration to Thomas Draper Campbell, who later became a dominant figure in the South Australian dental and anthropological community. Ramsay Smith was born on 27 November 1859 in Aberdeenshire, Scotland. His father, William Smith, was interested in science and assembled an excellent collection of Stone Age materials. His son apparently inherited this aptitude for science.

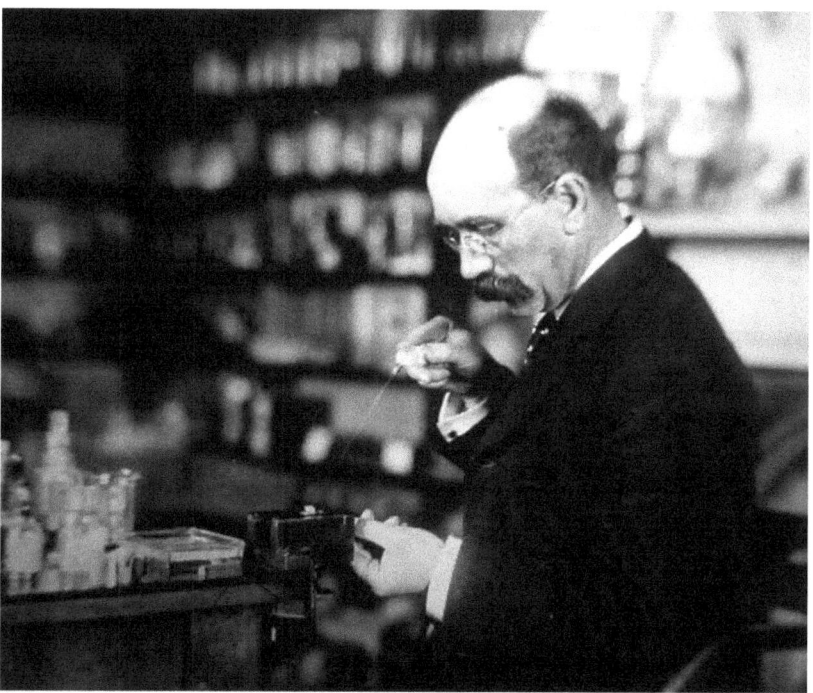

Figure 1.2
William Ramsay Smith at work

Ramsay Smith was a conscientious scholar. He commenced an Arts course at Edinburgh University in 1877, supported by a scholarship, and in 1878 he was elected president of his University's Philosophical Society. At the age of 24 he enrolled for medical studies in Edinburgh, supporting himself by teaching natural history and zoology. In 1888 he graduated with a BSc degree, was appointed the Senior Assistant Professor of Natural History, and organised the largest biological laboratory in the UK. It is a measure of his intellect that his first textbook, *Manual of Practical Zoology*, was published in 1887 while he was still an undergraduate. In 1892 he completed his medical studies after demonstrating Anatomy from 1890–92 and was soon appointed examiner for the Royal College of Physicians, Edinburgh.

After declining a hospital appointment, Ramsay Smith undertook three years as a private practitioner at Rhyl on the coast of North Wales. He considered that private practice was the best basis for later specialisation. While at Rhyl he accepted an appointment as Physician at the Adelaide Hospital, later the Royal Adelaide Hospital. It is interesting to note that by 1896, the year he left the UK, Ramsay Smith had published some 57 works, including three textbooks, articles on zoology and natural history, papers on anatomy, medicine and pathology as well as reports for the Fishery Board of Scotland.

Ramsay Smith's appointment to the Adelaide Hospital was occasioned by the crisis brought about by a dispute between the Chief Secretary, the Hon JH Gordon, and the Board of the Adelaide Hospital over the appointment, resignation and dismissal of nursing staff. J Estcourt Hughes described the now famous "Hospital Row" in his history of the Royal Adelaide Hospital (Hughes, 1967). As a result of this appointment, Ramsay Smith was considered to be somewhat of a strikebreaker and was subsequently ostracised by the medical profession, expelled by the South Australian Branch of the British Medical Association, and accused (but exonerated) of incompetence by a group of house surgeons who later resigned or were dismissed. Ramsay Smith went on to become a leading figure in the medical and scientific world of early South Australia. His many appointments included pathologist to the Adelaide Hospital, Chairman of the Central Board of Health, City Coroner, Inspector of Anatomy and Superintendent of the University School of Anatomy.

Apparently Ramsay Smith developed a keen and scholarly interest in Australian Aboriginal people from his arrival in Adelaide. This interest is apparent in his address to the Australasian Association for the Advancement of Science, later to become ANZAAS (Smith, 1907). His introduction to this address provides an insight into the intense interest in Aboriginal people and the scientific opinions at the time:

> I will endeavor, therefore, to set forth briefly the place of the Australian aboriginal in recent research in anthropology, and to outline what has been done, what is being done, and what still requires to be done in order to settle problems that are calling for solution. As almost every part of the anatomy of the aboriginal is being examined and re-examined with the view of discovering keys that will open up the secrets of human origin and racial affinities, I will try to indicate to scientific workers how they may aid by observations.

The paper outlined many aspects of physical anthropology with reference to the author's own observations of skeletal material. His detailed descriptions of supernumerary teeth and other aspects of dental morphology is evidence of his interest and expertise in these topics.

Ramsay Smith contributed substantially to public health medicine, providing numerous government reports on a variety of topics. He was well known as an anthropologist and devoted many years to the study of Australian Aboriginal people. In this field, his best-known works are *In Southern Seas* (Smith, 1924a) and *Myths and Legends of the Australian Aborigines* (Smith, 1930). In recent years it has been generally accepted that the latter work was largely appropriated without acknowledgement from Aboriginal philosopher and writer David Unaipon (1872–1967). At the time of his death on 28 September 1937 at the age of 77 years, Ramsay Smith had several books, numerous scientific publications and dozens of government reports to his credit. However, his reputation suffered from 1903 after being charged with misusing human remains and he was temporarily suspended from coronial duties (James and James, 2001).

Ramsay Smith showed an interest in dental anatomy, dental pathology and anthropology, although these interests do not appear to be adequately acknowledged by his biographers (Southcott, 1986; Elmslie and Nance, 1988). Shortly before 1907, the year when the Odontological Society of South Australia was formed (later the Australian Dental Association South Australian Branch), he published his first article on a dental subject - *Some rare abnormalities of teeth* (Smith, 1906) - in which he described eleven teeth with unusual crown or root morphology. The first paragraph of this paper is informative:

> When making inquiries into the dentition of Australian aboriginals and South Sea Islanders, I took occasion to show some interesting

teeth to Professor Watson, of the Adelaide University, and Mr Crank, D.M.D. In the course of our examination, Dr Crank produced several teeth which I had asked him to present to odontological collections; and Professor Watson thought it was a pity they should go undescribed, seeing that they presented some very rare abnormalities, and he made me promise to prepare a description for publication. The following is the result.

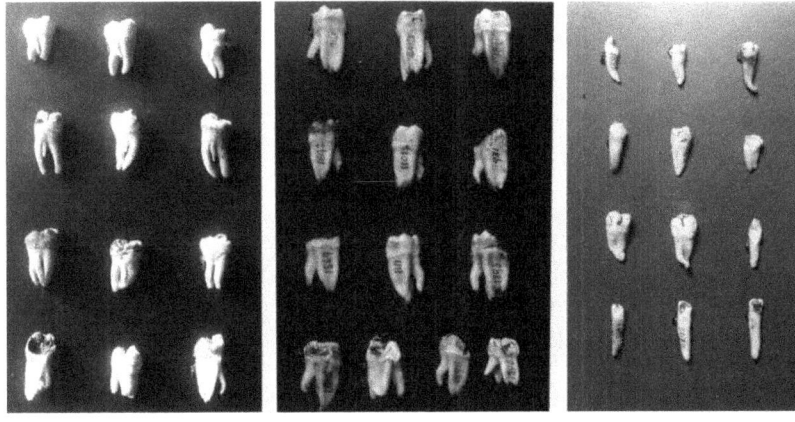

Figure 1.3
Specimens from The Ramsay Smith Bequest

Over the following years, Ramsay Smith was guest speaker at Odontological Society meetings on many occasions, his topics including the structure and development of teeth, dental malformations, dental anthropology and other related topics. He was obviously respected by the members of the Society, who elected him an Honorary Member in 1910. His lectures to the Society were well received and some were subsequently published (Smith, 1921, 1922, 1924b).

He also acted as a consultant on dental matters and often gave opinions on dental anomalies. His papers on dental topics resulted from this interest: some of them include illustrations and references to specific dental specimens, many of which are located in the collections at the School of Dentistry, The University of Adelaide. It is probable that his final paper on a dental subject was presented in 1930 at the 7th Australian Dental Congress - it was titled *A medico-dental study (tooth in bronchus)*.

A manuscript by Ramsay Smith titled *Studies in Odontology* is located in the School of Dentistry, The University of Adelaide. It illustrates his expertise in dental anthropology and pathology and consists of eight typed chapters based on lectures he gave to the Odontological Society. The chapters contain numerous references to individual specimens of teeth in the collection that the Australian Dental Association received in February 1937. This collection of 150,000 teeth is known as the Ramsay Smith Bequest. It is now held in the School of Dentistry but unfortunately is no longer intact as requested by the donor.

Thomas Draper Campbell 1893–1967

After the First World War, anthropological studies were in recess but two collaborators initiated a resurgence of interest and together they were responsible for establishing the reputation of The University of Adelaide as a centre for research in physical anthropology. One, Thomas Draper Campbell, was a dental graduate of 1921, and the other, Frederic Wood Jones, was an English anatomist appointed to the Chair of Anatomy in The University of Adelaide from 1920–27.

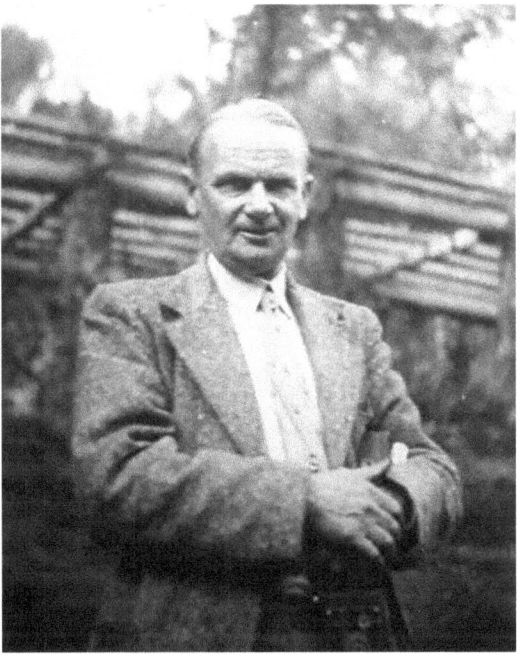

Figure 1.4
Thomas Draper Campbell

To appreciate Campbell's achievements it is necessary to consider the times in which he lived and the personalities and events that influenced his career. Draper Campbell was born in Millicent in the south-east of South Australia in March 1893, the son of Walter, a storekeeper, and Lucy. As a child, Draper, a name he received from his paternal grandmother Jane Draper, got to know the countryside of the south-east well and he developed interests in the history and geology of the region that he retained all his life.

After moving to Adelaide in 1907, Campbell was educated at Prince Alfred College and then completed the training in dentistry conducted by the Dental Board. He was registered as a dentist in 1917 and served in the Australian Army Medical Corps Reserve (Dental Unit) as an Honorary Lieutenant. As a member of the Odontological Society, Campbell and others formulated the content of the future university course in dentistry that was established in 1919. Campbell himself was one of the original six who graduated with the new BDS degree in 1921. Immediately he commenced work as a house surgeon at the Dental Department of the Royal Adelaide Hospital and became its Superintendent a few years later in 1926. Although he maintained his clinical skills throughout his life, particularly in oral surgery, Campbell's main interests were clearly academic and his first university appointment came three years after graduation when he became Lecturer in Dental Anatomy.

Apart from completing his dental degree he undertook the extensive observations required for a doctoral thesis and presented them in a style that became a standard for later works. He also studied at the Elder Conservatorium in 1919, gave several papers to the Odontological Society between 1920 and 1925, became a fellow of the Royal Society of South Australia in 1922 and in 1924 was appointed an Honorary Curator at the South Australian Museum.

By then he was already highly qualified, having received his DDSc degree in 1923 for anatomical and anthropological studies. His thesis, titled *Dentition and Palate of the Australian Aboriginal*, became the first Keith Sheridan Foundation publication of The University of Adelaide (Campbell, 1925). It is interesting to recall the words of his preface: "The subject of Dentition can no longer be considered one of only incidental interest, but must and will take its place as an important branch of the science of Physical Anthropology."

Campbell's work received excellent reviews from around the world. For example, in 1926 a reviewer for the *British Dental Journal* stated, "Considered both as a contribution to dental anatomy and to anthropology this book is of permanent importance". Sir Arthur Keith from the Royal College of Surgeons in the *Journal of Anatomy* stated, "His monograph in its methods, scope, statement and exhaustiveness is a model which other workers will do well to copy" (Keith, 1926). The *British Medical Journal* suggested that "[the book is] one which will satisfy the requirements of the scientific dentist and expert anthropologist for many years to come" (1926). Judging from the fine reviews the book received and the continuing citations it still enjoys, there is no doubt that this example of meticulous, detailed and disciplined scientific study was important in establishing dental anthropology as a modern science that has become one of the major sub-disciplines of physical anthropology and human biology. The *Dentition and Palate of the Australian Aboriginal* marked the beginning of Campbell's career as an anthropologist of note.

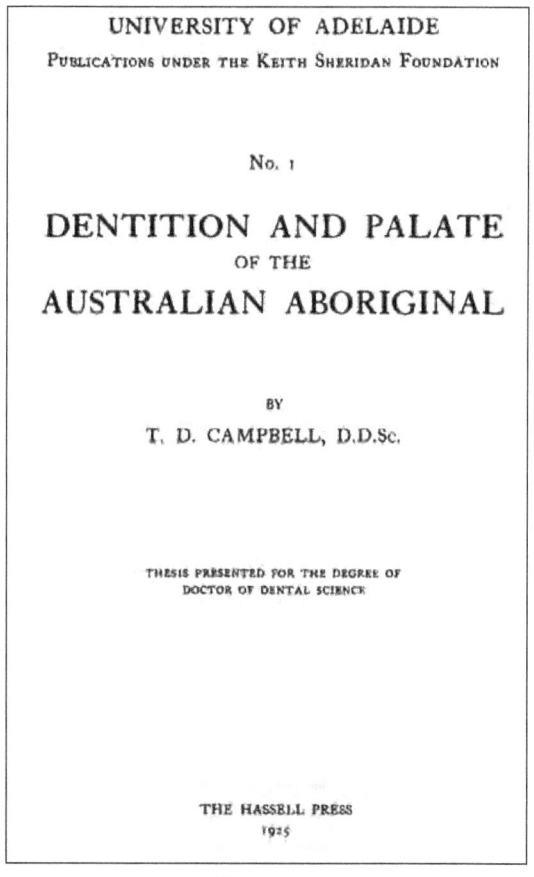

Figure 1.5
Campbell's first major publication in dental anthropology

Before Campbell's work, there were few detailed studies of the dentition or palate, most of those available being based on descriptions of a few teeth from fossil hominids. By reporting on a large sample of teeth and jaws, Campbell was able to bring new insights to the emerging discipline of dental anthropology. There is little doubt that his clinical experience as a dentist allowed him to focus on the relationships between form and function rather than limiting his observations to descriptions of morphological features.

In many respects the *Dentition and Palate of the Australian Aboriginal* was a landmark study covering a wide range of topics including metric and non-metric characters of the dentition and palate, occlusion and eruption of the teeth, the temporomandibular articulation, tooth wear, pathology and Aboriginal attitudes to dental disease. Many statements by Campbell anticipated future research and concepts regarding dental form and function and their relationship to dental health. He expanded his understanding of these topics later with observations made during a series of field trips.

In the concluding words of his address to the Australian Society for the Advancement of Science, Ramsay Smith stated his hope that anthropological research would flourish in South Australia (Smith, 1907):

> If, however, by anything I have said I have succeeded in making some people repentant over lost opportunities, and resolved to do something to help Australia - and especially South Australia - to take her proper place in anthropological research, then I am content.

Perhaps these words inspired Campbell to undertake many field trips to remote parts of Australia, culminating in his leadership of the first expedition to Yuendumu in 1951.

What were the influences that guided this young man into anthropology? Who were the personalities of the time who may have served as role models? What was the scientific atmosphere of Adelaide in the early part of the 20th century?

Frederic Wood Jones 1879–1954

Frederic Wood Jones was a comparative zoologist of note and also a competent anthropologist. His term in Adelaide encompassed the years during which Campbell studied dentistry and completed the research for his doctorate. Wood Jones was appointed to the Elder Chair of Anatomy at The University of Adelaide in 1919, a position he held until 1927. He came to Adelaide with a distinguished reputation following teaching posts in medical schools in England and service in the Royal Army Medical Corps. Upon his appointment, Wood Jones immediately assumed a productive role in the scientific activities of the state. He was particularly interested in Aboriginal people as a humanitarian and also because of his interest in anthropology. MacCallum (1983) highlighted his many other achievements.

The influence of Wood Jones on Campbell is clearly evident in the following tribute (Campbell, 1936):

> The advent of Professor Wood Jones was an important factor in making the early twenties another outstanding time mark in anthropological interest in the State. It was largely due to Wood Jones' infectious enthusiasm and methods of critical observation that he was such a stimulating influence on workers about him.

Later the two undertook field studies and published together (Wood Jones and Campbell, 1924a, 1924b, 1925).

This period, the 1920s into the 1930s, must have been especially stimulating and exciting for an energetic and inquisitive young scientist like Campbell. Besides Wood Jones, there were many other prominent Adelaide figures interested in anthropology, their names including Herbert Hale (Director of the South Australian Museum), Sir John Cleland (pathologist, botanist and State Coroner), Cecil Hackett and James Hugo Gray (physical anthropologists), Thomas Harvey Johnston (botanist), Robert Pulleine (physiologist), Frank Hone (medical practitioner), Bernard Cotton (zoologist), Norman Tindale (ethnologist), and Harold Davies (Aboriginal songs and music). One can well imagine the atmosphere of scientific enquiry and debate these men must have created, an atmosphere that we would have difficulty in duplicating today. His experience during this period convinced Campbell that anthropological research should be multi-disciplinary, a view that was well ahead of then contemporary thinking but one that he held throughout his life. Indeed, he anticipated the discipline of biological anthropology by some 30 years.

Nurtured by this atmosphere, Campbell and Wood Jones were instrumental in establishing the Board for Anthropological Research at The University of Adelaide in 1926, the same year in which Campbell and Pulleine founded the Anthropological Society of South Australia. Thus, within four years of graduation as a dentist and within two years of his doctorate, Draper Campbell was firmly established in the forefront of Australian anthropology and was becoming well known overseas.

Percy Raymond Begg 1898–1983

Percy Raymond Begg was another Adelaide dentist, later orthodontist, who became interested in the dentition of Australian Aboriginal people through his studies of skeletal material from the pre-European period. He trained as an orthodontist in the United States at the Angle School of Orthodontia, becoming versed with the theories and methods of Edward Angle. Subsequently, he practised as the sole specialist orthodontist in Adelaide for many years. His early research work led to a thesis for his Doctorate degree that dealt with irregularities and malocclusions (Begg, 1935).

Later he continued his studies of the Aboriginal dentition and published a series of papers dealing with his theories on the aetiology of malocclusion (Begg, 1954). This series detailed his concepts of interproximal tooth wear in fully functioning dentitions as a causative factor for creating space within the dental arch. According to Begg, the lack of this wear in modern populations was responsible for tooth crowding and other malocclusions. His clinical treatment methods were based on these concepts, combined with the use of a light arch wire technique. Begg received widespread recognition for his teaching and his methods became known around the world as the Begg Technique. He received many honours during his life and maintained an enthusiastic following. He died in 1983.

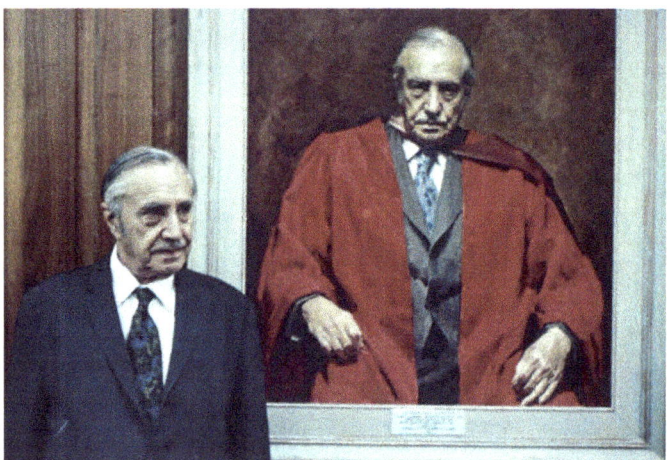

Figure 1.6
Percy Raymond Begg in front of his portrait that is displayed on the fourth floor of the Adelaide Dental Hospital building

Early expeditions 1923–1939

The Board for Anthropological Research, without doubt, was the dominant driving force that made Adelaide the leading centre of physical anthropology in Australia. Tindale (1986) and Jones (1987) have described the history and activities of the Board in detail. The field expeditions organised by the Board during the 1920s and 1930s produced a wealth of scientific material and ethnographic films of Aboriginal customs that are the envy of other institutions. Draper Campbell was closely involved with the organisation of these expeditions into Central Australia and he personally led eight of them. Table 1.1 lists the early expeditions of the Board, many of which included Campbell, and Figure 1.7 shows their locations.

Table 1.1 Early expeditions by researchers from The University of Adelaide showing the trip prefix, year and location[1]

Prefix	Year	Location	State
	1923*	Stuart Range and Mount Eba	South Australia
A	1925*	Wilgena	South Australia
B	1926*	Wilgena and Ooldea	South Australia
C	1927*	Macumba	South Australia
C	1927*	Alice Springs	Northern Territory
D	1928*	Koonibba	South Australia
E	1929	Hermannsburg	Northern Territory
F	1930*	MacDonald Downs	Northern Territory
G	1931*	Cockatoo Creek	Northern Territory
H	1932*	Mount Liebig	Northern Territory
I	1933	Mann Range and Ernabella	South Australia
J	1934*	Diamantina	South Australia
K	1935	Warburton Range	Western Australia
L	1936	The Granites	Northern Territory
M	1937	Nepabunna	South Australia
O	1939	Ooldea	South Australia

1 The Board for Anthropological Research was established in December 1926 after the success of the 1925 expedition to Wilgena that was then given the Prefix A. Warlpiri Aboriginals would have been encountered on expeditions H to Mount Liebig and L to The Granites. Data were obtained from the Archives of the South Australian Museum, file AA 346/03, listed on the Museum's web site and from Jones (1987).
* T Draper Campbell was a team member on these expeditions.

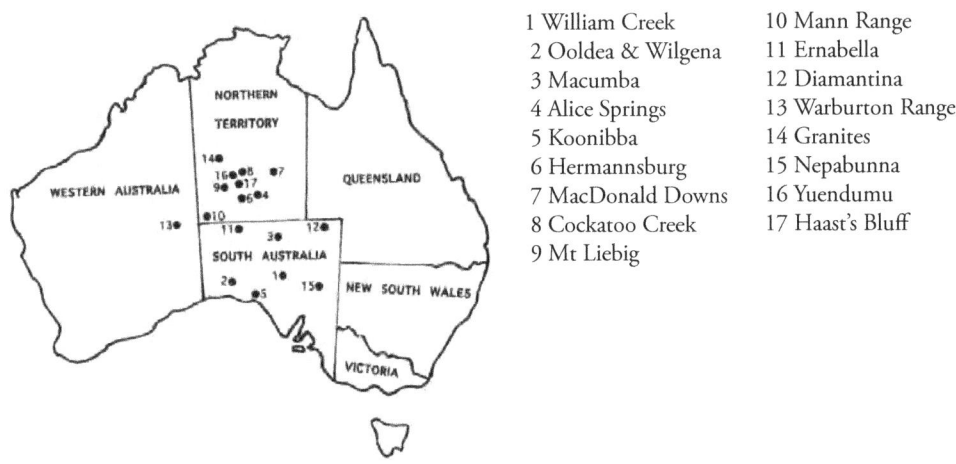

Figure 1.7
Map showing the locations of field expeditions sponsored by
The Board for Anthropological Research (redrawn after a map used by TD Campbell)

Campbell published extensively during this period, his papers covering a variety of topics including physical anthropology, dentistry, ethnology and stone tools. The papers describing the dentitions of Aboriginal people cemented Campbell's stature as a leading pioneer dental anthropologist and stimulated world interest in this emerging discipline. Between 1926 and 1938 nine of his publications dealt specifically with the dentition, most of which were published in the *Australian Journal of Dentistry* under the title "Observations on the teeth of Australian Aborigines", including Campbell and Lewis (1926), Campbell and Gray (1936) and Campbell (1938). His field observations during these expeditions to remote regions together with his experience as a dental clinician allowed Campbell to consolidate his views about the nature and causes of dental and oral disease in modern populations. In a scholarly series of landmark publications he drew the attention of the dental world to the relationship between dietary habits and dental disease, always referring to the excellent dentitions of nomadic Aboriginal people, well aligned and free of dental decay, which were in marked contrast to the degenerate and diseased dentitions of Europeans at that time (Campbell, 1939). His efforts were rewarded when he was admitted to the Doctor of Science degree in 1939, having submitted 37 original research papers for examination.

Staff of The University of Adelaide and the South Australian Museum carried out most research regarding Aboriginal peoples in the 1920s and 1930s. The Board-sponsored expeditions to various parts of Australia, from which numerous scientific papers resulted (over 200 in all fields of anthropology). In addition, an extensive series of cinematographic records was made depicting the customs and daily life of nomadic Aboriginal people. The earliest of these expeditions brought Europeans into contact with nomadic people of the interior for the first time (Figure 1.8).

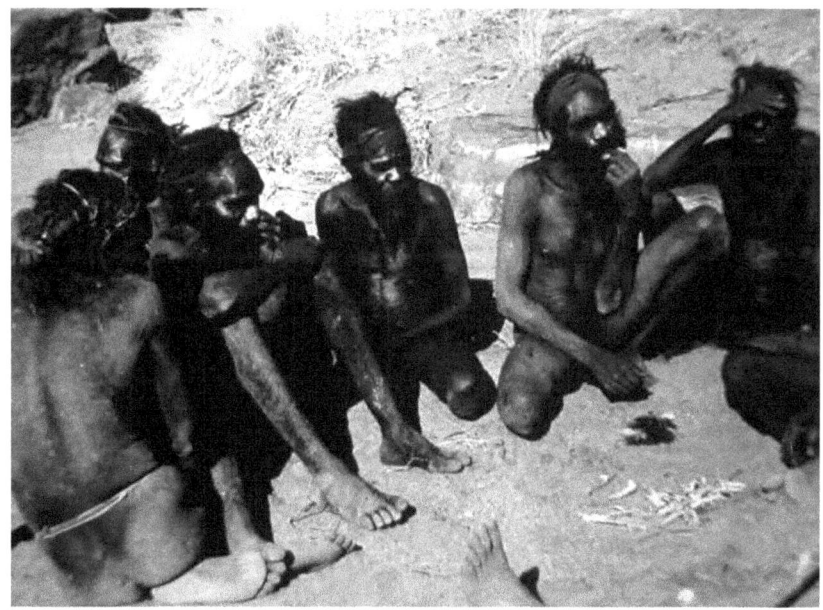

Figure 1.8
Early photograph of unidentified Aboriginal people by Campbell

International liaisons were now well established and many prominent scientists had visited Adelaide or would do so shortly, including Joseph Birdsell from the US and Aleš Hrdlička, the famous Czech anthropologist. There was hope for a Chair of Anthropology in Adelaide, but the first Chair was established in Sydney in 1926.

This decision was a savage blow for Campbell and his colleagues, who included The University's Vice Chancellor and Professors Cleland, Wood Jones, Kerr Grant and Harold Davies. It would take until 1973 for the creation of a Chair in Anthropology at The University of Adelaide. The main thrust of this new department was social anthropology and, furthermore, the research focus was far removed from Australia. It appeared that the efforts of Campbell for many years and others after his death had been in vain. In spite of having no official academic base or perhaps, as some would argue, because of it, the Adelaide group strove that much more and maintained an active and productive interest in anthropology for the remainder of Campbell's life and beyond. It was not until 1995 that a bequest from anatomist Professor Ray Last allowed physical anthropology to receive official recognition in The University of Adelaide with the establishment of the Wood Jones Chair of Anthropological and Comparative Anatomy and the appointment of the first professor, Maciej Henneberg.

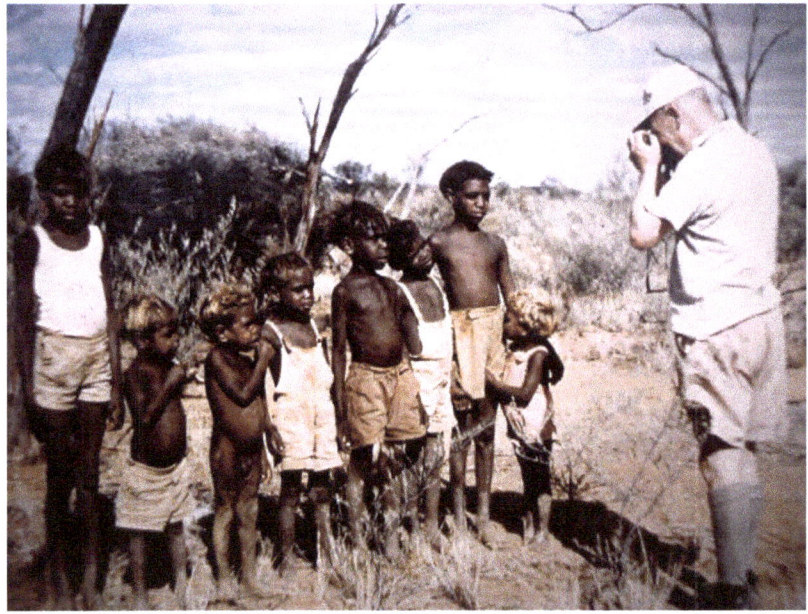

Figure 1.9
Campbell and unidentified children - from the 1950s (courtesy of PG Dellow)

It is a credit to the scientists of the 1920s and 1930s that the group of Adelaide anthropologists flourished to achieve a well-deserved international reputation. However, the Sydney anthropologists who held the purse strings of the Australian National Research Council provided little help. Local anthropologists such as JB Cleland and CP Mountford were refused funding and the Sydney board even insisted on copies of all field notes made by South Australians. Such was the lack of support from Sydney that the South Australians often funded their research from their own pockets with some help with transport from the State Government.

Campbell's fascination with anthropology never waned and in his later years, after retirement from the University, he worked with his friends Robert Edwards, then a Curator of the South Australian Museum, and geologist Paul Hossfeld, publishing with each (Campbell and Edwards, 1966; Campbell and Hossfeld, 1966). These years were fruitful as Campbell returned to his interests in the archaeology and geology of the south-east of the State, his notes and letters revealing details of his trips to the countryside of his childhood. Robert Edwards shared Campbell's interest in Aboriginal tools and together they spent many hours collating and surveying stone tools and attempting to fashion implements in the way Aboriginal people had for thousands of years. During this time he was a frequent lecturer on the pre-history of the south-east and he was much respected by the townspeople of the region.

Quite apart from his reputation as an anthropologist of note, Campbell's parallel dental career also flourished and he became the longest serving Dean of the Faculty of Dentistry, holding the position from 1939 until 1958. He maintained his clinical skills during his university appointment and lectured to the Australian Dental Association on many occasions, both locally and at national meetings. His subjects were varied and ranged from anatomy and anthropology through to surgery, pathology and dental health.

In 1951 he led the team of scientists to Yuendumu and over the next decade he directed several ethnographic films about the crafts and skills of the Warlpiri people, whom he greatly admired. His significant studies of Aboriginal camp sites and stone tools culminated in his 1963–65 investigation of archaeological sites for the Australian Institute of Aboriginal and Torres Strait Islander Studies, of which he was a founding member. Campbell's classification of stone tools influenced the typology used in Australia. A remarkable man and a great scholar, Campbell served as a mentor for Murray J Barrett, as they worked together at Yuendumu in the 1950s. His scientific writings, films and examples of innovative and meticulous investigation continue to influence the present day researchers in craniofacial biology at the School of Dentistry in The University of Adelaide.

References

Begg PR (1935). *Studies on the Aetiology of Irregularity and Malocclusion of the Teeth.* DDSc Thesis, The University of Adelaide.

Begg PR (1954). Stone Age Man's Dentition. *Am J Orthod* 40:298–312; 40:373–383; 40:462–475; 40:517–531.

British Dental Journal (1926). Review of *Dentition and Palate of the Australian Aboriginal.* XLVII: 645–646.

British Medical Journal (1926). Review of *Dentition and Palate of the Australian Aboriginal.* 1:869–870.

Campbell TD (1925). *Dentition and Palate of the Australian Aboriginal.* Adelaide: Hassell Press.

Campbell TD, Lewis AJ (1926). The Aborigines of South Australia: Dental observations recorded at Ooldea, South Australia. *Aust J Dent* 20:371–376.

Campbell TD (1936). Anthropology and the Royal Society. *Trans Roy Soc South Aust* 60:19–24.

Campbell TD, Gray JH (1936). Observations on the teeth of Australian Aborigines. *Aust J Dent* 40:290–295.

Campbell TD (1938). Observations on the teeth of Australian Aborigines. Cockatoo Creek, Central Australia. *Aust J Dent* 42:41–47.

Campbell TD (1939). Food, food values and food habits of the Australian Aborigines in relation to their dental conditions. Parts I – V. *Aust J Dent* 43:1–15; 45–55; 73–87; 141–156; 177–198.

Campbell TD, Edwards R (1966). Stone implements. In: *Aboriginal Man in South and Central Australia. Part 1.* Cotton BC, editor. Adelaide: Government Printer, pp. 159–220.

Campbell TD, Hossfeld PS (1966). Australian Aboriginal stone arrangements in North-West South Australia. *Trans Roy Soc South Aust* 90:171–176.

Curr EM (1886–7). *The Australian Race: its origin, languages, customs, place of landing in Australia, and the routes by which it spread itself over that continent.* Melbourne: J Ferres, Government Printer (4 vols).

Dampier W (1697). *A New Voyage Round the World.* London: J Knapton.

Darwin C (1859). *On the Origin of Species by Means of Natural Selection.* London: John Murray.

Dutton GPH (1978). *A Taste of History.* Adelaide: Rigby.

Eyre EJ (1845). *Journals of Expeditions of Discovery into Central Australia and Overland to King George's Sound. Volumes 1 and 2.* London: Boone.

Elmslie RG, Nance S (1988). *Smith, William Ramsay (1859–1937).* In: Australian Dictionary of Biography Volume 11. Melbourne: Melbourne University Press, pp. 674–675.

Flinders M (1814). *A Voyage to Terra Australis, Vols 1, 2 and Atlas.* London: G and W Nicol.

Hughes JE (1967). *History of the Royal Adelaide Hospital.* Adelaide: Board of Management, Royal Adelaide Hospital.

James R, James H (2001). Historical Perspective: Retention of Human Organs and the Dismissal of Ramsay Smith. *Pathology* 33:172–173.

Jenkin G (1979). *Conquest of the Ngarrindjeri: The Story of the Lower Murray Lakes Tribes.* Adelaide: Rigby.

Jones PG (1987). South Australian anthropological history: The Board for Anthropological Research and its early expeditions. *Rec South Aust Mus* 20:71–92.

Keith, Sir Arthur (1926). Review of *Dentition and Palate of the Australian Aboriginal.* Journal of Anatomy LX, IV:462.

Kirk RL (1985). *History of Physical Anthropology in Australia.* International Association of Human Biologists, Occasional Papers, Vol 1 No 5. Newcastle upon Tyne: International Association of Human Biologists.

MacCallum M (1983). *Jones, Frederic Wood (1879–1954).* In: Australian Dictionary of Biography, Volume 9. Melbourne: Melbourne University Press, pp. 510–512.

Smith WR (1906). Some rare abnormalities in teeth. *J Anat Physiol* 41:216–220.

Smith WR (1907). *The place of the Australian Aboriginal in recent anthropological research.* Adelaide: Australian Association of Advanced Science, pp. 1–22 plus 24 plates.

Smith WR (1921). Adventitious roots. *Aust J Dent* 25:203–205.

Smith WR (1922). Some legal aspects of dental practice. *Aust J Dent* 26:64-80.

Smith WR (1924a). *In Southern Seas: Wanderings of a Naturalist.* London: John Murray.

Smith WR (1924b). Peg-shaped teeth and dislocation of molars. *Aust Dent J* 5:451–457.

Smith WR (1930). *Myths and Legends of the Australian Aboriginals.* London: George G Harrap.

Southcott RV (1986). Medical Sciences. In: *Ideas and Endeavours - The Natural Sciences in South Australia.* Adelaide: Royal Society of South Australia, pp. 213-234.

Spencer WB, Gillen FJ (1899). *The Native Tribes of Central Australia.* London: McMillan and Co.

Stirling EC (1896). Anthropology of the Central Australian Aborigines. In: *Report on the Work of the Horn Scientific Expedition to Central Australia.* WA Horn, editor. London: Dulau and Co, pp. 1–517.

Stirling EC (1911). Preliminary report on the discovery of native remains at Swanport, River Murray; with an inquiry into the alleged occurrence of a pandemic among the Australian aboriginals. *Trans Roy Soc South Aust* 35:4-46.

Stuart J McDouall (1863). *J M'Douall Stuart's Explorations Across the Continent of Australia*: with charts, 1861–62. Melbourne: FF Bailliere.

Sturt CN (1833). *Two Expeditions into the Interior of Southern Australia, during the years 1828, 1829, 1830, and 1831: with Observations on the Soil, Climate and General Resources of the Colony of New South Wales.* London: Smith, Elder and Co. 2 Vols.

Sturt CN (1848–49). *Narrative of an Expedition into Central Australia, Performed under the Authority of Her Majesty's Government, During the Years 1844, 5, and 6: Together with a Notice of the Province of South Australia in 1847.* London: T and W Boone. 2 vols.

Taplin G (1879). *Folklore, Manners, Customs and Languages of the Aborigines of Australia.* Adelaide: Government Printer.

Tindale NB (1986). Anthropology. In: *Ideas and Endeavours – the Natural Sciences in South Australia.* Twidale CR, Tyler MJ, Davies M, editors. Adelaide: Royal Society of South Australia, pp. 235–277.

Wood Jones F, Campbell TD (1924a). Six hitherto undescribed skulls of Tasmanian natives. With an account of the palate and teeth. *Rec South Aust Mus* 2:459–469.

Wood Jones F, Campbell TD (1924b). Anthropometric and descriptive observations on some South Australian Aboriginals, with a summary of previously recorded anthropometric data. *Trans Roy Soc South Aust* 48:303–312.

Wood Jones F, Campbell TD (1925). A contribution to the study of eoliths: some observations on the natural forces at work in the production of flaked stones on the Central Australian tablelands. *J Royal Anthrop Inst* 55:115–122.

2
Yuendumu and the Warlpiri: Early History

Location and meaning of the word Yuendumu

Yuendumu is located near the south–eastern edge of the extent of traditionally owned Warlpiri land with Anmatyerre land to the east, Pintubi/Luritja land to the south and Kukatja land to the west. It is the largest community in Central Australia, with the exception of Alice Springs. The Community Government area comprises 22,242 sq km and Traditional Owners control the land. Entry permits are required by visitors intending to stay overnight or to visit for a greater period of time. Most Yuendumu residents are Warlpiri speakers with minor groups of Anmatyerre, Luritja, Kukatja and Pintubi speakers. It lies in true "Red Centre" country, experiencing the hot days and cold nights of inland Australia. Access is via about 140 km single lane bitumen Tanami Road with the remainder being formed dirt (Northern Territory Police, 2006).

The Warlpiri word "Jukurrpa" means dreaming and it is central to understanding Warlpiri culture and law. The place name "Yuendumu" is also associated with dreaming, as it is a derivative of the word "Yurntumulya', which means Dreaming Woman (Napaljarri and Cataldi, 2003). The Warlpiri call the area "Yurtumu" whilst the white administration, when creating a ration depot in 1946, decided to call it "Yuendumu'. A report from the Administration of the Northern Territory in June 1946 stated that the name had been chosen as it was "a native name for a line of hills in the immediate vicinity" (Carrington, 1946). This difficulty with language emphasises one of many divides that have separated Western culture from understanding and appreciating indigenous beliefs and cultures.

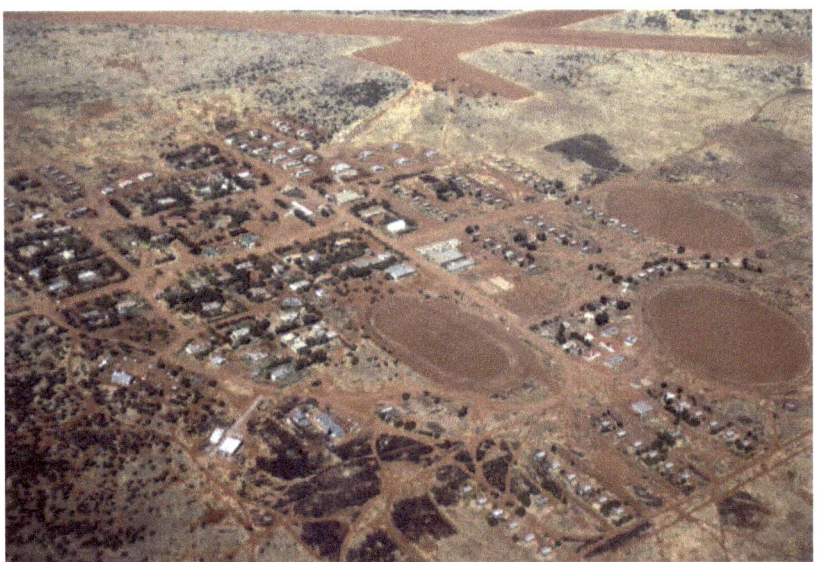
Figure 2.1
Aerial view of Yuendumu (courtesy of OzOutback Internet Services)

Few of the early European settlers would have bothered to learn the languages or make an attempt to understand the Aboriginal way of life. In some ways this is understandable because it would be difficult to decipher the complex relationships within and between groups of the indigenous population. An example of this can be seen when the concept of a community is considered. The Aboriginal people living at Yuendumu are usually referred to as Warlpiri people but other words such as Walbiri, Walpiri, Elpira, Ipara or Wailbri have been used that can cause confusion. Also the term Warlpiri is a collective word incorporating four separate social groups: Yalpari, Waneiga, Walmalla and Ngalia. It is questionable whether the Warlpiri living in the region before Yuendumu was established even had what could be called a community (Rowse, 1990) and this may have acted against the indigenous people of the region when they were confronted with the sustained contact of European settlement.

Expansion and conflict associated with European settlement

The expansion of the pastoral communities in the Victoria River district of the Northern Territory in the 1880s, plus the search for gold in the Halls Creek and

Tanami Desert areas in 1910 and the 1930s, provided a background in which displacement and conflict were common. From an Aboriginal viewpoint, the contacts with the European miners and pastoralists meant the end of Jukurrpa. Their cultural idea of Jukurrpa as a single means of explanation of the world they knew became lost in the "culture of the West". As Napaljarri and Cataldi (2003) noted in the introduction of *Warlpiri dreaming and histories,* it was:

> apparent that many Warlpiri people are much more clearly aware of the nature of cultural conflict and the nature of the two cultures than Europeans are. Such awareness is the privilege of the loser in this kind of conflict.

With both the law supporting the demands of white settlement, and the low opinion many of the settlers had of the Aboriginal population, it was not surprising that repression became central to government policies concerning the native population and the land they occupied. Resentment and distrust came to a head in the 1920s, leading to the Kimberley Massacre in Western Australia (1926) and the Coniston Massacre[1] in the Northern Territory (1928). The Kimberley Massacre did, to some degree, set the tone for the Coniston Massacre: if Aboriginal people committed a crime, the authorities sent armed men into the bush with the intention of arresting the culprits and bringing them to trial. After the Kimberley incident, the reality was that armed upholders of the law were likely to shoot indiscriminately at any Aboriginal person found in the vicinity of a crime and anyone else who happened to wander into it.

This indiscriminate killing of Aboriginal people and the lack of a conviction for the atrocities committed in both massacres provided a field day for newspaper editors who publicised the Coniston case in both the national and international press. Public outrage was so intense that important measures were established to ensure that no indiscriminate killing of native Australians would ever occur again, and that the injustices seen to be supported by the judicial system would not be permitted in the future. Possibly, nature also played a part in the fortunes of the Warlpiri.

---

1   Coniston is located in Warlpiri lands about 70 km to the east of Yuendumu. By 1928 white graziers had moved into the region. Warlpiri tribesmen killed a dingo hunter, Fred Brooks, at a soak 21 km south of Coniston Station. Constable Murray was sent from Alice Springs to arrest the murderers. On this and several subsequent occasions, police parties killed up to 100 Aboriginal people, although the official death toll was reported as 31. The Coniston Massacre lives on in the memories and ceremonies of the Warlpiri people to this day.

The worst drought on record occurred from 1924 to 1929. The drought forced people out of the desert to search for food and water amongst the mining and cattle interests. As Meggitt (1962) noted:

> The influx of so many hungry and unemployable Aborigines seriously embarrassed the cattlemen, who were themselves in difficulties, and relations between the two peoples soon became tense.

For the Warlpiri people who survived the Coniston Massacre, life in their traditional lands would never be the same. Some travelled north-east toward Tennant Creek, whilst others sought refuge in a north-westerly direction toward Mount Singleton, Mount Doreen, Granites and Tanami regions. Meggitt (1962) emphasises that:

> The shootings left the people with a long-standing distrust of Europeans and to an important degree reinforced the authority of the older men of the tribe who had previously tried to dissuade their juniors from becoming entangled with white men. The effects of this attitude are seen today in the continued adherence of many Walbiri to the traditional rules and values.

By the early 1930s, the Ngalia Warlpiri had drifted southwards in their traditional lands toward Haast's Bluff, bringing them into contact with the Lutheran missionaries of the Finke River Mission at Hermannsburg. Concerned for their welfare and not wishing to see further degeneration of the people of the desert, Pastor FW Albrecht made known to representatives of the government, including the Federal Minister of the Interior, the Administrator of the Northern Territory and the Chief Protector of Aboriginals, the true state of affairs concerning the Haast's Bluff Aboriginal population.

It was partly through Albrecht's intervention in indigenous affairs that the Federal Government eventually opened Yuendumu as a ration depot in 1946 (Rowse, 1990). Not only did Pastor Albrecht make known the plight of the Ngalia Warlpiri to government officialdom, he also broached the matter with Rev Dr EH Watson. Watson, who was the Baptist chaplain to the armed forces based in Alice Springs, had previously shown interest in promoting Baptist missionary work in Central Australia and, after Albrecht's approach, he decided to forward the matter to the South Australian Baptist Mission. In essence, the proposal was to set up a mission for the Warlpiri in the Haast's Bluff region, a proposal that relied heavily on Lutheran support.

Between 1942 and 1944, the South Australian Baptist Home Mission Department agreed in principle to set up a mission and to follow Pastor Albrecht's guide in the choice of location. The church sent Rev Laurie Reece to examine an area north of Coniston and west of Mount Singleton, covering some 600 miles over territory ministered by the Lutheran Church. He returned convinced that the establishment of a Baptist mission was going to be an essential factor in serving the needs, spiritual and otherwise, of the people in the region.

Conflict between European pastoral interests and Warlpiri needs

One of the many decisions facing the government in dealing with the displacement of the Warlpiri people was whether to issue rations to them in containment or reservation areas. Professor JB Cleland from The University of Adelaide, concerned over what he saw as a degeneration of Aboriginal values caused by dominant white mining interests, recommended establishment of a reserve between Mount Doreen in the north and the Granites in the west. Chief Protector Dr CE Cook rejected this recommendation because the location impinged on an established mining camp lease drawn up in the 1920s. The owners of that lease, William and Doreen Braitling, also objected to Cleland's proposal. Cook upheld their opposition because the proposal placed restrictions upon and limited the Braitling's access to a water hole called "Chilla Well". TGH Strehlow, one of the first Northern Territory patrol officers, also proposed the establishment of a reserve to encompass the Warlpiri homelands in the Davenport Ranges. Cook rejected this too on the basis that such a reserve would benefit few of the Warlpiri people. It became a conflict between the needs of the Warlpiri people and European interests. The latter were concerned with the maintenance and development of existing pastoral leases as well as establishing lucrative mining enterprises. The European interests won the day.

Such proposals did not alter the need for some form of assistance to the Warlpiri. Sometimes patrol officers would note that people in particular need were receiving various degrees of unsupervised welfare from the mining communities. They included the very elderly, who remembered the old days in their desert homeland and found it difficult to accept their present displacement, and the younger generation born after displacement with fewer ties to the land. As early as 1933, certain licences enabled mining lease holders to employ Aboriginal workers and, whilst this alleviated some of the distress, it often created added problems when entitlements under the Aboriginal Ordinance Act 1918 were not given to Aboriginal workers. Those who did supply rations to the needy did so with government subsidies.

In the reports from the patrol officers between the years 1940-1944 it was evident that indigenous living conditions had deteriorated with few opportunities for the native population to live consistently off the land. In this period, patrol officer Strehlow's comments concerning degeneration and disease at Mt Doreen gave Albrecht the ammunition needed to influence action on behalf of the South Australian Baptist Home Mission. Rev Laurie Reece returned from his exploration of the Mt Doreen and Granites region in 1944 angered at the treatment of the local Aborigines by the leaseholders William and Doreen Braitling. With bad feeling between the leaseholders and the local Warlpiri, the Braitlings made Reece's survey even harder because they regarded the best water hole for many miles (Vaughan Springs) as out of bounds to both the Warlpiri people and any future Baptist mission. Preventing the Warlpiri people from using the water at Vaughan Springs was in fact a violation of Section 24 of the Crown Lands Ordinance that gave Aboriginal people the right to gather food and water on pastoral leases (Rowse, 1990).

Establishment of Yuendumu (Rock Hill Bore) Settlement in 1946

Reece's report stimulated action by the Administrator who, whilst agreeing with the principle of establishing a Baptist mission in the Mount Doreen area, stated that the Baptist Home Mission would have to negotiate directly with the Braitlings (Rowse, 1990). Despite the Braitling's opposition, the Federal Government established a ration and welfare depot in 1946. Originally known as Rock Hill Bore, the Native Affairs Branch subsequently renamed the site Yuendumu (Figure 2.1).

The establishment of Yuendumu did alleviate, to some extent, the pressures experienced by the Haast's Bluff ration depot. This depot had been established in 1942 as a means of halting the eastward drift of the Warlpiri people toward the townships along the Stuart Highway (Meggitt, 1962). It also provided some respite to the Warlpiri people in the Mount Doreen area. Although the Native Affairs Branch gave it the status of an "Aboriginal Reserve', the Lutheran Church at Hermannsburg ran and managed it. The creation of Yuendumu acted as a magnet for the Warlpiri people in the Mount Doreen and Granites areas, and as people migrated toward this supply source it became more of a settlement than a distributional centre. Once food and warm clothes were available on a regular basis to the needy, reliance on Yuendumu increased and few would have wanted to return to the rigours of living off the land permanently. However, by the end of 1946, traditional, long-standing tribal feuds between the 400 Warlpiri people living at the Settlement were re-emerging. The threat of bloodshed was so real that the authorities decided to separate the warring factions and form a further Aboriginal Reserve at Hooker Creek. By 1951 approximately 150 Warlpiri had arrived there from Yuendumu and the Granites. Meggitt (1962) observed:

> Thus, by 1955 about two-thirds of the tribe lived on settlements under the direct supervision of N.A.B. officers; almost all the other Walbiri lived on cattle stations, where patrol officers visited them regularly to investigate their welfare.

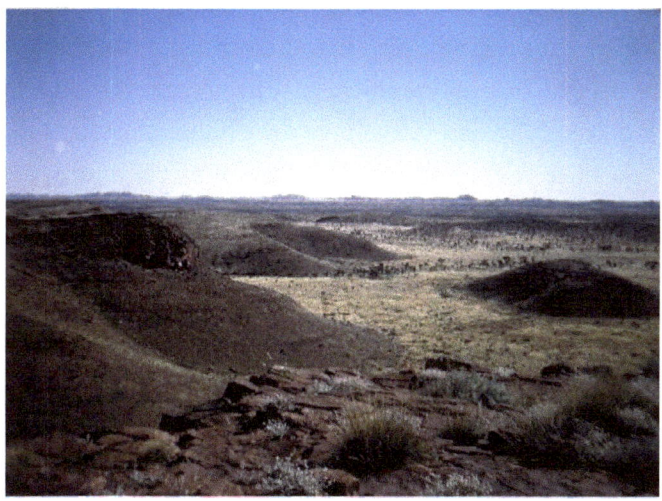

Figure 2.2
Yuendumu environs

In August 1946, the Federal Baptist Home Mission Board appointed Rev Laurie Reece and Rev Phillip Steer as the first Baptist missionaries to Yuendumu. Jordan (1999), writing about the Baptist ministry and its work amongst the indigenous peoples of Central Australia, makes the point that from the moment the first missionaries arrived at Yuendumu on 13 February 1947 the following factors became very evident:

From its inception, Yuendumu was a government settlement and not a mission, with the responsibility for policy and daily affairs being that of the government. Thus the missionaries were required to operate within the bounds of such policies as assimilation. However the Baptists were involved in much more than meeting spiritual needs. They helped supply clothing and medical supplies, taught sewing, commenced and ran the first store, helped build and often staffed the hospital, commenced a kindergarten, and commenced the first school.

Reverends Reece and Steer held relatively short ministries at Yuendumu. In April 1950, the Rev Tom Fleming and his wife Pat commenced a ministry that lasted 25 years. They eventually handed over their ministry to the Rev Ed Kingston in June 1975.

The establishment of Yuendumu as a ration station in 1946 would have made life considerably easier for the Warlpiri who did not have either employment or the protection of the mining or pastoral interests. They received food and clothing, and in return were expected to work in developing the Settlement for community living. As time passed, they became familiar with cooked meals and were paid part of their wages in cash. By 1969 a pattern had been established where the inhabitants fed and clothed themselves through purchases at the local store. Once this had occurred the government could well have thought that the Aboriginal people had reached a level of assimilation in being able to live as members of permanent settled groups, and to accept the controls imposed upon them by their European supervisors. Middleton and Francis (1976) make the point that:

> the manner of settlement administration produced a passive, dependent attitude among the Aborigines … Not only does the atmosphere of the "total institution" inhibit the development of initiative, experiment and responsibility; it also promotes the resentment and resistance of the inmates towards the European staff.

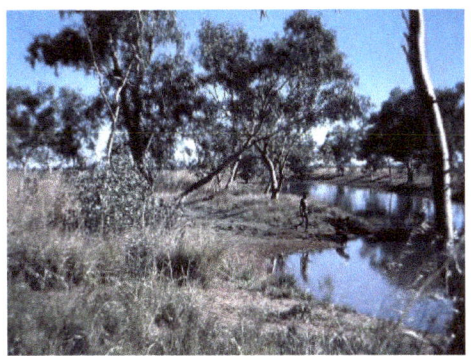 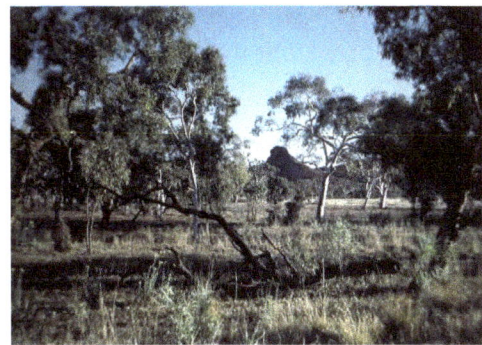

Figure 2.3
Yuendumu environs – water and greenery in a good season

In many ways, the Aboriginal people must have felt that they were being stretched between two worlds, the world they knew before European influence (the world of Jukurrpa) and the world they experienced after. Even after Yuendumu's establishment, it was not uncommon for small family groups to leave the Settlement for varying lengths of time to develop outstations located in Warlpiri land some distance away where they would live partially off the land in the traditional way.

Previously the Warlpiri traditional and nomadic life of hunting and food gathering was governed by their surroundings, the climate, geography and the availability of favourable flora and fauna. Considerable time, effort and skill were required to survive under harsh conditions, vast distances, infrequent rainfall and low food productivity (Campbell and Barrett, 1954). Commenting on this situation, Barrett (1968) noted that:

> they did not have the means or the knowledge to alter their
> environment to any marked extent. Consequently, they had to adapt
> their mode of life to their surroundings as they found them.

Food might not have been plentiful in the arid interior but it was extensive in variety. Mammals, birds, reptiles, insects and honey, usually acquired from the native bees or from storage sacs in the honey ants, were favoured foods. Added to these selections was a large variety of plants and plant products. Most methods used in the preparation of food were simple. Much was eaten raw, but when cooked it was often over an open fire or the food was buried in the hot ashes after the fire had subsided. After a successful hunt, the Warlpiri people singed kangaroos in an open fire and then cooked under ashes and hot earth. After cooking, they sectioned the game for distribution with the sharp edge of a boomerang or a stone knife. The Warlpiri people had no eating utensils and ate their food using only teeth and hands.

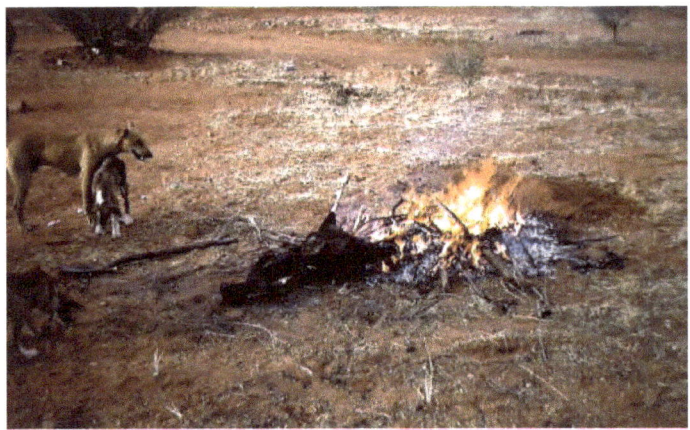

Figure 2.4
Camp dogs watching a kangaroo cooking

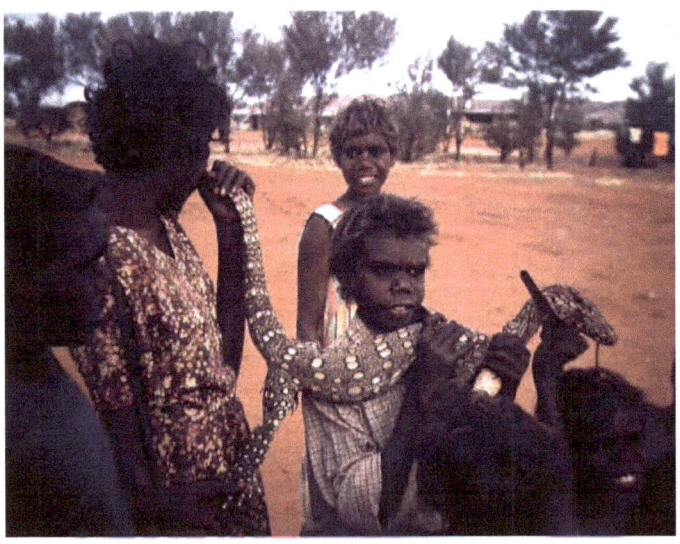

Figure 2.5
Unidentified Warlpiri children with a goanna

Because of the isolation of Australia from the rest of the world, the indigenous inhabitants had a manageable range of communicable diseases, which meant they were free from many of the serious illnesses that plagued European communities. Middleton and Francis (1976) remarked that, in general, the adult population experienced good health, unlike many of their children who, from the age of around six months, did not receive the proper sustenance for growth with consequential high infant mortality rates. Furthermore, they had no immunity to the diseases introduced by European settlers, smallpox and respiratory disease being the most prevalent, which proved fatal to them. Even after European foods were introduced on a regular basis, health did not necessarily improve with inadequate variation and poor diet often leading to malnutrition and vitamin deficiency. This was often compounded by the land surrounding the settlements being denuded of the flora and fauna that could have been used to supplement any food deficiency. Apart from dietary deficiencies, crowding, poor hygiene and sanitation would have contributed to the spread of disease, particularly viral and bacterial infections.

Baptist ministry of the Reverend Tom and Pat Fleming

When Yuendumu was established, many Aboriginal people had experienced contact with European culture to varying degrees. Because European authorities were prepared to set up ration depots in the more desolate areas of Central Australia, the most needy groups of Aboriginal people would have decided whether to accept the assistance or not. Circumstance would have argued for acceptance. But the point has been made that relationships between the indigenous and the white populations were, at times, less than cordial, particularly for those Warlpiri people with long memories. To accept anything from white hands without paying for it in some way or another was going to be difficult. In his assessment of the suitability of Yuendumu as a research centre, Barrett (1968) made the following observations:

> The settlement is relatively isolated geographically. Its population consists of a fairly static, self contained group of people, almost free of non-Aboriginal admixture. In their general mode of life and methods of food preparation and eating habits they are at an intermediate stage of transition from their previous hunting and food-gathering existence to the adoption of a civilised way of life.

> The key words "fairly static" and "self contained" indicate a degree of permanency amongst the Aboriginal population, a fact crucial to any future study which had as its core the notion of observing physical differences in human beings undergoing fundamental transitional changes from one lifestyle to another.

Physical characteristics of the Warlpiri

Somatometry

Many early mariners, inland explorers and anthropologists had described the metric and non-metric characters of Australian Aboriginal people from different regions of the continent. However, it was not until Andrew Abbie, Professor of Anatomy at The University of Adelaide, summarised the results of his field expeditions to ten Aboriginal communities in the 1950s–1960s that knowledge of the age changes in a range of anthropometric variables and indices emerged (Abbie, 1975a, 1975b, 1975c). Abbie's data cover a wide range of observations, both metric and non-metric. The results cemented his previous view that Aboriginal people from widely separated regions display physical homogeneity (Abbie, 1968).

Abbie's surveys 1950-1960

Abbie's surveys had the advantage of providing observations obtained from children and adults living in South Australia, Western Australia, Northern Territory and Queensland. For the growth study, he obtained 38 measurements from 445 males and 424 females ranging in age from newborn to 20 years. He pooled data and formed it as a single cross-sectional sample, presenting results in tables and growth charts for each variable (Abbie, 1975a). He measured adult Aboriginal people at Yuendumu, Haast's Bluff, Yalata, Maningrida, Beswick and Kalumburu (Abbie, 1975b). For the statistical analysis, he pooled data from 205 males and 150 females, ranging in estimated age from 21 to more than 60 years. He reported some selected measurements and indices for smaller sub-groups of Aboriginal adults from four different regions. The main disadvantage of these studies arises from the cross-sectional nature of the data, the very low subject numbers for most age groups and the difficulty in performing statistical analysis. For example, only 23 males and 27 females represented the adult Warlpiri people from Yuendumu and Haast's Bluff. Most age groups had less than ten subjects. Abbie (1975c) provided a detailed account of the non-metric characters of Aboriginal people but we do not consider this topic further here.

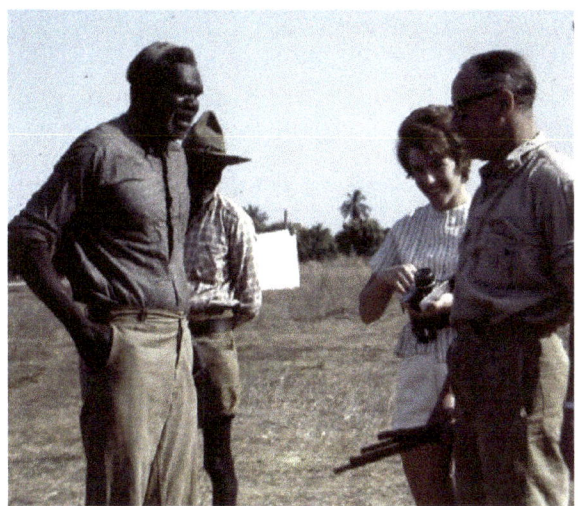

Figure 2.6
Professor Andrew A Abbie at Kalumburu,
Western Australia, 1963

Establishment of studies concerning dental features and craniofacial growth 1951-1971

Between 1951 and 1960, the field expeditions to Yuendumu by the dental researchers were concerned primarily with dental features. However, researchers realised that the inclusion of selected general body measurements and assessments of skeletal maturation would facilitate the analysis and understanding of the processes involved in craniofacial growth and development of the jaws and dentition. Consequently, on each visit from 1961, researchers obtained a number of somatometric records from each subject examined. These they entered into computer data files for future descriptive and correlative studies.

Serial records: mixed longitudinal data

The accrued data were mixed longitudinal, that is, subjects were examined on one or more annual visits up to a maximum of 10, allowing a reliable basis for determining the growth patterns of the measurements obtained (Table 2.1). Some of these results have been published previously, particularly for stature and weight (Barrett and Brown, 1971; Brown and Barrett, 1971, 1972, 1973a, 1973b; Brown and Townsend, 1982). Statistical analyses for most of the somatometric data relating to growth patterns of the Warlpiri children and the physical characteristics of young adults have not been published previously. These are included in Appendix B to present the first growth tables for a number of variables and to provide a basis for comparison with the cross-sectional results derived from the pooled sample of individuals measured about one generation previously (Abbie, 1975a, 1975b). In addition, our analyses form a reference standard for future growth studies of Warlpiri children living under changed environmental and nutritional influences.

Table 2.1 Yuendumu subjects with recorded birthdates: distribution by sex and number of serial records

Number of serial records	Males		Females	
	Subjects	Records	Subjects	Records
1	45	45	45	45
2	21	42	21	42
3	5	15	10	30
4	12	48	8	32
5	17	85	8	40
6	14	84	6	36
7	8	56	9	63
8	16	128	15	120
9	13	117	9	81
10	3	30	3	30
Total	154	650	134	519

Computer analysis of data

The number of serial records for individual subjects varied from 1 to 10 (Table 2.1). In total, researchers made 650 recordings for 154 males and 519 recordings for 134 females. Only subjects with known birth dates were included in the sample. The mixed longitudinal data were analysed by computer using the method proposed by Solow (1969) and described by Brown and Barrett (1971). The analysis uses multiple interpolations to provide estimates of the growth achieved at monthly intervals between the first and last recordings for each subject. With breaks in the sequence of observations for a subject, resulting in missing data points, the values before and after the breaks were treated as separate data sets. When sample size permitted, the measures of skewness showed that most distributions did not depart significantly from normality. The mean values were then accepted as the 50th centiles. The 10th and 90th centiles at each age were constructed as deviations from the mean using multiples of the standard deviations. As suggested by Tanner *et al.*, (1966), some visual smoothing of the standard deviation curves was carried out before calculating the final centiles. This compensates for irregularities in centile curves constructed from actual standard deviations.

Table 2.2 Summary of selected variables measured in young adults from Yuendumu (recorded age = 20 years)

Variable	Males (N=20)		Females (N=34)	
	Mean	SD	Mean	SD
Stature (cm)	172.8	6.6	162.8	4.9
Weight (kg)	60.8	11.1	48.6	5.7
Weight/stature (gm/cm)	362.0	57.6	299.0	-
Radius length (cm)	27.4	1.2	25.0	1.3
Head length (cm)	20.4	0.7	19.0	0.5
Head breadth (cm)	14.1	0.4	13.7	0.4
Head circumference (cm)	58.0	1.8	54.4	1.1
Cephalic index (%)	69.9	2.5	72.4	2.9
Bizygomatic diameter (cm)	14.1	0.5	13.0	0.4
Bigonial diameter (cm)	10.3	0.7	9.8	0.4
Morphological face height (cm)	11.8	0.5	10.8	0.4

Table 2.2 shows a summary of the analyses with respect to young adult males and females with recorded age of 20 years. Means, standard deviations and centiles are included in the more comprehensive tables listed in Appendix B.

The differences in mean values between those in Table 2.2 and those reported by Abbie for young adults are marginal and could reasonably be explained by experimental error including differences in measurement techniques and sample sizes, or possibly generational change. In relation to the latter, we cannot rule out a secular change between generations (Barrett and Brown, 1971; Brown and Barrett, 1973a).

Abbie's summary provides a useful description of the metric characters and growth patterns of Aboriginal populations, considered as a single homogeneous group (Abbie, 1975a):

> Aboriginal growth unfolds in a highly distinctive pattern, obviously strongly determined genetically, practically achieved - except in absolute dimensions - by the onset of puberty and, apparently, impervious to the influence of a wide diversity of environments.

> The pattern leads to a lean slender physique, with long head and face (but prominent cheek bones), short neck and relatively short trunk, narrow shoulders and hips and long slender extremities - especially the inferior - and more particularly in the distal segments.

The cephalic index in our study falls well within the dolichocephalic range, being substantially less than 76 per cent in males and females, not only in the young adults but also from age 5 years. Our study supports Abbie's observation of prominent cheek-bones and this requires further comment. This feature combined with a relatively narrow face at the gonial regions is emphasised by the difference between the mean bizygomatic and bigonial diameters - 3.8 cm in males and 3.2 in females. This facial morphology is reflected in the underlying relative breadths of the upper and lower dental arches and a form of dental occlusion that that was termed "X-occlusion" by Barrett (1953) in an exhibit of dental casts. A more functional description is "alternate intercuspation" or anisognathism, a condition that develops with divergent growth of the maxillary and mandibular dental arches. It is more prevalent in males than females (Barrett, 1969; Brown *et al.*, 1987; Brown 1992). So-called X-occlusion is discussed further in Chapter 3.

Other studies from the Adelaide group offer more detailed descriptions of craniofacial morphology in the Warlpiri Aboriginal people (Brown, 1965; Barrett *et al.*, 1965; Brown and Barrett, 1964). In profile, the Aboriginal face displays marked alveolar prominence or prognathism (Figure 2.8). This is accompanied by relatively large tooth diameters and a marked forward migration of the upper and lower dental arches during facial growth. The prognathism is confined to the alveolar region and is not evident in the basal jaw region as also remarked upon by Abbie (1975c).

Growth patterns, velocities and parameters

The Yuendumu mixed longitudinal data also allowed the calculation of growth velocities including the magnitude and the timing of peak adolescent growth (Brown and Barrett, 1973b). For stature, the peak adolescent velocity of 9.8 cm/year occurred in boys at 13.7 years whereas in girls the relevant values were 8.3 cm/year at 12.0 years. Dimensions of the face displayed similar ages for the adolescent growth spurt.

Brown and Townsend (1982) completed a more detailed analysis of adolescent growth patterns in which they calculated the growth parameters by curve fitting using the method outlined by Preece and Baines (1978). This method is robust and provides a very accurate fit to growth data through the derivation of five curve coefficients. The study only selected children with known birth-dates and six or more successive measures of height. The coefficients can calculate several biological parameters descriptive of adolescent growth. These include the peak height velocity (PHV), the age at PHV, the age at take-off into the adolescent spurt and the height at take-off (Table 2.3). The values obtained for PHV and the age at PHV are similar to those derived by using mixed longitudinal data as described previously.

Table 2.3 Biological growth parameters derived by the Preece-Baines model 1 for Aboriginal children (PHV = peak height velocity)

Biological parameters	Aboriginal boys N=39		Aboriginal girls N=23	
	Mean	SD	Mean	SD
Adult height (cm)	172.1	5.8	162.9	4.6
Age at take off (yr)	10.6	1.4	8.8	1.5
Age at PHV (yr)	14.0	0.8	11.9	1.1
Height at take off (cm)	136.0	8.5	129.1	5.2
Height at PHV (cm)	157.1	6.3	147.9	4.8
Velocity at take off (cm/yr)	4.4	0.8	5.0	1.2
Velocity at PHV (cm/yr)	10.3	1.2	8.4	0.9
Height increase take off to PHV (cm)	21.1	3.8	18.8	3.1
Height increase PHV to adult (cm)	15.0	2.9	15.0	2.1
% Adult height at take off	79.0	3.9	79.3	2.5
% Adult height at PHV	91.3	1.7	90.8	1.3

A further advantage of the Preece-Baines method is that mean constant curves for height attained and height velocity can be calculated to provide more graphic comparisons of subjects within and between groups or populations (Figure 2.7).

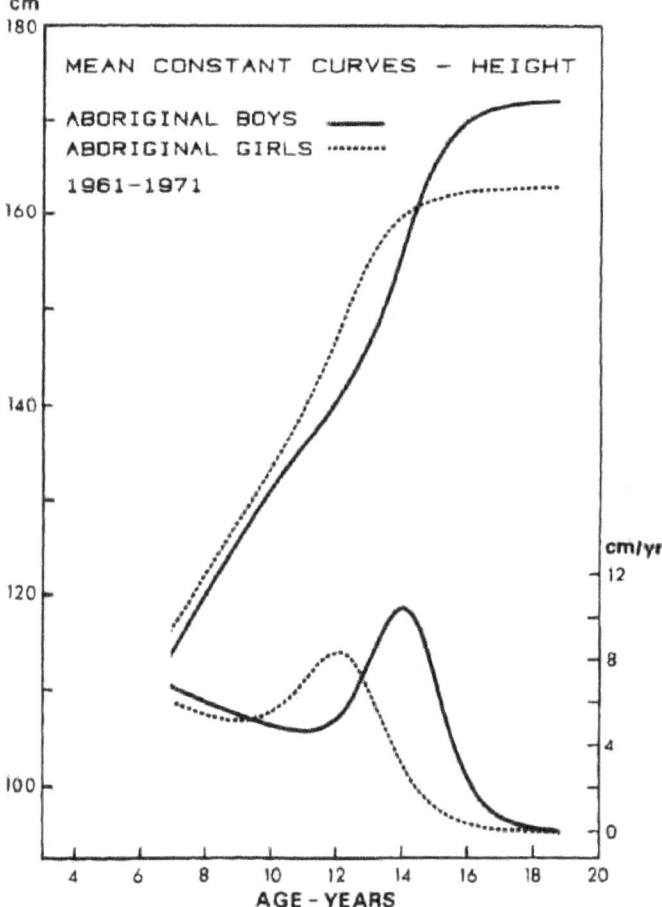

Figure 2.7
Mean constant curves for height and height velocity in Warlpiri boys and girls

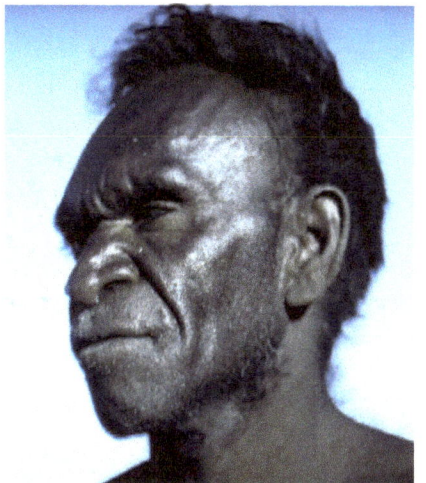 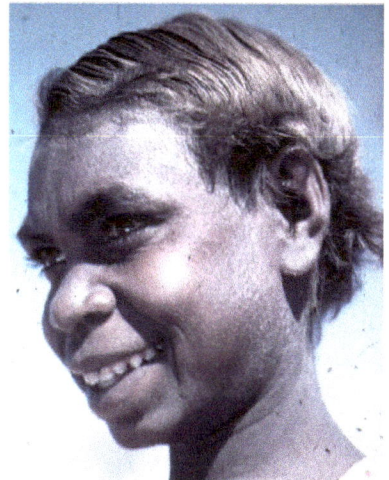

Figure 2.8
Unidentified Warlpiri man and woman showing distinctive facial characters

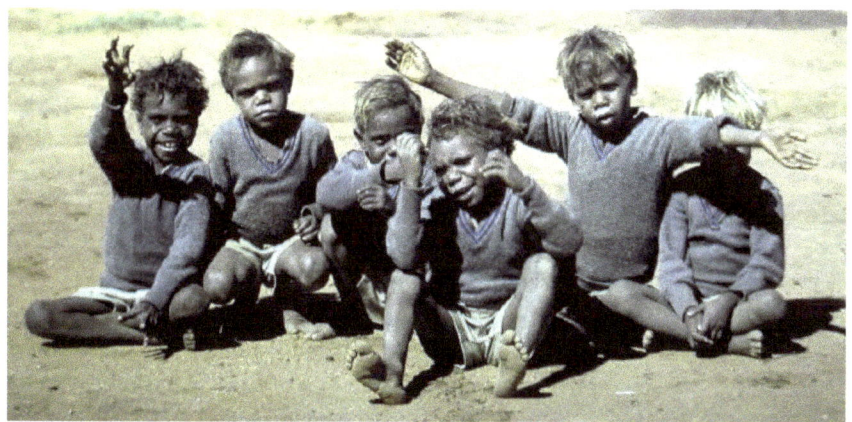

Figure 2.9
Unidentified Yuendumu schoolboys

Dentition

Numerous publications from the Adelaide group have described characteristics of the Warlpiri dentition. Of particular relevance are the collected papers of Barrett (1976) dealing with tooth size, dental arch size, tooth eruption, dental occlusion and tooth wear, and the papers by Townsend and others listed in Chapter 9. Chapter 5 also reviews some aspects of these topics.

References

Abbie AA (1968). The homogeneity of Australian Aborigines. *Arch Phys Anthrop in Oceania* 3:223–231.

Abbie AA (1975a). The Aboriginal growth pattern. In: *Studies in Physical Anthropology. Research and Regional Studies Vol 2.* Canberra: Australian Institute of Aboriginal Studies 5:1–48.

Abbie AA (1975b). Metrical characters of adult Aborigines. In: *Studies in Physical Anthropology. Research and Regional Studies Vol 2.* Canberra: Australian Institute of Aboriginal Studies 5:76–103.

Abbie AA (1975c). Non-metrical characters of Aborigines. In: *Studies in Physical Anthropology Research and Regional Studies Vol 2.* Canberra: Australian Institute of Aboriginal Studies 5:104–115.

Barrett MJ (1953). X-Occlusion. *Dent Mag Oral Top* 70:279. Report of an exhibit at the Thirteenth Australian Dental Congress, University of Queensland, Brisbane, June 1–5, 1953.

Barrett MJ (1968). Features of the Australian dentition. *Dent Mag Oral Top* 85:15–18.

Barrett MJ (1969). Functioning occlusion. *Ann Aust Coll Dent Surg* 2:68–80.

Barrett MJ (1976). *Dental Observations on Australian Aborigines. Collected Papers and Reports 1953–1973.* Adelaide: Faculty of Dentistry, The University of Adelaide.

Barrett MJ, Brown T (1971). Increase in average height of Australian Aborigines. *Med J Aust* 2:1169–1172.

Barrett MJ, Brown T, Macdonald MR (1965). Size of dental arches in a tribe of Central Australian Aborigines. *J Dent Res* 44:912–920.

Brown T (1965). *Craniofacial Variations in a Central Australian Tribe. A Radiographic Investigation of Young Adult Males and Females.* Adelaide: Libraries Board of South Australia.

Brown T (1992). Developmental, morphological and functional aspects of occlusion in Australian Aboriginals. *J Hum Ecol Special Issue* 2:73–75.

Brown T, Barrett MJ (1964). A roentgenographic study of facial morphology in a tribe of Central Australian Aborigines. *Am J Phys Anthropol* 22:33–42.

Brown T, Barrett MJ (1971). Growth in Central Australian Aborigines: Stature. *Med J Aust* 2:29–33.

Brown T, Barrett MJ (1972). Growth in Central Australian Aborigines: Weight. *Med J Aust* 2:999–1002.

Brown T, Barrett MJ (1973a). Increase in average weight of Australian Aborigines. *Med J Aust* 2:25–28

Brown T, Barrett MJ (1973b). Dental and craniofacial growth studies of Australian Aborigines. In: *The Human Biology and Aborigines in Cape York.* Human Biology Series. Kirk RL, editor. Canberra: Australian Institute of Aboriginal Studies, 5:69–80.

Brown T, Townsend GC (1982). Adolescent growth in height of Australian Aboriginals analysed by the Preece-Baines function: a longitudinal study. *Ann Hum Biol* 9:495–505.

Brown T, Abbott AH, Burgess VB (1987). Longitudinal study of dental arch relationships in Australian Aboriginals with reference to alternate intercuspation. *Am J Phys Anthropol* 72:49–57.

Campbell TD, Barrett MJ (1954). *So They Did Eat.* Adelaide: Board for Anthropological Research, The University of Adelaide.

Carrington VG (1946). *Report on the Administration of the Northern Territory for The Year Ending 30th June 1946.* Canberra: Australian Institute of Aboriginal and Torres Strait Islander Studies.

Jordan I (1999). Ministry among Indigenous People. Brief History of Baptist Ministry to the Indigenous People of Central Australia. http://www.bwa-baptist-heritage.org/bap-ab.htm

Meggitt MJ (1962). *Desert People: A study of the Wailbiri Aborigines of Central Australia.* Sydney: Angus and Robertson.

Middleton MR, Francis SH (1976). *Yuendumu and it Children. Life and Health on an Aboriginal Settlement.* Canberra: Australian Government Printing Service.

Napaljarri PR, Cataldi L (2003). *Warlpiri Dreamings and Histories Yimikirli.* Walnut Creek, California: Alta Mira Press, pxxiv.

Northern Territory Police (2006). *Description of Yuendumu.* http://www.pfes.nt.gov.au/

Preece MA, Baines MJ (1978). A new family of mathematical models describing the human growth curve. *Ann Hum Biol* 5:1–24.

Rowse T (1990). Enlisting the Warlpiri. *Continuum: Aust J Media Cult* 3:5.

Solow B (1969). Automatic processing of growth data. *Angle Orthod* 39:186–197.

Tanner JM, Whitehouse RH, Takaishi M (1966). Standards from birth to maturity for height, weight, height velocity and weight velocity: British children, 1965. *Arch Dis Child* 41:454–613.

3
Yuendumu:
The Longitudinal Project 1951-1960

Anthropology in Adelaide pre-Yuendumu

The arrival of Frederic Wood Jones in Adelaide caused a great deal of excitement when he became Curator of the South Australia Museum in 1919. He was a dominant figure in medical science and anthropology and "was a gifted comparative anatomist and illustrator, as well as a fluent orator and writer" (Southcott, 1986). At the time, there was an enthusiastic group of men from several disciplines pursuing their interests in the physical and cultural anthropology of Central Australian Aboriginal people. Wood Jones succeeded Archibald Watson in 1920 as the Elder Professor of Anatomy at The University of Adelaide.

Since the settlement of South Australia there had been numerous studies of Aboriginal people, particularly by staff of the South Australian Museum. Tindale (1986) provided an excellent summary of previous anthropological research in the 19th and 20th centuries, including an extensive list of references. Among the group of Adelaide scientists in the 1920s was Thomas Draper Campbell, then a dental surgeon aged 27 years. Clearly influenced by Wood Jones, Campbell joined him on field expeditions.

Two significant events occurred in 1926: the formation of the Anthropological Society of South Australia by Wood Jones, Campbell and John B Cleland; and the establishment of the Board for Anthropological Research, following a recommendation by Wood Jones to the Council of The University of Adelaide. Wood Jones resigned the same year to accept a professorial appointment at the University of Hawaii. However, his enthusiasm and activities while in Adelaide served to focus attention on this city as the Australian centre for physical anthropology.

Jones (1987) described the formation of the Board for Anthropological Research and the field investigations of staff from the South Australian Museum and The University of Adelaide up to the outbreak of World War II. The purpose of the Board was to approve expeditions to observe and document Aboriginal groups, and to sponsor them and to support them financially to a limited extent. Campbell was a leading figure in pre-war field expeditions and he published extensively on dental and anthropological subjects (see Chapter 1).

The main objective of the Board's expeditions in the pre-war years was to gather records of Aboriginal people still following a nomadic hunter-gatherer way of life. The data were descriptive and, of necessity, cross-sectional in nature. It was not until the 1960s that access to computers made longitudinal studies and more sophisticated statistical analyses feasible. By then the nomadic life style was rapidly disappearing among Aboriginal groups as they gradually moved onto government settlements. Campbell's background in dentistry, however, enabled him to explore the relationships between dental conditions and food habits, environment and cultural influences. He was able to contrast the well-formed Aboriginal dentitions with the degenerate and diseased dentitions of European Australians. This topic and the reasons for such contrasts were to occupy Campbell's interest and his teaching all his life.

Campbell was always a meticulous observer and recorder of Aboriginal people and their cultures. Consequently, he became one of the pioneer ethnographic filmmakers, filming Aboriginal nomads, their lifestyles, subsistence techniques and ceremonial activities. He first operated a movie camera in May 1926 at Ooldea in South Australia. Later, between 1930 and 1937, he and other members of the Board's expeditions made 47 films of Aboriginal life at Cockatoo Creek, Mount Leibig, Mann Range, Ernabella, Warburton Range and the Granites. Most, if not all, of the recordings were made using 400 feet, 16 frames per second, movie film. Many of these documentary films were used in anthropological teaching at overseas universities. Campbell continued his activities as a film ethnographer at Yuendumu in the 1950s and 1960s.

As a scientist with an innovative mind he was one of the first to emphasise the significance of biological adaptability, thereby extending his concept of anthropology beyond mere description. Campbell also had a genuine admiration and respect for the Aboriginal people he met and he openly admired their skills and intellect. As a measure of their respect for Campbell, the Aboriginal population of Yuendumu, to whom he was known as *Tjangala*, exhibited much sadness in 1967, when it was learnt that "old fella Tjangala bin finished up" (Brown, 2001).

Dental Anthropology at Yuendumu

During the Second World War, there was a hiatus in anthropological research sponsored by the Board. Not until 1951, when Campbell led the first team visit to Yuendumu, did field research recommence. The second half of the 20th century saw significant changes in the personnel, objectives and methodology of research in dental anthropology. Campbell had eight years left before retirement in 1958, and it was important that what had been established should be allowed to prosper and develop. From that time, Campbell produced a series of ethnographic films sponsored by the Board for Anthropological Research. Murray Barrett and John Simpson were the cinematographers for these films. The best known of these is probably the 1953 documentary *So They Did Eat* which depicts the daily search for food and water by nomadic Aboriginals (Campbell *et al.*, 1954) Another made in 1958 and entitled "*Nabarula*" gives a brief outline of the life of an Aboriginal girl from childhood to adulthood. Others in the series preserved the craft-making skills of the Warlpiri by documenting the making of the boomerang, the woomera, palya (spinifex gum), spears, hair string and axes. Campbell's final film, "*Ngoora*", was produced in 1965 and it shows an enactment of the movement of a small group of Aboriginal people to a new camping site. He published only two papers relating to dental topics in the 1950s (Campbell and Barrett, 1953; Campbell 1956). After his retirement from the university, Campbell continued his interests in Aboriginal crafts and the archaeology and geology of the southeast region of South Australia. During these years, he visited old quarries and published papers dealing with stone implements and crafts.

Murray Barrett saw the advantages of visiting Yuendumu on a regular basis to chart dental development in young Warlpiri children and, being a specialist prosthodontist, to study dental occlusion and masticatory function in an ethnic group recently congregated on a Government Settlement. This marked the beginning of the longitudinal dental study that he led until his death in 1975. The first expedition to Yuendumu in August 1951 was particularly important for Barrett in a number of ways. It gave him the opportunity to work within an interdisciplinary environment with scientists of the calibre of Campbell, Abbie, Mountford, Cleland and Tindale. It was also his introduction to the Warlpiri people and he quickly formed a personal attachment to them and their culture, which was to last for the rest of his life. Finally, this period of working in a remote region provided him with first hand experience of the problems associated with both the organisation and the difficulties incurred in gathering data in the field.

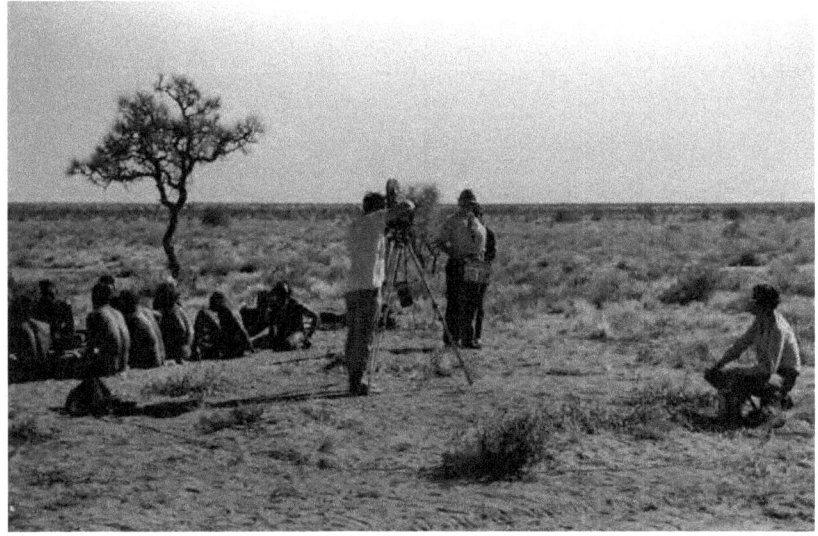

Figure 3.1
Murray Barrett filming at Yuendumu

The Board for Anthropological Research always assigned an alphabetic prefix of one or two letters for each expedition that it sponsored. The 1951 Yuendumu visit was assigned the prefix letter P. It was Barrett's custom to add a serial number for each subject examined so that the 10th subject examined in 1951 was registered as P10. In addition to this identification, each subject would also be given a permanent dental or "delta" number that would remain with him or her throughout the longitudinal study. The dental models that were cast in a dental stone were also inscribed with this information as well as the date of examination. For example, if subject number 586 in the longitudinal study was examined on three occasions there would be three sets of dental casts inscribed as follows: Δ 586 AL 86; Δ 586 AP 71; Δ 586 AS 27. In this way, the subject and all associated records would be uniquely cross-referenced according to the subject's dental number and the expedition serial number.

At the time the dental casts were obtained, Barrett would complete a thorough oral and dental examination, charting teeth present and recording the findings on charts together with the date of examination, gender and any dental anomalies such as agenesis of teeth, enamel hypoplasia, instances of tooth evulsion or other soft or hard tissue abnormalities. Birth dates, either recorded or estimated, genealogical relationships, and other relevant information would also be entered on the data sheets. In the 1960s these data sheets were redesigned and expanded to include cross-referencing to the wider range of physical examinations undertaken in those years. Photographs of the subjects were also obtained.

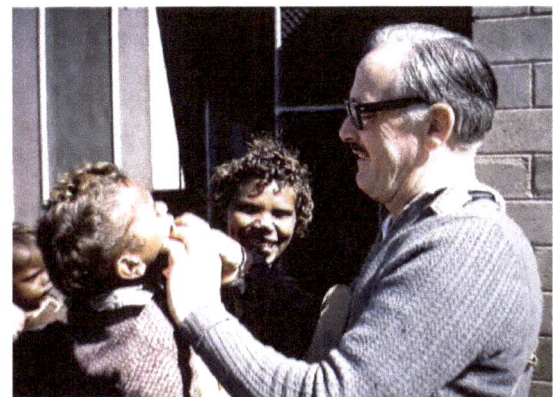

Figure 3.2
Murray Barrett examining Anthony Jampijinpa Egan with Jeannine Nungarrayi Egan watching

During the second visit to Yuendumu in May 1952, Barrett and Campbell set the pattern for research that would continue to dominate throughout the 1950s. Central to this visit was the decision to concentrate attention on children and young adults. Looking through notes of the projects in 1952 it becomes evident that the first four objectives were to examine children and adults who had recently arrived at Yuendumu, to examine the eruption of teeth in infants, to obtain impressions and casts of children and young adults, and to observe and document an unusual relationship of upper and lower teeth in young adults. Barrett initially named this morphological feature "X Occlusion" until a more descriptive term could be found (Barrett, 1953a). Certainly, the idea to obtain dental impressions of children had been put into practice in 1951 and it was most likely that Barrett saw the potential for further examinations and dental casts of the same individuals. This decision was the basis of a fundamental aspect of the anthropological research at Yuendumu, the development of longitudinal study programmes.

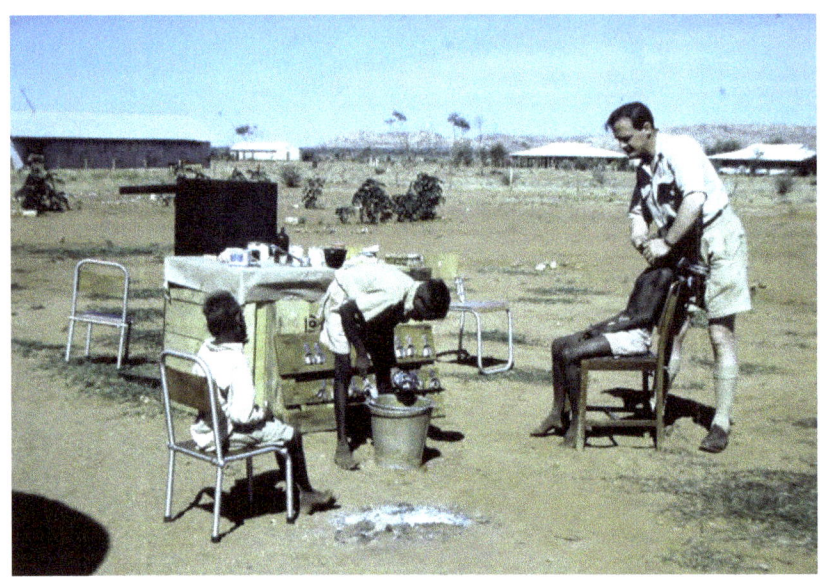

Figure 3.3
Murray Barrett obtaining dental impressions in the early 1950s

Another topic of research during the 1952 visit was to determine the dietary habits of the indigenous population of Yuendumu. Campbell and Barrett believed that knowledge of food habits and food preparation would add to their understanding of Aboriginal people's dental conditions, explain how they differed from modern European dentitions, and clarify the factors contributing to observed dental characteristics. To address these issues, observations were made on matters such as dietary patterns, native foods compared with store-bought provisions, methods of food preparation, eating habits, and food intake, including information on calories, proteins, fats and carbohydrates. Investigating dietary habits provided the researchers with insights into the reasons for changes in the dentition upon transition from a nomadic hunter-gatherer way of life to the more sheltered existence at Yuendumu. As Campbell and Barrett (1953) observed:

> this change may be summed up as follows. The native diet under natural conditions contains a wide range of food materials. Habits of preparation, cooking - when carried out - and consumption ensure the retention of protective substances, minerals and roughage. On the other hand, the newly-acquired routine diet contains white flour and white sugar as its staple items …The present routine diet

is overbalanced with refined carbohydrates; possibly has vitamin deficiencies and is certainly limited in roughage ... The meals served at the settlement and food they prepare from rations require little or no mastication. Food items consumed in their old native habits - to which they now only occasionally revert - were mostly of a type conducive to marked attrition of the teeth and natural detergence. These factors were undoubtably important in maintaining a sound healthy dentition.

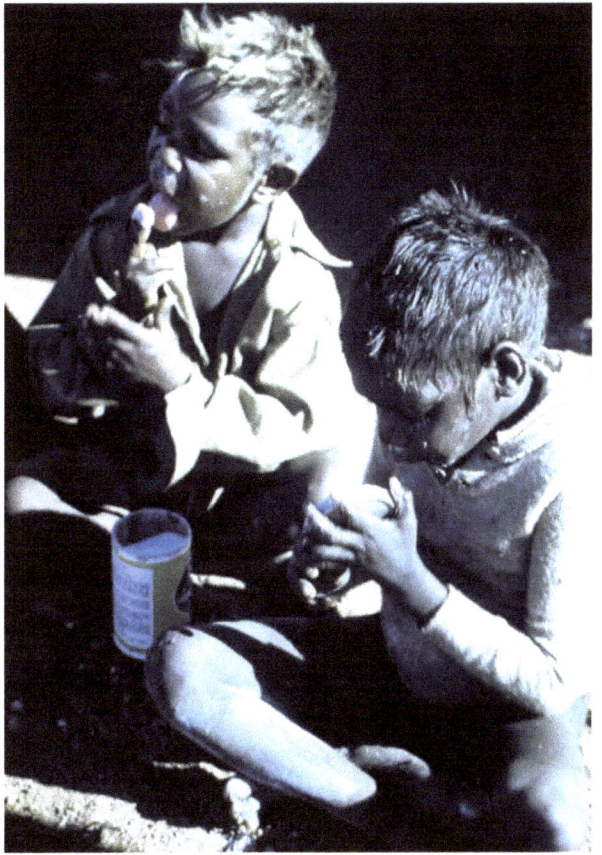

Figure 3.4
Children licking condensed milk from their fingers

The belief that the adoption of the Yuendumu lifestyle could be detrimental to the continued general and dental health of the Warlpiri stimulated two further avenues of research. As a traditional nomadic lifestyle was conducive to healthy and fully functional dentitions, the researchers considered it necessary to first define a healthy dentition and determine how it was maintained. The second aim was to discover to what extent changes in food habits caused deleterious dental consequences over time. This was particularly relevant when comparisons were made between the dentitions of the Yuendumu Aboriginal people and those familiar to the researchers in European Australians.

Expeditions and locations

The pattern of Campbell and Barrett's research was established for the remainder of the 1950s. While Campbell concentrated on recording the crafts and daily life of the Warlpiri, Barrett continued with a variety of topics within the general discipline of dental anthropology. The Board for Anthropological Research sponsored many expeditions to Aboriginal settlements during these years (Table 3.1) and Barrett led or joined ten visits to Yuendumu in the 1950s. On all of these he obtained dental casts from new subjects and also from subjects he had already enrolled in the longitudinal study. However, there were other expeditions to Yuendumu by other scientists, for example staff from the South Australian Museum, Abbie, Packer and their team of anatomists, and others from The University of Adelaide.

Barrett was particularly interested in functional dental occlusion, that is, the way in which upper and lower teeth meet not only in static relationships but also during mastication of various foods. It was important to obtain permanent and durable casts of the subjects' dentitions for later research into growth, age changes and tooth wear from abrasive elements in cooked food. Obtaining impressions and making dental casts became a major priority and, as each year passed, better materials and techniques were adopted to produce very accurate and durable casts. When mixing impression powder and dental stone, precise water/powder ratios were adopted as well as methods of vibration to reduce air bubbles being trapped when pouring dental stone into the impressions. When the dental models were firmly set, they were matched against the intraoral examination to verify teeth present and then securely packed for transport to Adelaide, where the excess plaster around the periphery was trimmed in a standard way and a plaster base was added.

Table 3.1 Expeditions to Yuendumu and other locations between the years 1951 -1959[1]

Trip	Destination	Date	Team leader	Team members	
P*	Yuendumu	1951	Campbell TD	Abbie AA Barrett MJ Campbell DJ Fry HK Kerr DIB Mountford CP Walsh GD	Adey WR Crosby ND Cleland JB Hill B LeMessurier HD Tindale NB Wherrett G
Q*	Yuendumu	1952	Campbell TD	Barrett MJ	
R	SA, WA, NT, Melville Islands	1953-1955	Birdsell JB	Tindale NB Birdsell E	Bartholomew GG Epling PJ
T*	Yuendumu	1953	Campbell TD	Barrett MJ	Simpson JM
U*	Yuendumu	1954	Barrett MJ	Lawton GH Simpson JM	Whitford CW LeMessurier HD
V*	Yuendumu	1955	Barrett MJ	Cran JA Packer AD	Dellow PG Walsh GD
W*	Yuendumu	1956	Campbell TD	Barrett MJ	Dellow PG Schultz RA
X*	Yuendumu	1956	Campbell TD	Barrett MJ	Cran JA
Y	Haasts Bluff	1956	Abbie AA	Cleland JB, Kempster P Casley-Smith JR Walsh GD	Heithersay GS Packer AD Tindale NB
Z	Mt Blyth and Giles, WA	1957	Tindale NB	Johnson JE Macdougall WB	Macauley R Warne S
AA	Yuendumu	1957	Packer AD	Kent P	Walsh GD
AB	Haasts Bluff	1957	Abbie AA	Packer AD, Cleland JB Walsh GD, Stocker EO Tindale NB	Butdz-Olsen O Kempster P Casley Smith J
AC*	Yuendumu	1957	Campbell TD	Barrett MJ Meadows AW	Cran JA Poidevin LOS
AD*	Yuendumu	1958	Campbell TD	Barrett MJ	Beyron HL
AE	Yalata	1958	Packer AD	Kempster P	Walsh GD
AF	Koonibba	1958	Campbell TD	Barrett MJ Reade PC	Cran JA Thomson KW
AG	Maningreda	1959	Abbie AA	Frowde G Packer AD	Kempster P
AH	Yuendumu	1959	Campbell TD	Cran JA Kay LJ	Horsnell AM Reade PC

1 The table shows the alphabetic prefix assigned by the Board for Anthropological Research for each visit and the leader and membership of each team. Barrett obtained impressions on trips marked with an asterisk.

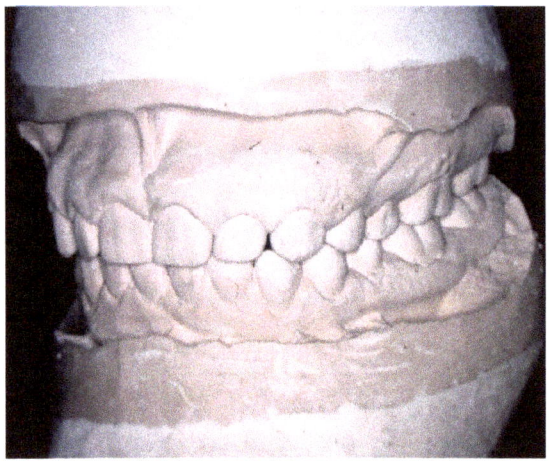
Figure 3.5
Dental casts of an adolescent Warlpiri male illustrating
a normal, healthy and functional dentition

Where possible, the upper and lower dental models of a subject were registered in what is often termed "intercuspal occlusion", referring to the way in which upper and lower teeth meet when the jaws are brought together from a resting position. For some subjects, this position was registered with a wax wafer bite record in which shallow impressions of the subject's teeth were made when intercuspal occlusion was assumed. From the bite registrations, the dental models could then be brought together to duplicate the jaw positions. In later years Barrett occasionally obtained more extensive jaw recordings to permit him to mount the dental models of a subject on an anatomical articulator, a device that could reproduce jaw movements. To study the physiology of mastication, researchers obtained movie films and still photographs of subjects chewing a variety of foods.

X-occlusion

A morphological feature of the dentition described as "X-occlusion" by Barrett (1953a) was referred to briefly in Chapter 2. Barrett's initial description of X-occlusion was as follows:

> The teeth on one side only show occlusal relationships conforming to text-book centric occlusion, but the lower jaw is in lateral relationship to the upper. When such unilateral interdigitation is established, the

cusps and depressions of the teeth on the opposite side of the arches are not interlocked - there is an obvious buccolingual discrepancy. These casts are not an isolated case, but illustrate a type of occlusion, which has been observed in a number of living subjects and in skull material. Although the occlusal relationships do not conform to textbook "normal" occlusion, for the aboriginal in his native environment they must be considered within the normal.

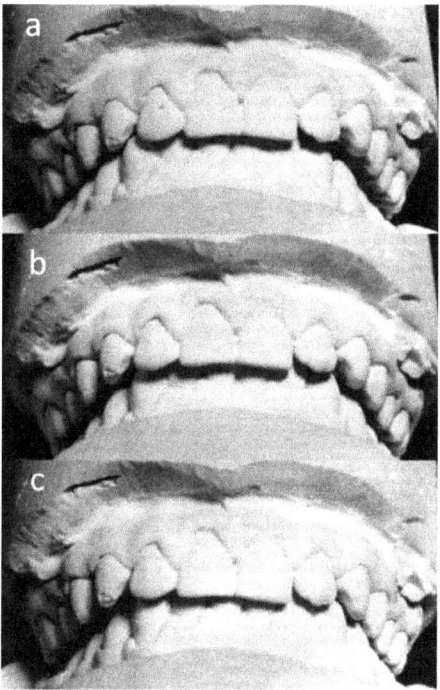

Figure 3.6
X–occlusion: dental models showing
a) occlusion of the teeth on the right side only
b) in the central position where there is no maximum posterior tooth contact on either side
c) occlusion of teeth on the left side only

The observation that the upper and lower teeth could meet in maximum contact on either left or right sides but not on both sides together was indeed a novel observation that departed radically from accepted definitions of how human teeth should meet in occlusion. It would be regarded as a malocclusion by orthodontists and in need of treatment if found in a European child. And yet in the Aboriginal people the presence of "X-occlusion" was no hindrance to mastication. Indeed, the reverse was true, as it afforded a much wider range of lateral jaw movements, which was advantageous when grinding and chewing the tough food of the nomadic hunter.

Subsequent to Barrett's early description, further studies of this type of occlusion brought to light many other aspects of dental occlusion and tooth wear in Australian Aboriginal people. Later in the 1950s Barrett published a detailed descriptive account of the ever-changing functional occlusion of Aboriginal people in which he described continuing occlusal tooth wear with age and the consequences seen in the dental occlusion (Barrett, 1958). Beyron (1964), using Barrett's film and dental records, used the term "incongruent occlusion" to describe the morphological feature. Subsequently, in a later article published six years before his death, Barrett (1969) detailed his further concepts of functioning dental occlusion in an environment that places heavy demands on the masticatory system. In this article he used the term "segmental occlusion" to replace the earlier "X-occlusion". Furthermore, he indicated that the Chicago anatomist Harry Sicher, in a personal communication during a visit to Adelaide, had suggested "alternate intercuspation" as a suitable descriptive label, one that has been adopted by the Adelaide group in more recent years. Barrett suggested that approximately 25 per cent of the Yuendumu population of all ages showed this type of occlusion to some extent, but it was not until a larger number of longitudinal casts and more sophisticated computer techniques were available that a detailed study of alternate intercuspation was completed.

The longitudinal study was based on the analysis of age changes in relative dental age breadths of subjects from Yuendumu. In total, 1,055 dental casts representing 92 males and 68 females with four or more serial casts were included (Brown *et al.*, 1987). Of these, 100 subjects had been examined on six or more occasions. The findings threw further light on alternate intercuspation and revealed much higher frequencies than the 25 per cent reported by Barrett (1969). A divergent pattern of growth of the maxillary and mandibular dental arches leading to alternate intercuspation was reported in 58 per cent of all subjects, 71 per cent of males and 40 per cent of females. The paper also cited authors who had noted alternate intercuspation in other ethnic groups. In summary, the authors concluded:

> During its development in the individual, alternate intercuspation is often associated with prolonged growth at the median palatal suture and remodelling of the dentoalveolar processes. In a broader biological context, it can be postulated that the trait represents a successful adaptation to the demands of vigorous mastication.

As a corollary, the narrow dental arches, interlocking cusps, and constricted chewing movements of many modern populations could be viewed as examples of inhibited dentoalveolar development.

In a later study of the Yuendumu dental models, Corruccini *et al.*, (1990) quantified occlusal relationships, once more describing alternate intercuspation. This form of occlusion, which can also be termed anisognathism, is characteristic of many herbivores that use wide jaw movements during side-to-side chewing of fibrous food.

Dental casts of young Warlpiri children were used to study the sequence and timing of tooth emergence (Barrett, 1957a). If a child was too young for dental impressions, a direct oral examination would usually provide adequate information. Tooth emergence was defined as the stage when any portion of the emerging tooth was visible in the mouth. This was earlier than the stage of full emergence, when occlusal contact was established with the opposing teeth. Occasionally lateral jaw radiographs were obtained to assist in the investigation of tooth formation and emergence, more so in the 1960s than earlier. An important aspect of this study was to examine the replacement of deciduous teeth by permanent successors. Fortunately, accurate records of birth dates were available for most of the young children. These had been documented by the nursing staff of the Yuendumu hospital, by the Settlement staff and by Pat Fleming, the wife of Baptist missionary Tom Fleming. Pat was a meticulous keeper of records and therefore a source of detailed information about Yuendumu and the Warlpiri families. The dental team often relied on her knowledge and by this means it was possible to cross-check different sources of birth records and family relationships. Although a preliminary report was published by Barrett (1957b), it was not until adequate numbers of dental casts had accrued in the longitudinal study as it progressed into the 1960s that definitive studies on tooth emergence could be undertaken and subsequently published (Barrett *et al.*, 1964; Barrett, 1965; Barrett and Brown, 1966; Brown 1978; Brown *et al.*, 1979).

Although the two principal projects of the Adelaide dental teams during the 1950s were Barrett's collection of models and dental examinations and Campbell's production of his series of documentaries on Warlpiri customs and crafts, there was always time for a variety of other interests. One of these concerned the collection of native foods for grit content analysis. By an examination of the debris incorporated in foodstuffs, much of it being incorporated during the cooking of food in earth ovens, it was possible to identify the abrading agents responsible for the drastic reduction of enamel and dentine in teeth. Researchers obtained still photographs of the many food sources at the Warlpiri - cereals, fruits and meats - and movie films of subjects chewing various foods.

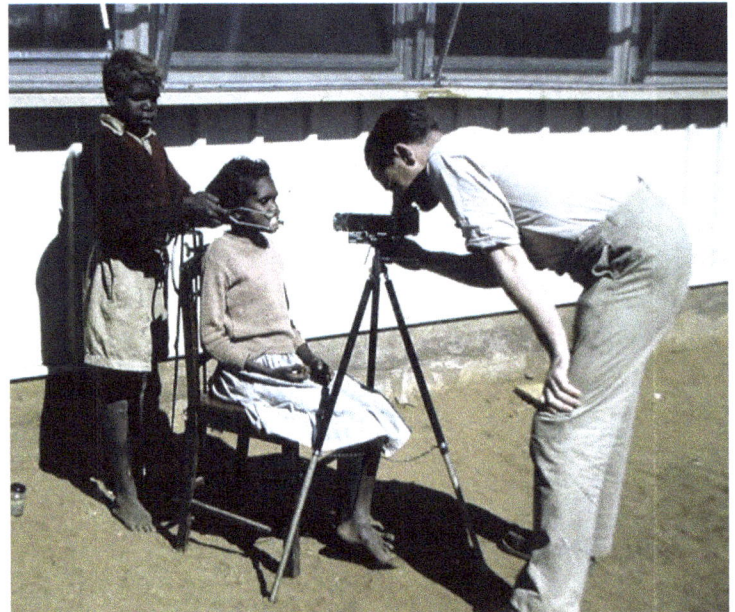

Figure 3.7
Murray Barrett taking a photograph of an unidentified young girl's mouth with a helper retracting her lips

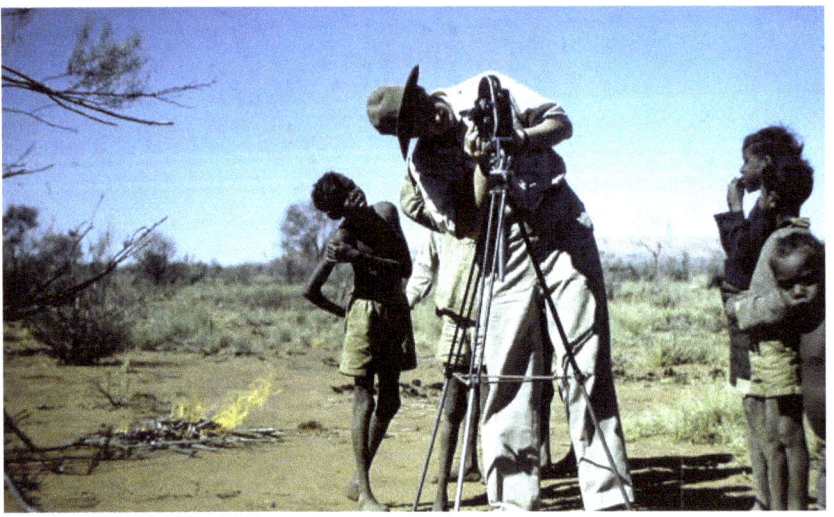

Figure 3.8
Murray Barrett preparing a movie camera to film the cooking of a kangaroo over a fire in the background

Organisation, equipment and supplies

Photography was an essential method of recording material and a typical list of photographic gear to take on each trip would be:

> One large and one small tripod, one 16mm movie camera, one 18mm movie camera, one 35mm colour camera, one 35mm B.W. camera, one electronic flash, one black bag, one case for carrying cameras, an exposure meter, a Vielswich attachment, a series of reflectors, films for all the cameras, photofloods and photo mirrors. (Barrett, 1953-1957)

Barrett took advantage of his presence at Yuendumu to make tape recordings of many Warlpiri song cycles. This custom of his continued throughout his visits to Yuendumu, resulting in a valuable collection of material that was eventually housed at the Australian Institute of Aboriginal and Torres Strait Islander Studies in Canberra. The song cycles of the Warlpiri are very complex, lengthy and often sung in an ancient form of their language. Mostly they are sagas of creation by mythical ancestors from the *Dreaming* but at times shorter songs about everyday topics such as birds singing were revealed to the recorder. Cycles handed down through oral tradition were usually only fully understood by older men as the younger ones were taught different sections over time. For this reason, Barrett would often gather a group of older Warlpiri together for coffee around the tape recorder. He would encourage them to record a song whereby one singer would commence with the others soon joining in, with sticks or boomerangs providing the rhythm. It is interesting to note that although the older men spoke little English, the dental people, with their miniscule knowledge of the Warlpiri language, found little difficulty in communicating. On the other hand, the children and young adults had a reasonable and in some instances fluent command of English.

It was usual for members of the dental teams to assist other researchers in Adelaide who were unable to make the journey to Yuendumu. Throughout the 1950s requirements were sought either in the form of specimens, including plants, animals, insects and Warlpiri weapons, information on genealogies or requests for Warlpiri language recordings and vocabulary notes. Dental anthropology might well have been the focus at this time but researchers also collected animals such as marsupial rats, mountain devils or other assorted small animals for the Zoology Department at The University of Adelaide. Often the researchers enlisted young children to look for desert wild life and there was much merriment when the successful searchers returned with their prized specimens. The Chemistry Department also had its wish list, with witchetty grubs and honey ants being in great demand, though no record exists as to why (Barrett, 1953-1957).

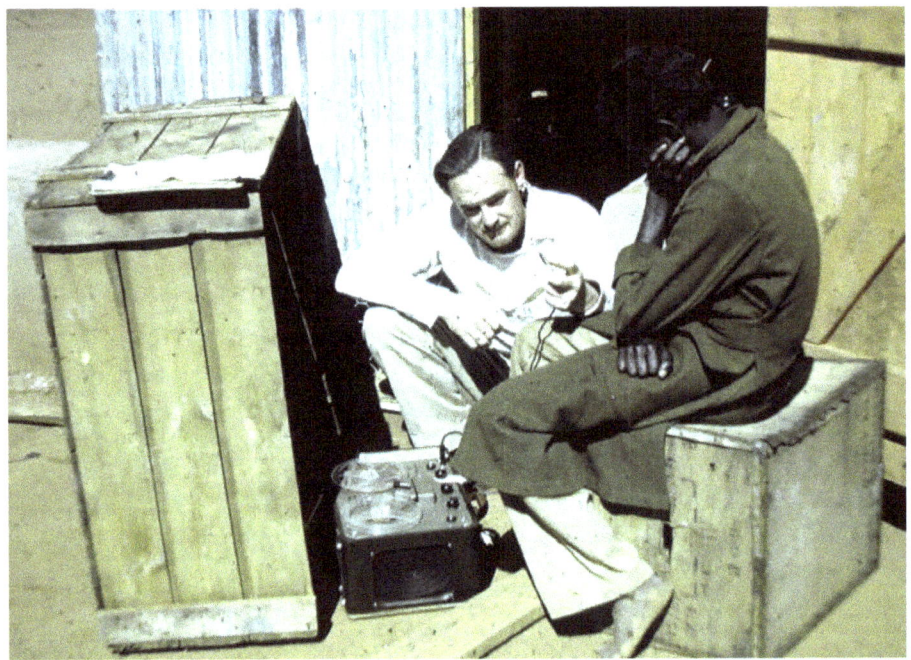

Figure 3.9
Murray Barrett recording an unidentified Warlpiri speaker

Campbell and Barrett were not the only dental staff from Adelaide to visit Yuendumu in the 1950s. Table 3.1 shows the team memberships on all expeditions sponsored by the Board for Anthropological Research. Dr Alexander Cran, a dental pathologist, joined the team each year between 1955 and 1959. Dr Peter Dellow participated in 1955 and 1956 as a photographer and Dr Peter Reade, Dr Judith Kay and Professor A M Horsnell, the newly appointed Dean of the Dental Faculty, joined the team in 1959. The dentists made a special visit to Koonibba, an Aboriginal settlement in South Australia, in 1958 and in the same year the Swedish dentist Henry Beyron joined Campbell and Barrett at Yuendumu. Several publications on diet, dental caries and oral conditions resulted from this additional research (Cran, 1955, 1957, 1959, 1960; Beyron, 1962; Reade, 1964, 1965).

Table 3.1 also lists visits to Yuendumu and other locations by non-dental teams from the South Australian Museum, led by Joseph Birdsell or Norman Tindale, and from the Department of Anatomy and Histology from The University of Adelaide, led by Andrew Abbie or Dudley Packer. Many publications resulted from these visits. Abbie's trip to Haasts Bluff in 1956 is noteworthy because one team member was Geoff Heithersay, a dentist (later an endodontic specialist) who subsequently published three papers dealing with the dentition and tooth wear in the Haasts Bluff Aboriginal people (Heithersay, 1959, 1960, 1961).

It is interesting to note the publications of Campbell and Barrett as the decade of the 1950s progressed. The early papers were concerned with descriptions of the dentitions, food patterns and changing environment at Yuendumu (Campbell and Barrett, 1953; Barrett, 1953a, 1953b; Campbell, 1956). Barrett's later publications dealt more with tooth eruption, mastication and dental occlusion (Barrett, 1957a, 1957b, 1958, 1960).

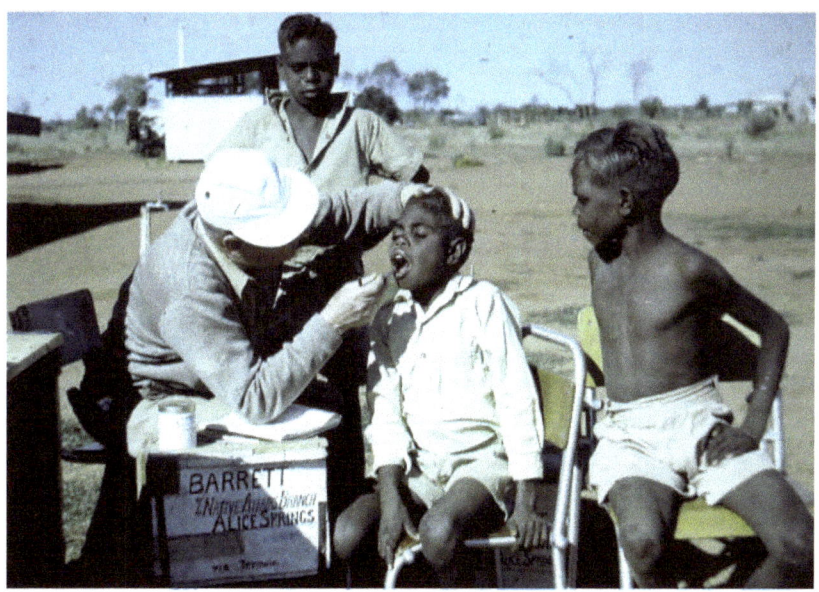

Figure 3.10
Murray Barrett examining an unidentified boy

Murray Barrett was a meticulous planner and organiser for the expeditions to Yuendumu, no doubt a valuable heritage from his service in the air force. He always spent considerable time listing the equipment and personal requirements that the researchers needed for each visit. Table 3.2 shows a typical list of supplies sent by rail to Barrett c/- Native Affairs Branch, Alice Springs, via Terowie, August 1953. Once delivered to Alice Springs, the consignment would go on to Yuendumu by road transport.

Much of this list details medical and dental equipment, clinical and laboratory dental materials, stationery and foodstuffs, including a bag of prunes (Barrett, 1953-1957). The prunes were rewards for the children for participating in the study. In later years, the list also included bags of dried apricots or pears. Most children happily participated in the study. Their visit to the workroom required absence from school for a period, a reward of dried fruit and the chance to help the dentist by cleaning the rubber bowls used to mix the alginate impression powder. There were always many jokes and happy faces on both sides.

Table 3.2 The list of supplies sent by rail and land transport to Yuendumu in 1953

Supplies		Box number					
Description	Quantity	1	2	3	4	5	6
Plaster	7lbs						7
Artificial stone	50lbs	7½	7½	18	18		
Zelex + Control + Alum	16lbs						16
Zelex balance	1		1				
Zelex bottles	2						2
Headrest	1		1				
Plaster bowls	2	2					
Spatulas	2				2		
Impression trays	21					1	20
Mirrors	2	2					
Probes	4	4					
Examination sheets	1 set					1	
Emergency gear	1						1
Compo knife	1				1		
Tray tags	14				14		
Razor blades	1 pkt			1			
Reflectors	2					2	

Table 3.2 cont. The list of supplies sent by rail and land transport to Yuendumu in 1953

| Supplies | | Box number | | | | | |
Description	Quantity	1	2	3	4	5	6
Retractors	6				6		
Dried fruit and nuts	4 pkts					4	
Numbering gear	1 set					1	
Note-books and pencils	3			3			
Gauze	2 yards						2
Plaster gauge	1						1
Barley	4 lbs						4
Spring balance	1					1	
Grinding stones	2					2	
Small scales	1 set					1	
Weights	1 set					1	
Aluminium foil	1 roll					1	
Prunes	1 bag					1	
Cellotape	1 roll	1					
Forceps	2	2					
Magnifying glass	1	1					
Calipers	2	2					
Face pencil	1	1					
Model shapes	5						5
Record cards	1 box						1
Stethoscope	1					1	
Binocular loupes	1					1	

It was important to foster good relationships with the authorities who had the power to sanction and support research applications or, if they felt it warranted, withdraw access permits to the Settlement. Examples of this correspondence include letters to the Administrator for the Territories, letters to Deputy Director Welfare at Alice Springs, letters to the Superintendent/Acting Superintendent at Yuendumu and letters to missionaries Tom and Pat Fleming. Much of the correspondence to the Flemings concerned transport arrangements and accommodation. The official approval for each planned visit to Yuendumu was given by The Board for Anthropological Research which, at its monthly general meetings, would have heard the reasons for each trip and, after agreeing to sponsorship, allocated a trip serial index number. Another feature of Murray Barrett's organisational ability was his careful filing of every document relating to the trip, and 35 years after his death it is still possible to discover information that many other people would have discarded as worthless. The Murray Barrett papers stored on the sixth floor of the Adelaide Dental Hospital are a valuable source of information. They illustrate not only the diversity of details considered for every field trip, but also the logistics necessary to maintain a group of researchers in the field for extended periods of time.

Amongst these papers is one that lists the personal gear recommended for the trip to Yuendumu in the winter of 1957. Each person should have "one cup, knife, fork and spoon, two towels, three sheets and two pillow cases, one tea towel and one blanket". Further recommendations, written in Murray Barrett's handwriting, include: "one packet of tea, three sock garters, one belt, either one windcheater or blue pullover, three pairs of shorts, one pair of trousers and four shirts" (Barrett, 1957c). This information provides an insight into what the male researcher might need, but does little to satisfy curiosity about what a female researcher might require.

Barrett always appreciated the help provided during field trips to Yuendumu. Many departments and individuals offered support, as the following acknowledgement from Barrett (1953b) reveals:

> This study forms part of the Adelaide University field research projects carried out under direction of the Board for Anthropological Research. The 1951 expedition was partly financed by a grant made from the Wenner-Gren Foundation for Anthropological Research, Inc. New York.
>
> The writer is indebted to the Department of Territories and officers of the Northern Territory Administration and Native Affairs Branch for approval and facilities provided on these visits to Yuendumu; also to the Commonwealth Office of Education for the assistance given in work on the Settlement school children. Analyses of water samples were made by the Engineering and Water Supply Department; this service was arranged by Mr. A. P. Plummer, B.D.S.
>
> To Mr. McCoy of the Native Affairs Branch at Alice Springs, and to

Messrs. Langdon, Stafford, Fleming and their families at Yuendumu, appreciation is expressed for the considerable local assistance given in this work.

As the decade ended, the dental researchers could be justifiably pleased with their progress. They had described characteristics of the Warlpiri people's dentition and published preliminary accounts of the food habits, water supplies and tooth emergence. Campbell had produced a number of documentary films and Barrett had extended his collection of serial dental models and continued his interest in functional dental occlusion. Good relationships had been established between the dental visitors, the staff at Yuendumu, the Baptist missionaries and, most importantly, the children and adult Aboriginal people of Yuendumu.

Impact of Barrett's visit to Scandinavia in 1960

The framework for the continuation of the Yuendumu study into the next decade and beyond came into focus after Barrett visited well-known researchers in Scandinavia in 1960. At this time, he met several experts in dental occlusion in Sweden, including Posselt, Seipel, Selmer-Olsen, Krough-Poulsen and Lundström. In Denmark, Barrett held discussions with PO Pedersen, who had studied Greenland Eskimos, Brill, a clinical prosthodontist interested in occlusion, and Björk, who was conducting an innovative longitudinal study of facial growth using metallic implants. These Scandinavian experts showed interest in Barrett's study of the Warlpiri and encouraged him to accumulate more records. Björk, then Professor of Orthodontics at the Royal Dental College in Copenhagen, made a particularly fruitful suggestion. He believed that a full understanding of dental occlusion and growth changes in the dental arches required a parallel study of general growth and, particularly, craniofacial growth. Barrett was convinced that he must extend the Yuendumu study to include observations of general growth patterns and changes in the jaws and craniofacial regions. He could not achieve this unless he obtained somatometric measurements and cephalometric measurements made from special radiographs to supplement the dental models. Thus, this formed the objectives for the field trips to Yuendumu in the 1960s. In 1960 Barrett enlisted Tasman Brown, who was also a student of Campbell's, as a new team member and the two researchers formed a productive liaison until Barrett's death in 1975.

References

Barrett MJ (1953a). X-Occlusion. *Dent Mag Oral Top* 70:279. Report of an exhibit presented at the Thirteenth Australian Dental Congress, University of Queensland, Brisbane, June 1–5, 1953.

Barrett MJ (1953b). Dental observations on Australian Aborigines – Yuendumu, Central Australia, 1951–52. *Aust J Dent* 57:127–138.

Barrett MJ (1953–1957). Yuendumu Correspondence and Notes. School of Dentistry, The University of Adelaide.

Barrett MJ (1956). Dental observations on Australian Aborigines: water supplies and endemic dental fluorosis. *Aust Dent J* 1:87–92.

Barrett MJ (1956). *Mastication – A Dynamic Process*. Adelaide: University of Adelaide. Film.

Barrett MJ (1957a). Serial dental casts of Australian Aboriginal children. *Aust Dent J* 2:74.

Barrett MJ (1957b). Dental observations on Australian Aborigines: tooth eruption sequence. *Aust Dent J* 2:217–227.

Barrett MJ (1958). Dental observations on Australian Aborigines: continuously changing functional occlusion. *Aust Dent J* 3:39–52.

Barrett MJ (1960). Parafunctions and tooth attrition. In: *Parafunctions of the Masticatory System (bruxism)*. Lipke D, Posselt U, editors. *J West Soc Perio* 8:133–148.

Barrett MJ (1965). Dental observations on Australian Aborigines. *Mankind* 6:249–254.

Barrett MJ (1969). Functioning occlusion. *Ann Aust Coll Dent Surg* 2:68–80.

Barrett MJ, Brown T (1966). Eruption of deciduous teeth in Australian Aborigines. *Aust Dent J* 11:43–50.

Barrett MJ, Brown T, Cellier KM (1964). Tooth eruption sequences in a tribe of Central Australian Aborigines. *Am J Phys Anthropol* 22:79–89.

Beyron H (1962). Investigation of the occlusion and mastication of Australian Aborigines: Survey of lecture (Undersuckning Hos Australiska Urinvanare). *Svensk Tandläkare–Tidskrift* 55:43.

Beyron H (1964). Occlusal relations and mastication in Australian Aborigines. *Acta Odontol Scand* 22:597–678.

Brown T (1978). Tooth emergence in Australian Aboriginals. *Ann Hum Biol* 5:41–54.

Brown T (2001). Thomas Draper Campbell: Pioneer Dental Anthropologist. In: *Causes and Effects of Human Variation (2001)*. Henneberg M, editor. The University of Adelaide: Australian Society for Human Biology, pp. 1–11.

Brown T, Abbott A, Burgess VB (1987). Longitudinal study of dental arch relationships in Australian Aboriginals with reference to alternate intercuspation. *Am J Phys Anthropol* 72:49–57.

Brown T, Jenner JD, Barrett MJ and Lees GH (1979). *Exfoliation of deciduous teeth and gingival emergence of permanent teeth in Australian Aborigines*. Occasional Papers in Human Biology. Canberra: Australian Institute of Aboriginal Studies, 1:47–70.

Campbell TD (1956). Comparative human odontology. *Aust Dent J* 1:26–29.

Campbell TD, Barrett MJ (1953). Dental observations on Australian Aborigines: A changing environment and food pattern. *Aust J Dent* 57:1–6.

Campbell TD, Barrett MJ (1954). *So they did eat*. Adelaide: Board for Anthropological Research, The University of Adelaide. Film.

Corruccini RS, Townsend GC, Brown T (1990). Occlusal variation in Australian Aboriginals. *Am J Phys Anthropol* 82:257–265.

Cran JA (1955). Notes on the teeth and gingivae of Central Australian Aborigines. *Aust J Dent* 59:356–361.

Cran JA (1957). Notes on the teeth and gingivae of Central Australian Aborigines. *Aust Dent J* 2:227–282.

Cran JA (1959). Relationship of diet to dental caries. *Aust Dent J* 4:182–190.

Cran JA (1960). Histological structure of the teeth of Central Australian Aborigines and the relationship to dental caries incidence. *Aust Dent J* 5:100–104.

Jones PG (1987). South Australian anthropological history: The Board for Anthropological Research and its early expeditions. *Rec South Aust Mus* 20:71–92.

Heithersay GS (1959). A dental survey of Aborigines at Haast's Bluff, Central Australia. *Med J Aust* 1:721–729.

Heithersay GS (1960). Attritional values for Australian Aborigines, Haast's Bluff. *Aust Dent J* 5:84–88.

Heithersay GS (1961). Further observations on the dentition of Australian Aborigines at Haast's Bluff. *Aust Dent J* 6:18–28.

Reade PC (1964). Infantile acute oral moniliasis. *Aust Dent J* 9:14–16.

Reade PC (1965). Dental observations on Australian Aborigines, Koonibba, South Australia. *Aust Dent J* 10:361–370.

Southcott RV (1986). Medical Sciences. In: *Ideas and Endeavours – the Natural Sciences in South Australia.* Twidale CR, Tyler MJ, Davies M, editors. Adelaide: Royal Society of South Australia, pp. 213–234.

Tindale NB (1986). Anthropology. In: *Ideas and Endeavours – the Natural Sciences in South Australia.* Twidale CR, Tyler MJ, Davies M, editors. Adelaide: Royal Society of South Australia, pp. 235–277.

4
Yuendumu:
The Longitudinal Project 1961–1971

Initial preparations

Murray Barrett returned from his sabbatical leave in Europe with renewed enthusiasm and a clearer idea of how he wished the Yuendumu study to progress. Extension of the research to include general and craniofacial growth would require additional funding and personnel. The researchers needed specialised equipment and to learn and test new research techniques before the next visit to Yuendumu in 1961. The number of academic staff members involved in the research projects soon increased from one to two: Murray Barrett, the Reader in Prosthetic Dentistry, and Tasman Brown, who had recently joined the staff as Lecturer in Dental Anatomy. Technical staff and occasionally students joined the principals on field trips to Central Australia. In later years, many postgraduate students and visitors from overseas made substantial contributions to the research objectives.

In the early 1960s, the main source of financial support was grants from research funds of The University of Adelaide. Transport of equipment and supplies to Alice Springs was generously provided through the auspices of the Commonwealth Minister for Shipping and Transport. Support was freely given by Government officials from South Australia and the Northern Territory. As always, the Baptist missionaries at Yuendumu offered accommodation to the principals and provided living quarters for others in the team. At this time, funding for the research was minimal and Barrett's team often relied on the generosity of others. For example, Brown recalls his first visit to Yuendumu in 1961 when he, Ross Macdonald and

Peter Reade shared the tray of the Settlement truck with a group of Warlpiri people returning from Alice Springs.

In 1963, however, financial support was greatly increased and made more secure after Barrett and Brown sought and gained research funding from the United States Department of Health, Education and Welfare in the form of a Public Health Service Research Grant approved by the National Institute of Dental Research, Bethesda, Maryland. Included was funding for car hire during the weeks of field work - no more reliance on the Yuendumu truck! The approved period was for seven years from April 1964 to March 1971. Research Grant DE 02034-07 allowed for the continuance and fulfilment of Barrett and Brown's vision to collect dental and growth records longitudinally for Warlpiri children through childhood and adolescence to young adulthood. It was largely through the financial support from the US Government that the project would later provide anthropologists, anatomists, geneticists and dentists from many countries with a unique and invaluable Australian research resource.

In preparation for the 1961 field trip, the first in the new expanded phase of the study, the researchers bought or borrowed anthropometric measuring instruments, and Brown, who was to be in charge of somatometry in the field, practised the techniques for making accurate and repeatable body measurements. They followed the standard text on anthropometry (Martin, 1957) for the definitions and measuring techniques. Table 2.2 lists the variables selected for study.

Radiographic cephalometry is a technique used by orthodontists, oral surgeons and craniofacial surgeons to produce standardised radiographs of the head from which measurements can be obtained for diagnostic and research purposes. This method predates the more recently developed techniques for constructing three-dimensional images from computer-tomography scans of the head. For the Yuendumu research, the researchers acquired a portable radiographic machine together with a cephalostat to position the head in a standard position and posture. A facility for changing film cassettes and developing test radiographs in the field was designed and built. The use of high-speed intensifying screens in the film cassettes reduced radiation exposure to a minimum – no more than a single small intraoral dental radiograph. At all times, the researchers used monitor badges to test for any scatter radiation. This was always below measurable levels.

The acquisition and testing of equipment and familiarisation with new techniques proceeded throughout 1960 until the two principals were satisfied that they could schedule a field trip to Yuendumu for the following year. They invited another staff member, Peter Reade, to join the team. He had previously joined Campbell and Barrett on field trips in 1958 and 1959. A fourth member, Ross Macdonald, joined the team as a student member.

The Warlpiri and their kinship system

At this time, the Warlpiri population formed a fairly static and self-contained group that was almost free of non-Aboriginal admixture. Culturally, the group was still traditionally orientated and economically it was at an early stage of transition from a food gathering and hunting type of society to a more settled existence centred around the government and mission facilities at Yuendumu. The relative geographical isolation of Yuendumu provided a unique opportunity to study a group of people who had not yet been influenced by European culture to any great extent.

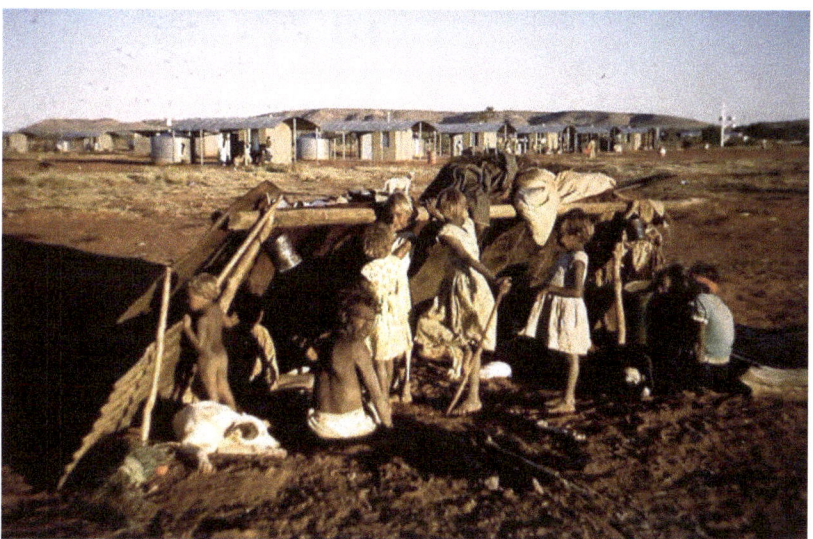

Figure 4.1
A typical shelter on the outskirts of Yuendumu. A group of European-style houses, provided by the Welfare Branch, with verandahs and water tanks typical of the late 1960s, are in the background

The Aboriginal people lived in rough shelters in the mulga scrub about a mile away from the Settlement compound and their camps were usually scattered over a wide area. Their shelters were often simple windbreaks or humpies built of natural material. Some were more complicated but were crude "houses" built of native timber covered by sheets of iron or canvas. A few people had purchased tents to live in. The Settlement compound consisted of about a dozen houses for the administrative staff and their families, a small hospital, three school buildings, a large dining hall and kitchen, and a number of stores and workshops.

The kinship system in many Aboriginal societies governs almost every aspect of social interaction. It specifies which male and female may form a union; unauthorised departures from this determination are usually punished severely. The system determines the kinship of any male or female offspring. It also prescribes how members of different kinships relate to each other particularly in ceremonial activities that the kinship system dominates.

Table 4.1 Spellings used for the Warlpiri kinship names

Genealogy*	Code*	Meggitt (1962)	Welfare	Fleming	AIATSIS**
Napnga	1F	Nabanangga	Nabanangga	Nabanangga	Napanangka
Japnga	1M	Djabanangga	Jabanangga	Jabanangga	Japanangka
Nungar	2F	Nungarai	Nungarai	Nungarai	Nungarrayi
Jungar	2M	Djungarai	Jungarai	Jungarai	Jungarrayi
Napalt	3F	Nalaldjari	Nabaljari	Nabaldjari	Napaljarri
Japalt	3M	Djabaldjari	Jabaljari	Jabaldjari	Japaljarri
Naprti	4F	Nabangari	Nabangadi	Nabangadi	Napangardi
Japrti	4M	Djabangari	Jabangadi	Jabangadi	Japangardi
Napur	5F	Naburula	Nuburula	Nabarula	Napurrula
Jupur	5M	Djuburula	Juburula	Juburula	Jupurrula
Nangal	6F	Nangala	Nangala	Nangala	Nangala
Jangal	6M	Djangala	Jangala	Jangala	Jangala
Nakam	7F	Nagamara	Nagamara	Nagamara	Nakamarra
Jakam	7M	Djagamara	Jagamara	Jagamara	Jakamarra
Nambit	8F	Nambidjimba	Nambajimba	Nambidjinba	Nampijinpa
Jambit	8M	Djambidjimba	Jamajimba	Jambidjinba	Jampijinpa

* The genealogy index and code used in the Yuendumu study
** Australian Institute of Aboriginal and Torres Strait Islander Studies

Meggitt (1962) described the complicated matrilineal system of family relationships in Warlpiri society. Each Warlpiri belongs to one of eight female or eight male groups, known by their kinship or moiety, locally called "skin" names.

For the Yuendumu study, the researchers recorded each subject in the genealogy index with their given name, any nicknames, their numeric identifier, an abbreviated skin name adapted from the local spellings, and a code consisting of skin name and sex as in 1F (Napnga : Female). Researchers linked each person by cross-indexing with family siblings and other relationships, including new ones that developed over time. Skin names for females began with the English phonic N and males J. English spellings of the kinships names are phonetically based and although they vary somewhat between different sources, the groupings are identical (Table 4.1).

Life at the Settlement during the longitudinal study

The children attended school each day and had their meals in the dining hall. Younger children attended kindergarten classes. Mothers brought their babies and toddlers to the hospital each morning for special meals and Aboriginal people who felt ill received treatment. The older people came in from their camps twice a day for meals in the dining hall.

Unfortunately, there was very little work for the Aboriginal people. Cattle stations employed young women occasionally as domestic aids; a few of the men worked as roustabouts. A few men worked at a copper mine at Mt Hardy. From Monday to Friday, all those who attended the kitchen received a midday meal of hot stew. Twice a week the staple food rations were issued at the Settlement store.

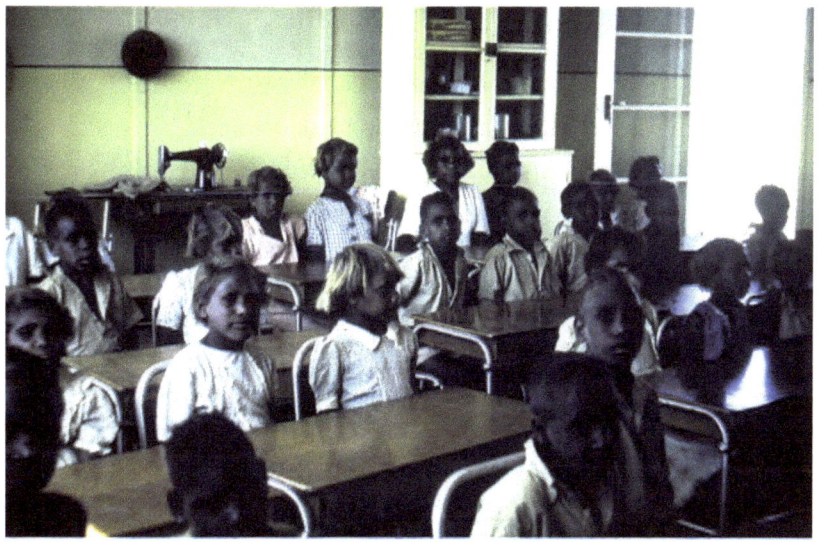

Figure 4.2
Inside a school room at Yuendumu during the 1950s

Occasionally, one or more of the families without aged or very young members, journeyed afield for a weekend, several days, or sometimes several weeks. The reasons varied: to seek other food supplies, to hunt wild dogs, or to visit some neighbouring group of Aboriginal people. A few families established semi-permanent camps some distance from Yuendumu, usually near a reliable source of water.

This brief general outline of life at the Settlement suggests that at that time, the mode of living was in marked contrast with the nomadic life of the past, when most of each day involved the quest for food. The men hunted, the women were the food gatherers. They traversed their tribal territory continuously in search of food and water. In the arid regions of Central Australia, especially during periods of prolonged drought, this often involved travelling long distances under conditions of high daytime temperatures and limited water supplies.

Water supplies

Much of the vast central area of Australia is a region of low average water precipitation with high evaporation (Barrett 1956b). Except immediately after heavy rainfall, when growth is rapid and abundant and food supplies temporarily increase, desert conditions prevail. During the brief times of plenty, nomadic Aboriginal peoples would make the most of it (Campbell and Barrett, 1953). But good seasons were offset by long periods of dryness, sometimes of prolonged drought, when the Aboriginal people, as well as animal and bird life, were forced to the range country where there were waterholes, springs and soaks.

In this unproductive environment, over long generations Aboriginal people developed an intense degree of nomadism, the only mode of life by which they could secure water and food supplies. Maintaining their material existence was a continuous, arduous task, as Campbell and Barrett (1953) describe:

> Yet so intimately was he part of, and in harmony with, his surroundings that the economics of making a living was an art in which centuries of experience had made him extremely proficient. It enabled them to survive successfully for a very long time in this strange, arid country.

It has appeared that Aboriginal people adapted themselves physiologically to minimise water loss when occasion demanded. Of more importance is the evidence that they practised water discipline and limited their water consumption to the bare necessities.

Life on the Yuendumu settlement consisted of having food provided – in sufficient quantity and variety, such as it was, to maintain bodily existence moderately well and with a plentiful supply of water that was readily available from the bores at Yuendumu. The water was lifted by windmill or petrol-driven motor pump to an elevated tank of 22,750 litres capacity. The overflow drained into a ground-level stock tank holding 113,750 litres. A shortage of water occurred from time to time owing to inadequate storage, the breakdown of the motor pump or a lack of wind to drive the windmill. To overcome these problems and to provide more water for a larger vegetable garden, the authorities drilled a second bore in the centre of the settlement compound in 1953. However, granite prevented penetration beyond eight metres. They then made a third drilling to a depth of approximately 28 metres, about 22 metres from the original bore, which gave a plentiful supply of water. The addition of two additional elevated tanks increased storage capacity.

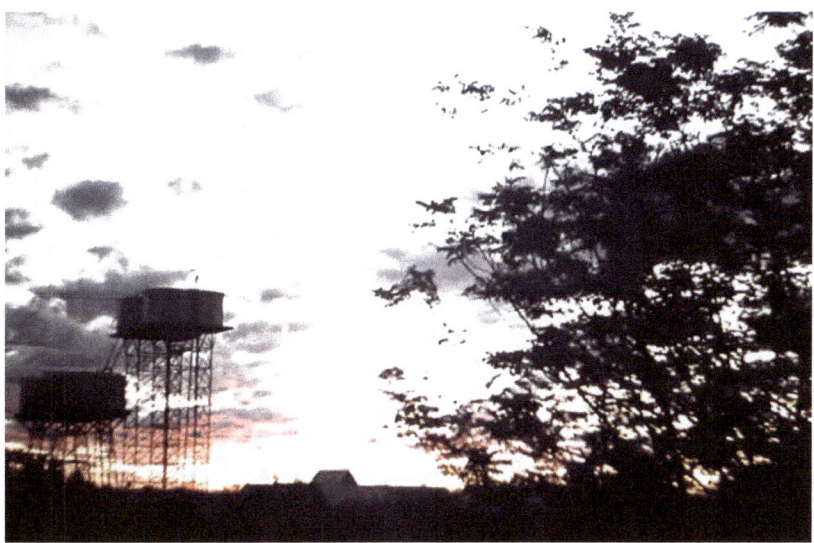

Figure 4.3
The Yuendumu water towers

The Warlpiri people had unrestricted use of the tank taps for their drinking water and the women carried water supplies back to their camps, using a variety of containers. From observations of the activities of family groups, buckets of water routinely sat on the ground at teatime while the damper loaves were cooking, and the young children gathered around for a drink. Water not used at teatime was stored in containers and secured on top of the humpies or windbreaks, or hung from a branch in a nearby tree to be out of reach of very young children and dogs. At Yuendumu, the Aboriginal people drank more water than the white inhabitants of the Settlement and, according to a senior teacher, the children who attended school drank much more water than the white children, particularly during the summer months.

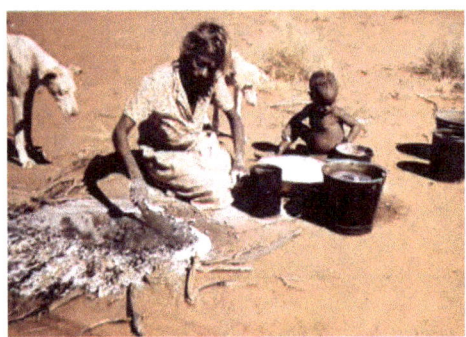 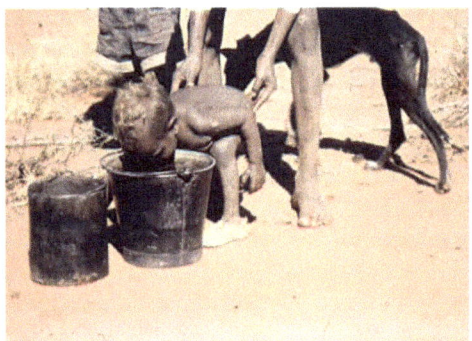

Figure 4.4
An unidentified woman preparing damper and a child drinking from a bucket

Bore water content

The average fluoride content of samples tested from the Yuendumu Settlement bore water during the 1950s and early 1960s was 1.5 parts per million (1.5 mg/L), much higher than the recommended levels. The present Australian recommendation for the level of fluoride in city water supplies is between 0.6–1.1 mg/L (Australian Research Centre for Population Oral Health, 2008).

In 1955, researchers noted mottled enamel in 30 per cent of the permanent teeth of 158 Aboriginal people aged from approximately six to 20 years (Barrett, 1956a). Most affected teeth occurred in the younger children and were in the categories "very mild" to "mild". None of the older Aboriginal people examined showed mottling. At the time, because of the relatively short period since the Government had established the Settlement, and the nomadic custom of some Warlpiri families, it was difficult to establish whether the children had been exposed to continuous use of the bore water and the ingestion of excess fluoride. Further study was required to determine the relative importance of other variables, such as food deficiencies and childhood diseases, as the causes of malformed enamel. However, the high level of fluoride was thought to inhibit the cariogenic effect of the increasing amount of carbohydrate food that was being consumed by the Warlpiri.

In 1970, researchers conducted a further oral health study to assess the state of oral hygiene and estimate the prevalence of oral mucosal and periodontal diseases, dental caries and developmental enamel defects among the Warlpiri (Barrett and Williamson, 1972). Since 1965, a different bore had been used for the main drinking supply and analyses of samples on three annual visits showed a consistent fluoride content of 0.4 parts per million (0.4mg/L), which was confirmed by the Water Resources Branch of the Northern Territory Administration. About 30 per cent of the Aboriginal people examined showed dental fluorosis assessed as "moderate" or "severe", but the prevalence of dental caries was low. These findings are consistent with what could be expected from exposure to high amounts of fluoride in the bore water before 1965 when the children's permanent teeth were developing.

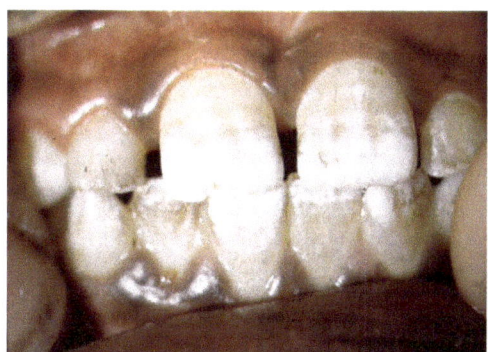 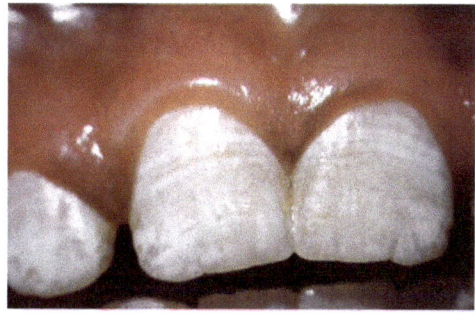

Figure 4.5
Examples of dental fluorosis

Changing food habits

While marriage and other social customs and beliefs were practised and maintained with the preservation of something of the previous tribal life, in this changed environment there was little incentive to continue or revert to the old mode of daily life. With the introduction of higher wages in 1969, the money income of the community increased suddenly and substantially. About 80 per cent of the welfare payments were spent in the local canteen, approximately two-thirds on food and one-third on clothing and other items. In the year following the wage increase, the canteen turnover increased ten-fold (Brown and Barrett, 1973a).

Because of higher incomes, most Aboriginal people preferred to purchase food from the canteen and have meals in their own houses or camps rather than in the communal dining hall. Educational programmes that taught them how to budget, how to balance their food purchase, and health and nutrition, influenced some of the younger people. However, most of the older people had little understanding of the nutritive values of various European foods and the relation between food and health. In these years there was a marked increase in the purchase of low-protein foods, including flour, sugar, bread, canned foods, biscuits and soft drinks. There is little doubt that the Warlpiri preferred meat above other foods and they would purchase meat when money was available for this expensive item.

Aims of the project

The specific aims of the work that was in progress in the early 1960s or proposed for the following years, were listed under five headings: dental morphology, tooth formation and eruption, size and shape of dental arches, the mode of tooth occlusion, craniofacial morphology, and growth changes in the craniofacial structures of the Warlpiri participants. When adequate records had accumulated, researchers would turn their attention to skeletal maturation, general body growth and genetics.

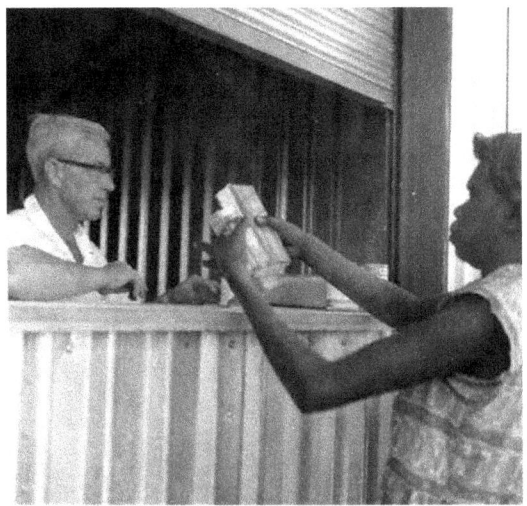

Figure 4.6
Tom Fleming at the Yuendumu store

The research plan was to continue working on the considerable pool of data already available from a number of visits to Yuendumu since 1951 and to revisit the Settlement annually for further observations, particularly of subjects previously examined. Visits more frequently than once a year were impractical.

The long-term objective was to assemble a pool of data that researchers could use to determine the morphological characteristics, functional relationships, and the patterns of growth and development of the dental and craniofacial structures. Observations consisted mainly of general physical assessment, anthropometry, hand and wrist roentgenography for skeletal age assessments, dental examinations, the collection of dental casts, craniofacial roentgenography, and photographs. During each examination, researchers noted age, whether actual or estimated, and checked and rechecked familial relationships.

Studies in the early 1960s

Initial investigations of metric characters of the teeth, dental arches, face and skull commenced in the early 1960s and results were published soon afterwards, including studies of craniofacial variations (Brown, 1965), dental observations including mesiodistal crown diameters of deciduous teeth (Barrett *et al.*, 1963a), mesiodistal crown diameters of permanent teeth (Barrett *et al.*, 1963b), prognathism (Barrett *et al.*, 1963c), the size of dental arches (Barrett *et al.*, 1965a), and a study of facial morphology (Brown and Barrett, 1964).

Morphological characteristics of the Australian dentition, metric and non-metric, had been studied in skull material from widely separated regions of Australia (Campbell, 1925). The main objective of the project at Yuendumu was to determine the variations in dental morphology shown by a single tribe of Australian Aboriginal people. Researchers had produced dental casts for most of the subjects and augmented them with field records of dental examinations and roentgenograms. Ongoing collection of genealogies would be useful in studying genetically determined differences in dental characters.

A longitudinal study of tooth formation and eruption was already in progress. The researchers intended to be compare the findings with those previously reported for North American white children (Fanning, 1961; Moorrees *et al.*, 1958, 1963; Garn *et al.*, 1956). Studies also existed regarding genetic polymorphisms in the sequence of tooth formation and eruption in North American white children (Garn et al., 1956, Garn and Lewis, 1957, 1963). Preliminary investigations of the gingival emergence of permanent teeth in Australian Aboriginal people revealed wide variations in tooth eruption sequence between individuals and provided evidence of eruption sequence polymorphism (Barrett, 1957a; Barrett *et al.*, 1964). Investigation of the relationship between stages of calcification, alveolar emergence and gingival emergence, as well as the chronology of tooth formation and eruption, also formed part of the longitudinal study.

The researchers obtained arch breadth and arch depth measurements from dental casts to determine the age differences and individual variations in the size and shape of dental arches (Barrett *et al.*, 1965a). Associated with this aspect of the study was the measurement of tooth dimensions to determine the relations between tooth size, crowding and spacing of teeth, and the size and shape of the dental arches. Serial dental casts obtained for the same subjects at different ages provide material ideally suitable for investigations of age changes (Barrett, 1957b).

More detailed investigation of the functional occlusal relations of the dental arches followed. Previous research had already paid some attention to the occlusion of teeth and patterns of mastication in Aboriginal people at Yuendumu (Barrett, 1953a, 1953b, 1956b, 1958, 1960; Beyron, 1964).

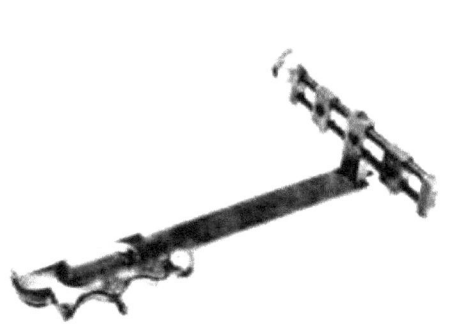
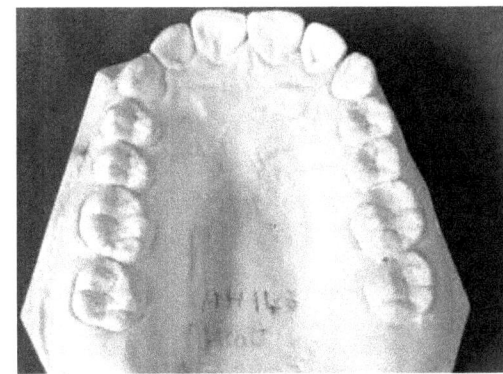

Figure 4.7
Instrument used for measuring arch breadth
and depth on dental models during the 1960s

To investigate patterns of child growth, researchers used a cross-sectional method during the first stage to determine norms for each age group. When sufficient data had accumulated, a longitudinal study of the growth changes in the craniofacial structures of the children at Yuendumu was possible. The researchers paid particular attention to the relationship between head growth and general physical maturation (Brown and Barrett, 1973b).

Carefully standardised lateral head and postero-anterior roentgenograms allowed researchers to obtain linear and angular measurements of various regions of the head indirectly from the films. In addition, researchers obtained a limited number of body measurements.

Age classification

Initially, few recorded birthdate records were available and the researchers adopted an alternative scheme of age classification based in the main on dental criteria (Barrett, 1953b). Table 4.2 shows the criteria for grouping the subjects by tooth emergence status and the names given the dental groups for reference. Grouping by this method was warranted on three counts. Firstly, the method does not rely on knowledge of chronological age, an advantage in the present study because there were no records of birthdates for a large per cent of the sample. Secondly, even though the researchers examined virtually the entire school population, the sample sizes when grouped by recorded or estimated chronological age were too small for comparison between groups. Thirdly, dental groups constitute comparable stages of dental development irrespective of chronological age. Beyond the stage when third molars had emerged, researchers grouped the subjects by estimating their ages from an assessment of their general physical appearance and sometimes with reference to the ages of their children. The use of hand roentgenograms offered an opportunity for the grouping of the children according to skeletal age. As the number of records increased over the years, it became possible to form groups of children with known birthdates for data analysis.

Table 4.2 Dental criteria for grouping subjects and dental code used for field sheets and computer input

Group	Criteria	Dental code
Infants	Primary dentition	21
Juveniles 1	Mixed dentition – early stage Primary canines and molars all present	31
Juveniles 2	Mixed dentition – late stage Some but not all primary canines or molars exfoliated	41
Adolescents	Permanent dentition Excluding third molars	51
Adults	Permanent dentition Including one or more third molars	61

Dental genetics

At that time, dental genetics was an area of research endeavour in urgent need of attention and the research team considered that the collection of dental casts would provide considerable material for an investigation of the variations in morphological characters of the dentition. Diminutive and peg-shaped maxillary lateral incisors were not uncommon in the Yuendumu population and several subjects showed congenital absence of lateral incisors. These and other dental and oral abnormalities warranted investigation.

There was also the opportunity to study familial trends in tooth formation and eruption and the genetics of craniofacial growth. Family studies, however, were complicated by polygynous unions and by the difficulty of distinguishing in family groups between actual and adopted children. There would be little progress in these aspects of the study until an additional investigator with special training in genetics could join the team. Besides being a geneticist, however, such a research worker needed to have a sound knowledge of kinship relations and the social structure of Australian Aboriginal communities. Accurate family data later provided a unique opportunity to examine genetic and environmental influence on morphological characters (Townsend, 1976).

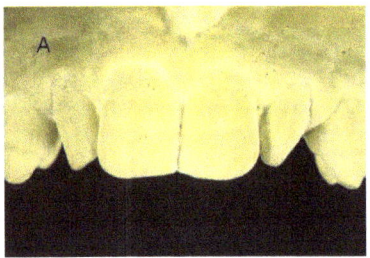
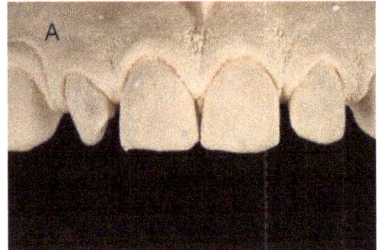
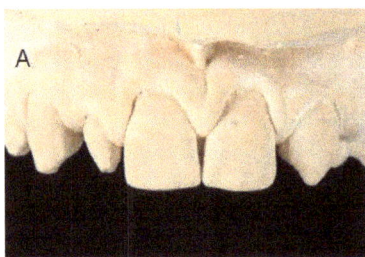
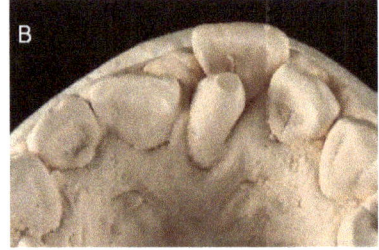

Figure 4.8
Examples of anomalies of the anterior teeth showing missing and peg-shaped lateral incisors (A) and a supernumerary tooth (B)

One of the particular advantages of the Yuendumu study was the "racial homogeneity" of the group compared with European society (Barrett et al., 1965b). With few exceptions, the subjects were of pure Aboriginal ancestry. Thus, there was no problem of selecting based on ethnic origin. Records of individuals of mixed ancestry were marked accordingly and excluded from the sample when analysing the data.

In selecting subjects there were two main objectives: first, to provide adequate sample numbers of males and females in each age group, and, second, to enrol as many young subjects as possible so that the longitudinal method of study could be used when sufficient data had accumulated. Willingness to attend offered no serious obstacle because the Aboriginal people generally were most cooperative.

Annual Trips

Each year the annual trip to Yuendumu was precisely planned to the last detail. Months in advance, the Remington typewriter in the laboratory pounded out many letters to government departments, the Flemings and various service providers. It was imperative that no delays occurred in transporting the boxes of equipment and supplies to the Settlement and that the project ran efficiently from the first day of the team's arrival. The postal service was the only means of communication between Adelaide and Yuendumu and sometimes letters took over a week to arrive at their destination. Email technology had not yet been invented!

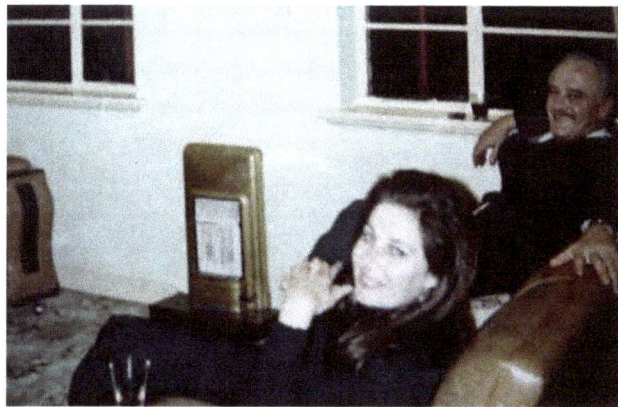

Figure 4.9
Sandy Pinkerton and Murray Barrett

Meticulous packing for the field visit needed to provide for every requirement ranging from spare parts for the equipment to cushioned pink pads to protect the dental models on their homeward journey. After all, Yuendumu was over 1800 km (1130 miles) from Adelaide and there could be no last minute purchase for an item forgotten. The introduction of computers in 1962 facilitated preparations considerably. They became more important and then essential as the study progressed and data processing facilities improved. Computer-generated class lists, data forms ranging from tooth emergence to family history and box inventories were prepared to streamline the collection of records from the school children and adults. Research assistant Sandra Pinkerton, who became very adept at using computer technology to generate any forms or lists that were required before each field trip, carried out these essential tasks.

Table 4.3 Team members of the Yuendumu field trips 1961–1971

Trip	Destination	Date	Team leader	Team members	
AJ	Yuendumu	28 December 1960 – 20 January 1961	Barrett MJ	Brown T	Reade PC Macdonald MR
AL	Yuendumu	2 – 21 August 1962	Barrett MJ	Fanning EA Macdonald MR Reynolds L	Brown T Davivongs V
AP	Yuendumu	4 – 19 May 1964	Barrett MJ	Brown T	Reynolds L Rao P
AQ	Yuendumu	17 May – 5 June 1965	Barrett MJ	Brown T Simmonds DW	Reynolds L Kuusk S
AS	Yuendumu	16 May – 4 June 1966	Barrett MJ	Reade PC Wright DWR	Beasley PRN Reynolds L
AU	Yuendumu	17 May – 1 June 1967	Barrett MJ	Brown T Kirkwood J	McNulty EC McLean R
AV	Yuendumu	17 May – 1 June 1968	Brown T	Clarke N Clarke H	Kuusk G Kuusk S
AW	Yuendumu	18 May – 7 June 1969	Barrett MJ	Brown T Ozaki T	Nugent MC Harrison N
AY	Yuendumu	19 May – 6 June 1970	Barrett MJ	Brown T Williamson J Townsend G Reynolds L	Ozaki T Lees G Lees E
AZ	Yuendumu	19 May – 5 June 5 1971	Barrett MJ	Brown T	Parker DAS Rollings T

The research team usually departed for Yuendumu during the The University of Adelaide inter-term break. Willing and enthusiastic local and overseas researchers interested in different scientific aspects of the project joined the team from time to time and ventured to the remote centre of Australia. Investigators Elizabeth Fanning, Peter Reade, Ed McNulty and Tadashi Ozaki all published scientific articles following their trips (Fanning and Moorrees, 1969; Reade 1964; McNulty *et al.*, 1968; Ozaki *et al.*, 1987).

In May 1970, two additional team members, John Williamson and Grant Townsend, were engaged in a separate epidemiological survey of oral and dental health. Murray Barrett also led special trips in 1969 and 1972. During these, Professor Beni Solow from The Royal Dental College, Copenhagen investigated craniofacial morphology and head posture in Australian Aboriginal people, and Professor William Proffit from The University of Kentucky studied the relationship between lip activity, tongue pressure and swallowing to dental arch form (Solow *et al.*, 1982; Proffit 1975; Proffit and McGlone 1975; Proffit *et al.*, 1975; Proffit 1978).

It was necessary for the team members to be aware of the culture at Yuendumu and to understand Warlpiri customs and beliefs, particularly those concerning teeth (Barrett, 1964). A sound knowledge of kinship relations and the social structure of Australian Aboriginal communities was also very important.

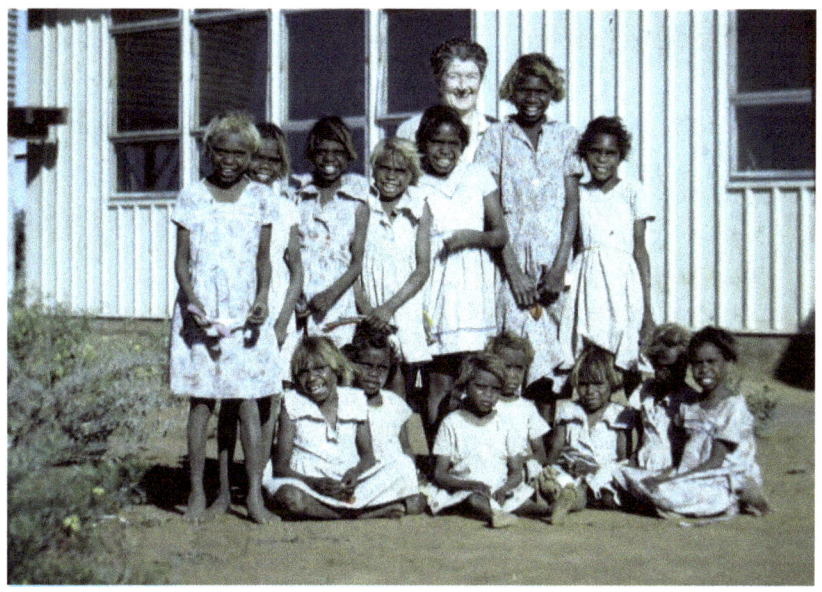

Figure 4.10
Pat Fleming with a class of pupils from Yuendumu School c1965

The Work Schedule

After arriving in Alice Springs, the first task was to collect and fuel the hire-car that Barrett had previously ordered. This was always a station wagon capable of carrying team members and some supplies. Next stop was the general store to purchase perishables for the first few days as well as canned food and other requirements. Murray Barrett always had a bottle of brandy on his list, purely in case of snakebite he insisted. Also on the list was "one bag of snakes", a sweet that remains a favourite of Australians both young and old.

Car and supplies secured, the team would head for Yuendumu some 285 km northwest from Alice Springs. A few kilometres out of the city the Tanami Road branched off to the left heading for the old gold mine at The Granites and then on to the West Australian border. The trip to Yuendumu would take 5–6 hours depending on road conditions after the bitumen stopped a few kilometres along the Tanami Road. It would usually be a non-stop drive passing the tracks into Hamilton Downs and Milton Park stations. At about the halfway mark there would be the Napperby Creek crossing, invariably a dry creek bed. Members of the team who were travelling in the Central Desert for the first time, especially those from overseas, found it difficult to accept the vast distance along a dirt road - sometimes recently graded, sometimes not - where on either side there were only spinifex clusters and sparse mulga scrub set against the vivid background of red sand. From time to time, a rocky outcrop would break the monotony. A newcomer would sometimes express a feeling of apprehension in case of a breakdown on this lonely road. Murray Barrett would put fears to rest with an assurance that there was sure to be another traveller on the road within a day or two! Conditions are quite different now, with an extension of the bitumen, a roadhouse stop and numerous adventurous tourists heading for the Kimberley region of Western Australia via the Central Desert.

The team would arrive at Yuendumu late in the afternoon or early evening. Hosts Tom and Pat Fleming would greet them, having prepared a welcome dinner for the members. After dinner, there was time to catch up with all the local news and happenings at Yuendumu and the presentation of a gift to the Flemings by Murray Barrett. Work would start in earnest the next morning.

The team would unpack and assemble equipment in the work area that was Tom's Yuendumu church on Sundays. They used the two back rooms for dental impressions and radiography, and completed examinations and photography in the larger main room. Barrett, the team leader, would announce his team's presence to the Settlement Administration, the hospital staff and the schoolteachers. Usually Barrett would hold a session with Warlpiri elders to explain the purpose of the visit and to enlist assistance if required. This was always freely given. By 1961, the Warlpiri people knew the dental visitors well through the visits by Campbell and his colleagues over the previous 10 years. The elders regarded Campbell with considerable respect, a sentiment that Campbell and his successors always returned.

After the equipment had been tested and was fully functional, it was time to start the examinations. These would continue on weekdays for the duration of the visit, allowing a day or two to dismantle and store equipment and pack dental models and radiographs for safe transport to Adelaide. Barrett used the school class lists, prepared by Sandra Pinkerton in Adelaide, to select each examination session. He selected children according to age group. Sometimes a session would be devoted to the examination of adult men and women but there was always difficulty in finding them in spite of the directions of a Warlpiri informer that "he must be somewhere".

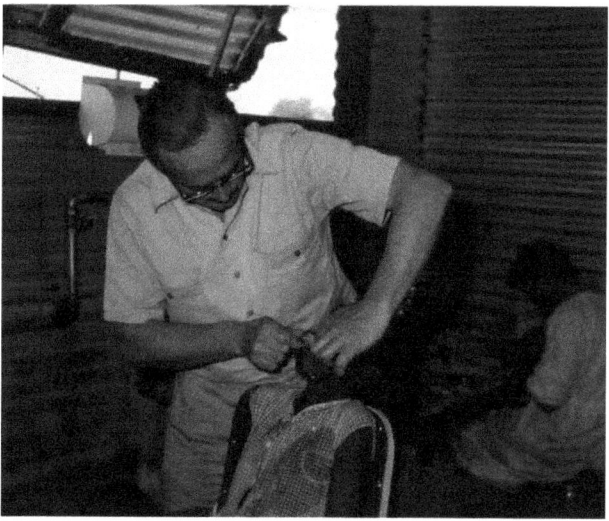
Figure 4.11
Murray Barrett obtaining a dental impression

Each examination session would include about 10–15 school children, who would be collected from school and taken to the examination room where Barrett would register them in the record book checking their name, age and family against information available in advance. They would receive a trip identification number and Barrett would complete his oral examination, noting any irregularities. The children would then move on to the other team members, who would complete their allocated tasks until they had examined all the children, after which they would be returned to school with pockets full of dried fruit.

A visual examination was made of the oral mucosa, the gingivae and the teeth, and the findings recorded on field record sheets. The team obtained stone casts of the dental arches for as many subjects as possible. In the 1960s the dental examination was extended to include standardised cephalometric roentgenograms and some oblique jaw roentgenograms. Researchers made a limited range of anthropometric observations, and obtained hand and wrist roentgenograms for skeletal age assessments in collaboration with the Department of Anatomy. The researchers took strict precautions to protect the subjects and investigators from the possible harmful effects of radiation.

Subject identification

Subjects were identified for cross-reference purposes by a general serial number recorded in a master register and on separate cards for each subject. These cards gave the name, estimated or recorded birthdates, dates of previous examinations, and family relationships. A register existed for each visit to the Settlement that recorded for each subject a serial number with an alphabetical prefix, specific to that visit. The team sometimes experienced difficulty in identifying the subjects at the time of the examination because many of them were known by several aliases. Reference to family relationships previously recorded helped to overcome this problem. To make sure that the research team could properly identify subjects, on return to Adelaide they compared the dental casts and photographs with those obtained previously.

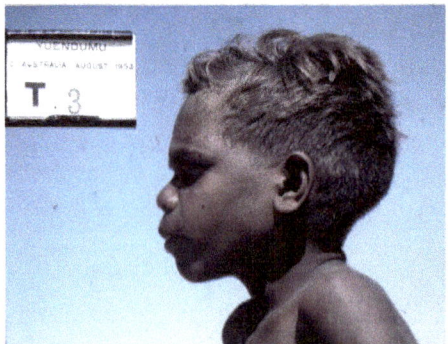

Figure 4.12
Harry Jakamarra Nelson in 1953 with his serial trip prefix and number

In addition to field record sheets, the researchers used other data sheets for further observations made on the dental casts and roentgenograms after returning to Adelaide. These they cross-referenced by the use of the general series and the specific register numbers.

The examination sessions were times of merriment for all involved. The children had a wonderful sense of humour. The team members were known by the kinship names that the Warlpiri had assigned them and everyone, including the school children, who would have known the classificatory kin system perfectly, soon knew these names. Hence, it was common for a Jakamarra team member to be told "that your wife" by a laughing child who pointed to a seven- or eight-year-old Napaltjarri schoolgirl, or "that your mother", pointing to a small Napanangka girl.

Hospital staff occasionally sent a patient for a hand or leg radiograph, usually after some trauma and a suspected fracture. The academic members of the team were dentally trained, so would also attend to any urgent dental problems, such as extraction of worn and painful teeth in older Warlpiri people.

Weekends were times of relaxation for the team, who would often join Tom and Pat Fleming on one of their visits to an outlying cattle station. On these occasions, Tom would often present lantern slides accompanied by biblical stories. On Sundays members would usually attend Tom's church service at Yuendumu. On weeknights the team would often gather for a chat with Tom and Pat, usually regarding Yuendumu or aspects of Aboriginal society generally. On special occasions, members would accompany a few of the Aboriginal elders to sites of rock paintings. These were very special privileges, as were the invitations to witness Warlpiri ceremonies held from time to time. The cooking and sharing of a kangaroo was also an impressive occasion to witness, as was the gathering of berries and witchery grubs by the women and children of Yuendumu.

Limitations of the study

The limitations of the study are obvious. The number of subjects available for study at Yuendumu was small compared with the numbers enrolled in growth studies in Europe and the United States. Under ordinary circumstances the Yuendumu population varied from 500 to 550, occasionally rising to 600 or more with the influx of visitors from neighbouring areas. Reasons for the influx included initiation activities when people visited from other areas such as Haast's Bluff (a four-day walk to the south) and Christmas festivities. However, the number of Aboriginal people in any particular age group was small. For example, from 30 to 40 young adult males was the maximum number that researchers could expect to be available for examination on a single visit. Because of temporary or permanent migration, subjects were not always available for repeat examinations on each visit to the Settlement. Another limiting factor was that actual ages were mostly unknown, except for children born at the Settlement after 1950 when the object of establishing and maintaining a comprehensive demographic record of the community began (Fleming *et al.*, 1971). Present statistics estimate the population to be around 800 (Australian Bureau of Statistics, 2008). Another limitation of the study was the lack of accurate information on the nutritional and health status of the Aboriginal people, although histories of illnesses were available from hospital records at the Settlement. However, these were far from complete. Later research by Middleton and Francis (1976) largely remedied this deficiency.

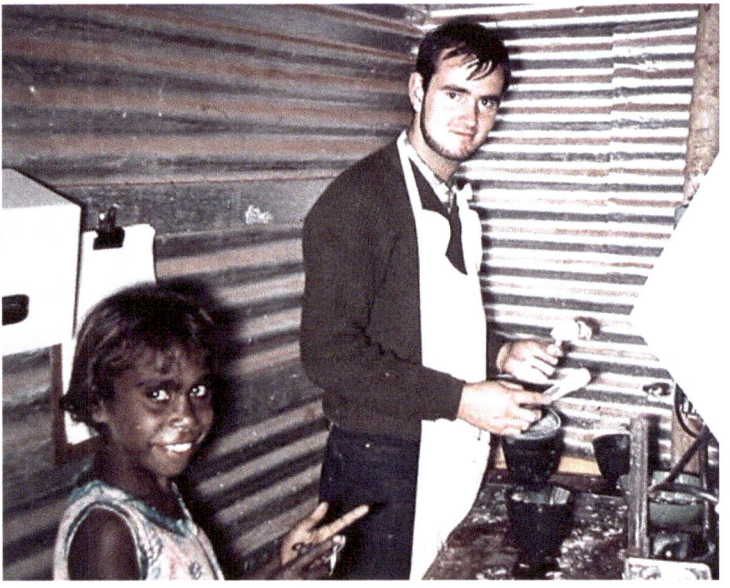

Figure 4.13
Senior dental student Harold Clarke producing dental models in the field at Yuendumu during the 1968 field expedition

Because of the complexity of the overall study and of the individual problems, the project contained sections, with each member of the team responsible for a clearly defined area of study. Close collaboration at each stage and the integration of findings were essential features of the research plan. The team attempted on each visit to record the full range of data for every subject called up for examination, but with the limited time available this was not always possible because of the difficulty of holding the subjects attention at the examination centre.

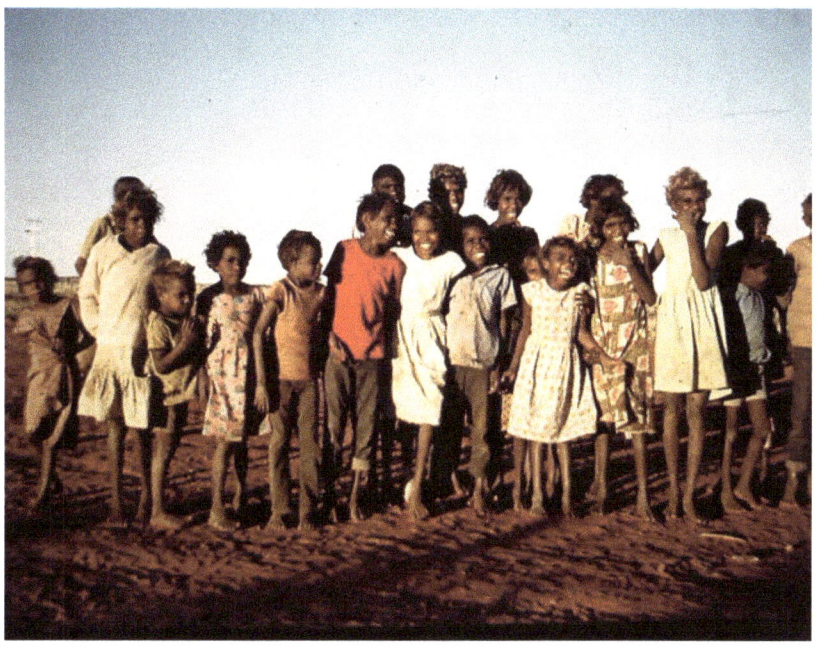

Figure 4.14
Raelene Napurrula Kennedy, Oscar Jungarrayi Wayne, Gavin Japaljarri Spencer, Alice Napanangka Granites, Chrissy Nampijinpa Fry, Bess Nungarrayi France, Clarrise Nampijinpa Fry, Violet Nampijinpa Brown in line to participate

Some of the difficulties due to limited staff and time were overcome by using the services of senior dental students during University vacation periods. The students undertook investigations of well-defined problems which formed part of the total study and which were within the scope of their competence and were capable of satisfactory conclusions within a reasonable time. An important side effect of this policy was the fostering of the students' interest in research.

Transition to computers

Analysis of the data from Yuendumu was laborious and time-consuming before 1962 when The University of Adelaide hired its first commercial computer system. Until then, the researchers used an electric Marchant calculating machine for statistical analyses. Relatively few publications had dealt with the topics the dental teams were researching in an Aboriginal population and there were no similar longitudinal programmes in progress. Therefore, the initial analyses were primarily descriptive in nature to gain information on the mean values and distribution of the variables of interest. Some preliminary bivariate analyses were possible but the limitations of the Marchant machine prevented the calculation of the large correlation matrices required for multivariate analysis.

In May 1962, the university hired and took possession of an IBM 1620 computer (Kidman and Potts, 1999). This computer and its associated peripheral equipment were available to university researchers but a programming and operation service was not available. Barrett and Brown immediately realised that if their research was to progress further, particularly with the load of increasing data, access to computer processing was essential. Consequently, they were among the first university staff trained in the programming and operation of the computer systems and were enthusiastic users of the newly installed mainframe computer available at The University of Adelaide.

A Thursday night session was reserved for dental researchers and Barrett and Brown used this session to great advantage, honing their elementary programming skills and learning to operate the card reader and output devices such as the electric typewriter, the chain line printer and the 80-column card output machine. Within a few months they were executing relatively sophisticated programmes including their first applications of multivariate analyses. There was considerable relief that computer processing of data would be a permanent feature of the Yuendumu project, as it has been in the years since the field trips ceased.

Specific application programs were coded in Fortran, a computer language whose name was derived from *The IBM Mathematical Formula Translating System*. The handwritten programs were then manually typed on a keyboard that in turn relayed the alpha-numeric characters to the punch machine that punched rectangular holes. This method was a vast improvement from the calculating machine that had previously taken long, arduous hours to analyse and produce basic results, and most of the analyses that were used in the longitudinal project would not have been possible without this new technology (Barrett *et al.*, 1966). Results arrived in a matter of minutes, the time a punch card deck progressed up the queue to the University mainframe computer.

The team transferred information from the record sheets to punch cards as soon as possible to expedite the processing of the data. Herman Hollerith first introduced punched cards in the 1880s, and his electric tabulation machine, which read, counted and sorted punched cards, was first used to great advantage by the US Census in 1890. It accomplished in one year what would have taken nearly ten years of hand tabulation. In 1928 IBM introduced the 80-column card with 12 punch locations.

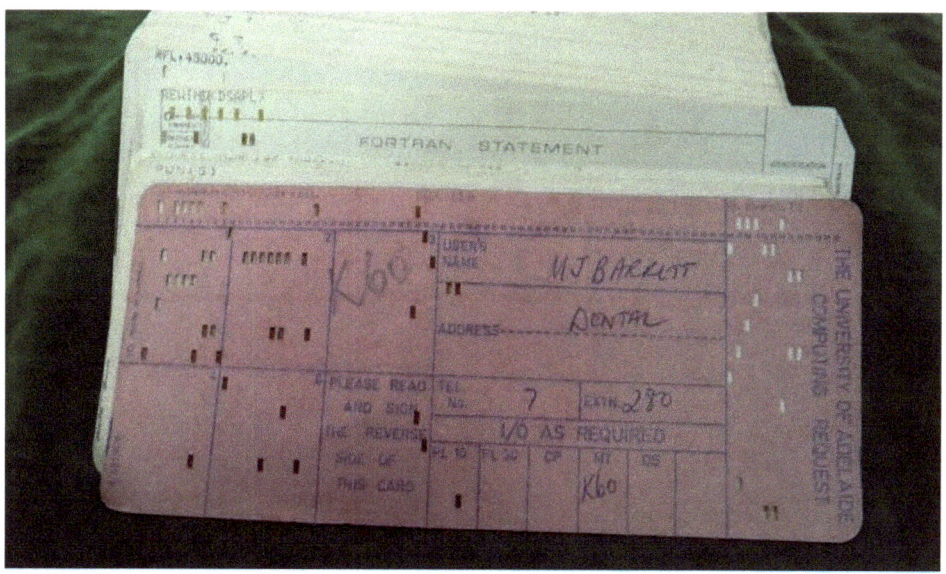

Figure 4.15
A typical punch card deck that was used for data processing by the only mainframe computer located on The University of Adelaide campus in the 1960s

As the computer was situated on the central campus, apart from the Dental School, many trips were made across Frome Road on a daily basis to deliver punched decks to the computer room. Repeated trips to check whether the output was ready or to resubmit the deck because of a programming or data error were numerous. A comma out of place in a punched card could guarantee further trips within the hour. The genealogy decks were so large that two 24 cm-long boxes were needed to contain them. Because of their uniqueness, it was always jokingly suggested that if an accident appeared imminent whilst walking across the road to the Computing Centre, the immediate response should be to throw the cards clear to avoid damage and the bearer was to make the supreme sacrifice.

The investigations during the visits (and those planned for the future) had been mainly observational and concerned with non-metric and metric characters. When sufficient data were accumulated in the long-term study, it was possible to use a longitudinal approach in the analysis. However, the longitudinal method required much time and there was the possibility that many of the subjects would not remain with the study. The team developed a methodology, including the planning of observations, estimation of the sources and magnitude of experimental errors (Barrett *et al.*, 1963a; Barrett *et al.*, 1963b; Dahlberg, 1940), and the selection of appropriate statistical methods, with the advice of specialists in biostatistics.

OSCAR

It was during this phase of the project that the University purchased an OSCAR F record reader from California. Its cost of AU$15,200 was equivalent to a family-sized Adelaide home in the late 1960s. OSCAR was used to obtain x and y coordinates directly from tracings or film projections of standardised cephalograms and dental casts. The coordinates were fed to a decimal converter and then output to punch cards for data analysis. This recorder eliminated systematic errors due to limitations in instruments and measuring methods. However, it could not reduce observer errors so the team always performed repeat or double determinations. Brown *et al.*,(1970) later formulated a technique for minimising and refining the discrepancies between two determinations of coordinates.

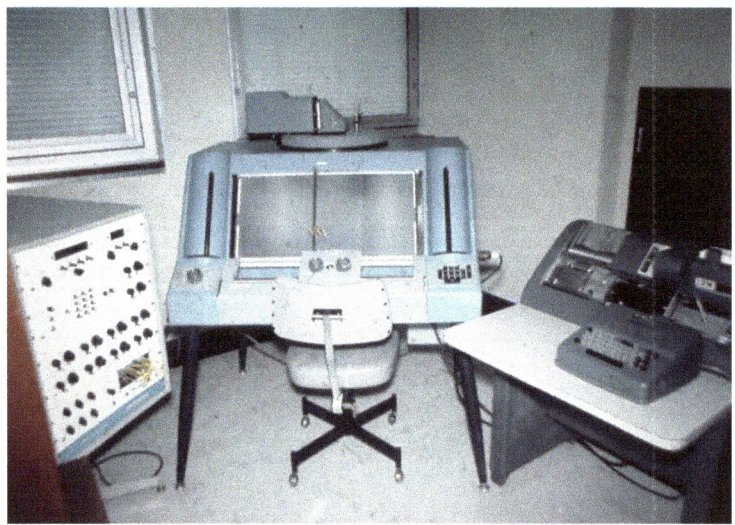

Figure 4.16
OSCAR – the record reader, decimal converter and card punch used to output coordinate data. Manufactured by Computer Industries Inc., Van Nuys, California

Although routine statistical methods formed the basis for a large part of the analytic procedures, attention was given to some of the developed applications of non-parametric and multivariate techniques to the type of data obtained in growth studies (Schull, 1962). Multivariate methods in particular seemed well suited for the analysis of interrelationships between dentofacial components, as they enabled the simultaneous study of a group of variables without needing prior assumptions of cause and effect among the variables (Brown *et al.*, 1965a, 1965b).

Later development of computer systems

The experience gained by programming and operating the IBM 1620 system gave Barrett and Brown the necessary skills to use the vastly superior computers that soon became available. The move to Control Data systems came first with data input and output by magnetic data tapes. Eventually, a campus-wide network of dumb terminals linked to a central mainframe computer brought access to powerful computing to the Dental School laboratory. This access was via a telephone connection at a slow Baud rate of 300. In recent years fast ethernet connections through cabling to powerful desktop computers have provided research personnel with considerable computer power.

Parallel with these changes, the team acquired more sophisticated analog-digital input devices to replace the slower OSCAR and programmed to output coordinate data for the analysis of radiographs and dental casts. There is no doubt that the Yuendumu project could not have developed as it did without access to computing facilities.

The collection

The available material in 1965 consisted of a total of 965 sets of dental casts representing 330 subjects; a total of 320 sets of lateral and postero-anterior skull roentgenograms representing 200 subjects; anthropometric observations of 200 subjects; oblique jaw roentgenograms of 150 subjects; intra-oral roentgenograms; standardised front view, oblique view and profile photographs; hand and foot roentgenograms; cinematographic records of mastication, and; genealogies.

At the conclusion of the field excursions in 1971, the study material accumulated consisted of 1717 sets of dental casts representing 446 subjects; relevant anthropometric data for all subjects enrolled in the study; 1169 sets of lateral and postero-anterior skull roentgenograms representing 288 subjects; oblique jaw roentgenograms; hand and wrist roentgenograms for approximately 250 subjects; standardised photographs of the subjects; over 850 family genealogies, and; other personal records (Brown and Barrett, 1973b).

During the 1960s, many visitors from across the world took advantage of the unique longitudinal data collection that was developing from the yearly trips to Yuendumu. Lasting collaborations began during this era with scientists from Japan, America and Scandinavia. The next phase of the study continued in Adelaide from the 1970s and beyond, as analyses of the vast collection of recorded information and "hard" records continued. International collaboration with researchers expanded and an increasing number of postgraduate students from Adelaide and overseas became regular participants in the Yuendumu study.

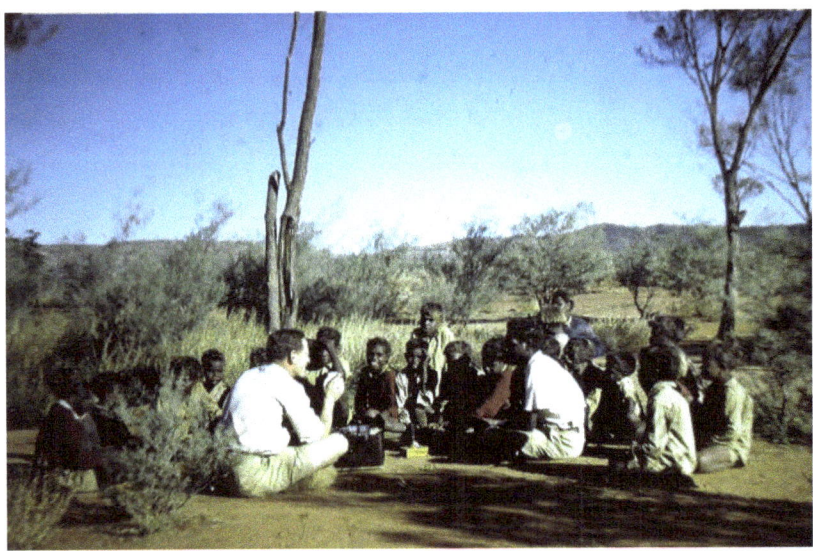

Figure 4.17
Murray Barrett recording a group of Yuendumu school children

References

Australian Bureau of Statistics (2008). National Regional Profile: Yuendumu (CGC, Local Government Area) http://www.abs.gov.au/ausstats/abs@.nsf/Latestproducts/LGA75000Population/

Australian Research Centre for Population and Oral Health (2008). *Fluoridation Atlas*. Department of Dentistry, The University of Adelaide. http://www.arcpoh.adelaide.edu.au/dperu/fluoride/fluoride_P1.pdf

Barrett MJ (1953a). X-Occlusion. *Dent Mag Oral Top* 70:279. Report of an exhibit at the Thirteenth Australian Dental Congress, University of Queensland, Brisbane, June 1–5, 1953.

Barrett MJ (1953b). Dental observations on Australian Aborigines: Yuendumu, Central Australia. *Aust J Dent* 57:127–138.

Barrett MJ (1956a). *Mastication – A Dynamic Process*. Adelaide: The University of Adelaide. Film.

Barrett MJ (1956b). Dental observations on Australian Aborigines: water supplies and endemic dental fluorosis. *Aust Dent J* 1:87–92.

Barrett MJ (1957a). Dental observations on Australian Aborigines: tooth eruption sequence. *Aust Dent J* 2:217–227.

Barrett MJ (1957b). Serial dental casts of Australian Aboriginal children. *Aust Dent J* 2:74.

Barrett MJ (1958). Dental observations on Australian Aborigines: continuously changing functional occlusion. *Aust Dent J* 3:39–52.

Barrett MJ (1960). Parafunctions and tooth attrition. In: *Parafunctions of the Masticatory System (bruxism)*. Lipke D, Posselt U, editors. Report in: *J West Soc Perio* 8:133–148.

Barrett MJ (1964). Walbiri customs and beliefs concerning teeth. *Mankind* 6:95–104.

Barrett MJ, Brown T, Luke JI (1963a). Dental observations on Australian Aborigines: mesiodistal crown diameters of deciduous teeth. *Aust Dent J* 8:299–302.

Barrett MJ, Brown T, Macdonald MR (1963b). Dental observations on Australian Aborigines: mesiodistal crown diameters of permanent teeth. *Aust Dent J* 8:150–155.

Barrett MJ, Brown T, Macdonald MR (1963c). Dental observations on Australian Aborigines: a roentgenographic study of prognathism. *Aust Dent J* 8:418–427.

Barrett MJ, Brown T, Cellier KM (1964). Tooth eruption sequence in a tribe of Central Australian Aborigines. *Am J Phys Anthropol* 22:78–79.

Barrett MJ, Brown T, Fanning EA (1965b). A long-term study of the dental and craniofacial characteristics of a tribe of Central Australian Aborigines. *Aust Dent J* 10:63–68.

Barrett MJ, Brown T, Macdonald MR (1965a). Size of dental arches in a tribe of Central Australian Aborigines. *J Dent Res* 44:912–920.

Barrett MJ, Brown T, Simmons DW (1966). Computers in dental research. *Aust Dent J* 11:329–335.

Barrett MJ, Williamson JJ (1972). Oral health of Australian Aborigines: survey methods and prevalence of dental caries. *Aust Dent J* 17:37–50.

Beyron HL (1964). Occlusal relations and mastication in Australian Aborigines. *Acta Odontol Scand* 22:597–678.

Brown T (1965). *Craniofacial variations in a Central Australian tribe*. Adelaide: Libraries Board of South Australia.

Brown T, Barrett MJ (1964). A roentgenographic study of facial morphology in a tribe of Central Australian Aborigines. *Am J Phys Anthrop* 22:33–42.

Brown T, Barrett MJ, Clarke H (1970). Refinement of metric data from cephalograms and other records. *Aust Dent J* 15:482–486.

Brown T, Barrett MJ (1973a). Increase in average weight of Australian Aborigines. *Med J Aust* 2:25–28.

Brown T, Barrett MJ (1973b). Dental and craniofacial growth studies of Australian Aborigines. In: *The Human Biology of Aborigines in Cape York*. Kirk RL, editor. Canberra: Australian Institute of Aboriginal Studies, Australian Aboriginal Studies No 44, pp. 69–80.

Brown T, Barrett MJ, Darroch JN (1965a). Factor analysis in cephalometric research. *Growth* 19:97–108.

Brown T, Barrett MJ, Darroch JN (1965b). Craniofacial factors in two ethnic groups. *Growth* 19:109–123.

Campbell TD (1925). *Dentition and palate of the Australian Aboriginal*. Adelaide: The University of Adelaide.

Campbell TD (1956). Comparative human odontology. *Aust Dent J* 1:26–29.

Campbell TD, Barrett MJ (1953). Dental observations on Australian Aborigines: a changing environment and food pattern. *Aust J Dent* 57:1–6.

Campbell TD, Barrett MJ (1954). *So They Did Eat*. Adelaide: Board for Anthropological Research, The University of Adelaide. Film.

Dahlberg G (1940). *Statistical Methods for Medical and Biological Students*. London: George Allen and Unwin, pp. 122–132.

Fanning EA (1961). A longitudinal study of tooth formation and root resorption. *N Z Dent J* 57:202–217.

Fanning EA, Moorrees CFA (1969). A comparison of permanent mandibular molar formation in Australian Aborigines and caucasoids. *Arch Oral Biol* 14:999–1006.

Fleming DA, Barrett MJ, Fleming TJ (1971). Family records of an Australian Aboriginal community. *Aust Inst Abor Stud* 3:15.

Garn SM, Lewis AB, Shoemaker DW (1956). The sequence of calcification of the mandibular molar and premolar teeth. *J Dent Res* 35:555–561.

Garn SM, Lewis AB (1957). Relationship between the sequence of calcification and the sequence of eruption of the mandibular molar and premolar teeth. *J Dent Res* 36:992–995.

Garn SM, Lewis AB (1963). Phylogenetic and intraspecific variations in tooth sequence polymorphism. In: *Dental Anthropology*. Brothwell DT, editor. Oxford: Pergamon Press, pp. 53–73.

Kidman B, Potts R (1999). *Paper Tape and Punched Cards: The Early History of Computing and Computing Science at The University of Adelaide*. Adelaide: The University of Adelaide.

Martin R (1957). *Lehrbuch der Anthropologie*. 3rd Edition. Saller K, editor. Stuttgart: Gustav Fischer.

Meggitt MJ (1962). *Desert People*. Sydney: Angus and Robertson.

McNulty EC, Barrett MJ, Brown T (1968). Mesh diagram analysis of facial morphology in young adult Australian Aborigines. *Aust Dent J* 13:40–446.

Middleton MR, Francis SH (1976). *Yuendumu and Its Children. Life and Health on an Aboriginal Settlement.* Canberra: Australian Government Publishing Service.

Moorrees CFA, Fanning EA, Hunt EE (1958). Formation and resorption of three deciduous teeth in children. *Am J Phys Anthropol* 21:205–214.

Moorrees CFA, Fanning EA, Hunt EE (1963). Age variation of formation stages for ten permanent teeth. *J Dent Res* 42:1490–1502.

Ozaki T, Kanazawa E, Sekikawa M, Akai J (1987). Three-dimensional measurement of occlusal surface of upper first molars in Australian Aboriginals. *Aust Dent J* 32:263–269.

Proffit WR (1975). Muscle pressure and tooth position: North American Whites and Australian Aborigines. *Angle Orthod* 45:1–11.

Proffit WR, McGlone RE (1975). Tongue-lip pressure during speech of Australian Aborigines. *Phonetica* 32:200–220.

Proffit WR, McGlone, RE, Barrett MJ (1975). Lip and tongue pressure related to dental arch and oral cavity size in Australian Aborigines. *J Dent Res* 54:1161–1172.

Proffit WR (1978). Equilibrium theory re-examined: To what extent do tongue and lip pressures influence tooth position and thereby occlusion? In: *Oral Physiology and Occlusion*. Proceedings of an International Symposium 1976. Newark, NJ, Perryman JH, editors. London: Pergamon, pp. 55–77.

Reade PC (1964). Infantile acute oral moniliasis. *Aust Dent J* 9:27–28.

Schull WJ (1962). The role of statistics in dentistry. In: *Genetics and Dental Health*. Witkop CJ, editor. New York: McGraw Hill Book Co.

Solow B, Barrett MJ, Brown T (1982). Craniocervical morphology and posture in Australian Aboriginals. *Am J Phys Anthropol* 59:33–45.

Townsend GC (1976). *Tooth Size Variability in Australian Aboriginals: A Descriptive and Genetic Study*. PhD Thesis, The University of Adelaide.

5
Occlusal Development and Function in the Warlpiri

A key outcome of the Yuendumu studies has been a new way of conceptualising what constitutes so-called normal occlusal development and function in humans. This new view has important implications for dentistry and the management of dental problems. This chapter provides an overview of some of the main findings arising from the studies of Yuendumu Aboriginal people and highlights their implications for dental science and practice.

Introduction

Anthropologists have extensively recorded population differences in the dentition in studies of comparative anatomy, human evolution and palaeo-pathology. Dentists must also consider the great variation in dental structures exhibited by members of a single population and by relatives within a family. The source of this variation is the interaction between genes and environment during the initial formation and subsequent growth of the masticatory structures. Even in the same individual, the arrangement of teeth within the dental arches and the manner in which they contact do not remain static throughout life but continually change in response to normal growth processes, environmental influences, dental treatment, pathology and ageing. Changes of this nature have particular relevance for the clinical dentist. Although significant advances in masticatory physiology have occurred in recent years, many concepts of dental occlusion retain an element of 19th century teleological thought. As Brace (1977) put it, "the idea of the perfect occlusion has shimmered in the imagination of the dental profession somewhat like the Holy Grail of Arthurian legend - the unattainable height of earthly aspiration".

Clinical dental practice places great emphasis on the correct interdigitation of upper and lower tooth cusps and on the significance of various jaw relationships and jaw movements. It is rather paradoxical that these concepts are based largely on observations of modern dentitions, which represent the end product of the selective pressures that have operated during human evolution. Many modern concepts of occlusion are untenable when applied to the dentitions of early humans or some present-day populations still living under environmental conditions similar to those prevailing during most of our existence.

In industrialised societies, cooking techniques, the use of eating utensils, and the ready availability of processed and refined foods have greatly reduced the demands placed on masticatory function. In contrast, under the harsh environmental conditions experienced by many earlier human populations, the ability to cope with masticatory stress had important survival value. Because of the natural variability referred to above, some individuals within a population adapted to their environment more successfully than others and were therefore more likely to survive and transmit their genetic endowment to offspring.

During hominid evolution, the masticatory structures have been subjected to selective pressures associated with the physical environment and requirements for the gathering, preparation and eating of food. Comparisons of skeletal material representing humans from prehistoric times through intermediate populations up to modern present-day societies reveal the extent of changes that have taken place in craniofacial morphology, particularly in the masticatory structures.

Because of their prime function in preparing food for ingestion, the teeth and jaws have been involved in these changes to a considerable extent. Generally, there has been a reduction in tooth size and decreased muscularity of the facial skeleton. Consequently, alveolar prognathism, which is a characteristic of most early populations, has reduced. The evolutionary process has also affected the morphological features of tooth crowns, the size and shape of the dental arches, the arrangement of teeth within the dental arches and the mode of dental occlusion. This has also affected the jaw musculature, temporomandibular joint system and masticatory function.

One of the most striking dental features of early humans is the almost universal presence of extensive occlusal and interproximal tooth wear. Wear of teeth, caused by the combination of vigorous jaw function and the inclusion of abrasive substances in food, commenced early in life, as soon as the deciduous teeth emerged, and continued until death. Up to a certain stage, tooth wear was a natural physiological event that had beneficial consequences for tooth occlusion and masticatory efficiency. However, when the extent or rate of wear exceeded the ability of the masticatory structures to adapt to the increased occlusal stress then the outcome was often degeneration or pathological change of one form or another. Under these conditions, the mode of dental occlusion continually changed throughout life - it was indeed a naturally functioning occlusion.

The adaptive ability of the individual subjected to severe occlusal stress was an important determinant of reproductive fitness. The human masticatory structures adapt to environmental stress in two main ways. Firstly, there is the somatic attribute of physiological plasticity, which enables the individual to adjust to changing functional demands. Examples of this mechanism for maintaining homeostasis in the masticatory system include, for example, the development of skeletal robustness, powerful jaw muscles and effective patterns of jaw movements in response to the demands for vigorous mastication. Adaptations to increased functional requirements in the dentition are also seen in the development of resilient periodontal and alveolar support, in the formation of secondary dentine in the presence of tooth wear and in remodelling of the articular surfaces of the temporomandibular joint. However, physiological plasticity has limits and excessive occlusal loads can result in degenerative and pathological events.

The second method of adapting to the environment is genetic, which is the agency for evolutionary change in the masticatory structures. A more favourable genetic constitution enables some individuals to cope with demanding environments better than others, possibly by enhanced physiological plasticity. On the other hand, susceptibility to debilitating conditions that interfere with masticatory efficiency, for example, gross malocclusion, dental decay, jaw pathology or degenerative disease of the temporomandibular joint, would be disadvantageous under harsh environments, leading to reduced reproductive fitness.

Technical advances such as the use of improved weapons and tools to obtain food and the development of more advanced methods for preparing and cooking food reduced the environmental stress on the dental structures of humans. Improvements in social organisation and the development of agricultural communities played a similar role. Heavy demands on the masticatory system are not characteristic of modern city dwellers and consequently dental efficiency has little survival value today. It is not surprising, then, that the dentitions of many present-day populations, compared with those of their ancestors who were nomadic food gatherers and hunters, display evidence of reduced masticatory function and efficiency together with an increased prevalence of malocclusions, dental decay, and periodontal disease. Moreover, the skill of the dental specialist has reduced the dependency of most present-day populations on a natural functioning occlusion for survival.

Morphology of the dental arches

In many respects, Australian Aboriginal people retain morphological and functional characteristics of the jaws and dentition that are closer to those of our late Pleistocene ancestors than are the features of many other modern populations. Begg (1954) elaborated on this concept in his classic paper "Stone age man's dentition", which formed the basis of the Begg philosophy of orthodontic treatment (Begg and Kesling, 1977).

The facial skeleton of the Australian Aboriginal person exhibits a morphology that correlates with the powerful and well-developed masticatory system (Figure 5.1). Alveolar processes of the maxilla and mandible are prominent. This results in the well-known mid-facial prognathism, which tends to be more striking in females. The palate is capacious but the body of the mandible is not particularly large so that the alveolar prominence gives a false impression of an underdeveloped chin. In contrast, the ramus of the mandible is broad, reflecting the powerfully developed masticatory muscles. The morphological characteristics of the Australian Aboriginal person allows the wide excursions of the mandible during the powerful grinding phase of the masticatory cycle.

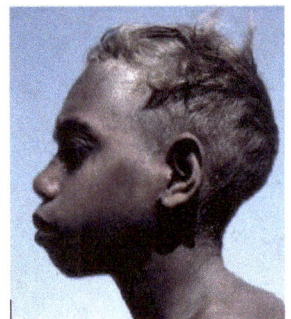 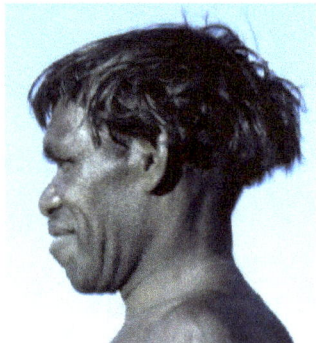

Figure 5.1
Unidentified juvenile and adult Warlpiri males showing characteristic facial morphology

Large teeth and well-formed dental arches characterise the dentition of Australian Aboriginal people (Figure 5.2). Dental crown diameters are considerably larger than in most other present-day populations, both in the deciduous and permanent dentitions (Townsend and Brown, 1979; Margetts and Brown, 1978). Regional variations in tooth-size are found throughout the continent and it is interesting that the ranges overlap those reported for Neanderthal specimens and in some instances even those of the earlier large-toothed Homo erectus dentitions (Brace, 1980; Smith *et al.*, 1981). As found in other populations, tooth diameters are larger in males than females. The permanent mandibular and maxillary canines exhibit greater sex differences in crown size than other teeth. Sex dimorphism is less marked in the deciduous dentition.

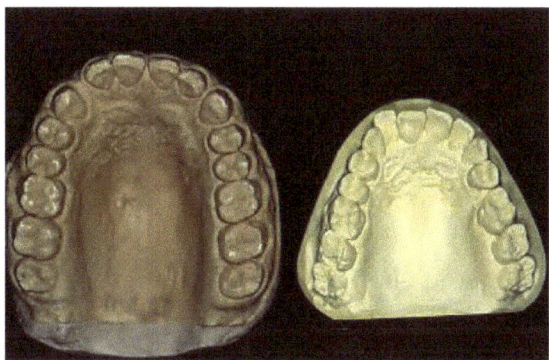

Figure 5.2
Maxillary dental models of Aboriginal and European Australians showing the marked differences in size and shape of the dental arch

Because of large tooth diameters, the dental arch dimensions are also large in Aboriginal people who display sex differences in both arch length and arch breadth. The arch dimensions are not static after eruption of the permanent teeth but undergo continual age changes consisting of a reduction in arch length, an increase in arch breadth and consequent modifications in shape. Usually the dental arches are spacious and symmetrical but tooth crowding and other occlusal irregularities are not infrequent.

Björk and Helm (1969) reported a detailed analysis of tooth crowding in several populations. The Aboriginal people studied by these authors were living under settlement conditions at Yuendumu and, in the absence of severe tooth wear, could be expected to show more tooth crowding than nomadic Aboriginal people.

Nevertheless, the findings (Table 5.1) indicate that some Aboriginal people, together with the South African Bantus, displayed considerably less malocclusion and tooth crowding than the other populations.

Table 5.1 Frequencies of malocclusion and tooth crowding in seven populations[1]

	Total malocclusions % subjects	Maxillary crowding % subjects	Mandibular crowding % subjects
Australian Aboriginals	53	11	21
Bantu	52	2	5
Quechua	78	26	33
Navaho	93	29	25
Chinese	67	25	28
Japanese	80	28	50
Danes	78	29	25

1 Data from Björk and Helm (1969)

A further comparison of the same group of Aboriginal people by Helm (1979) confirmed the earlier findings that Australian Aboriginal peoples often showed lower frequencies of tooth crowding than modern Danes and about the same as medieval Danish skulls from the 12th to 16th centuries (Table 5.2). These comparisons indicate that increased tooth crowding and malocclusion are the consequence of gradual transition from a lifestyle involving coarse food that needed vigorous mastication to the present use of refined and pre-processed foods.

Corruccini *et al.*, (1990) compared occlusal traits in a sample of older, previously nomadic, Aboriginal people living at Yuendumu with a sample of younger individuals who had grown up at the settlement. Interestingly, they found significant differences in incisor relationships, tooth alignment, and relative arch breadths between the two groups. However, the differences were relatively small compared with reports for other populations undergoing a transition to a westernised diet (Corruccini, 1984). One of the reasons for this may have been that the changes in dietary habits from one generation to the next at Yuendumu were not clear-cut.

During the 1960s, the Warlpiri at Yuendumu were at an early stage of transition from a nomadic hunter-gathering lifestyle. Some of the older individuals would have spent time working on cattle stations and eating western food before settling at Yuendumu. The younger Aboriginal people who were born and raised at Yuendumu were exposed to coarser and tougher native foods when these were available but they also had access to food from the canteen. It is possible that the rather subtle differences in occlusal variables between the older and younger Aboriginal people reflected gradual change in diet between generations.

Table 5.2 Frequencies of tooth crowding in Aboriginal Australians and modern and medieval Danes[1]

	Modern Danes % subjects	**Medieval Danes % subjects**	**Australian Aboriginals % subjects**
Maxilla or mandible	42	27	25
Maxilla	24	11	11
Maxillary incisor segment	17	10	10
Maxillary lateral segment	12	2	3
Mandible	33	23	18
Mandibular incisor segment	22	17	13
Mandibular lateral segment	23	13	10

1 Data from Helm (1979)

When living a hunter-gatherer lifestyle, the Warlpiri people retained most of their teeth in a state of functional activity throughout life. An exception to this was the ceremonial removal of a maxillary incisor in males or the occasional loss of teeth through trauma or disease. Dental caries was exceedingly rare by modern standards and even though a partial breakdown of the dentition occurred at times, particularly in old age, due to pulpal infections arising from occlusal wear processes, individuals still used the remaining teeth with reasonable effect.

Food habits and masticatory movements

Before European contact, Aboriginal people were nomadic hunters and food gatherers, a way of life conditioned by the country, climate and food resources available from time to time. Life was often very harsh, particularly in the desert areas of the continent where low rainfall often led to a scarcity of food and water. Consequently, much of their time was devoted to the daily quest for food, an exercise that demanded remarkable skills and knowledge of the land and its fauna and flora (Campbell *et al.*, 1954).

Typically, the Warlpiri people wandered their tribal territory in small family groups, stopping in one location only as long as the natural resources allowed before moving to a new campsite. The male was the hunter upon whose skill the group depended for large game. Women, accompanied by children, were responsible for gathering supplies of berries, seeds, edible roots, small reptiles and other desert foods, which they used to supplement family resources.

Methods of food preparation and cooking were primitive and did not appear to vary greatly from what was observed elsewhere throughout the continent. Many foods were eaten raw, particularly plant and plant products. Flesh foods received minimum cooking either on an open fire or, in the case of larger game, in a crude earth oven of hot sand and ashes. Seeds were ground between stones to a flour that was mixed with water to form a thick paste before cooking over hot ashes. Aboriginal people used no eating utensils but relied almost entirely on their teeth and hands. Preparation and cooking methods inevitably incorporated abrasive material into the food leading to the progressive tooth wear and changing occlusal relations that are characteristic of people living under these conditions.

It is interesting to note that dental decay in Aboriginal communities increased substantially with adoption of European food habits. Prevalences of up to 70 per cent in settlement dwelling people contrasted sharply with the situation seen in those living in a traditional manner, where decay affected only about 15 per cent of individuals (Brown, 1974).

Researchers have studied masticatory movements in the Warlpiri by direct observation and by the analysis of cinematographic records (Barrett, 1956). A detailed report on this topic by Beyron (1964) revealed a close relationship between the pattern of masticatory movements and occlusal conditions. Comparisons with findings reported for present-day Europeans indicated some striking differences between the two groups, particularly in the extent of mandibular excursions during mastication. The following description relies mainly on Beyron's work.

In Aboriginal people, movements of the mandible when the mouth is empty are generally free of the restrictions and asymmetry often observed in Europeans. For example, habitual opening and closing movements are smoothly executed without any marked deviation from the mid-line. Lateral excursions are wide in extent and can be made on either side with equal facility. A particular feature of lateral excursions is the intimate contact between opposing teeth on the working side; in many subjects, this contact extends from molars to the incisors. The extent of these working side contacts appears to increase with age, probably as a result of progressive occlusal wear, but even in young subjects the contacts are more extensive than in many present-day Europeans without wear. Contacts in the anterior region are also extensive in the protrusive position of the mandible.

The prehension and incision of food, which precedes masticatory grinding in preparation for swallowing, are important and powerful actions in Aboriginal people. For example, a large portion of meat is held in the hands and then gripped between the incisor and canine teeth. Incision of the meat is effectively executed by the vigorous use of numerous muscles, including those of the arms, jaws, neck and shoulders. The severed portion is then positioned between the tooth surfaces by lip and tongue musculature.

Chewing is performed alternately on right and left side with striking regularity, the food being passed to the other side by co-ordinated action of the cheeks, lips and tongue. Usually between two and four masticatory cycles, each about one second in duration, are executed on one side and then the food is passed to the other side for a similar number of cycles. The pattern is repeated until the food is ready for swallowing. The lips are mostly separated during mastication in Aboriginal people.

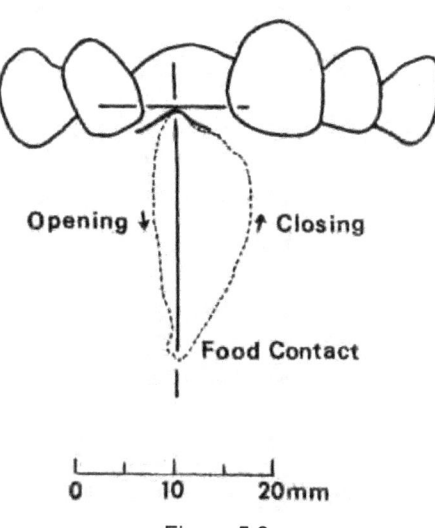

Figure 5.3
A typical chewing cycle in an Australian Aboriginal person. The path of tooth contact during empty grinding is shown at the top of the cycle (after Beyron, 1964).

The typical masticatory cycle shown in Figure 5.3 was constructed from cinematographic recordings of an Aboriginal person who had evulsion of the maxillary right central incisor. The cycle varies in size, shape and duration between subjects and within the same subject according to the type of food and the activity of the jaw musculature from time to time. However, for most subjects an individual pattern is distinguishable throughout several successive cycles.

A typical masticatory cycle commences with an opening phase in which the mandible moves away from tooth contact along a path close to the mid-line but gradually crossing to the masticatory or food side. The incisal point often moves towards the non-food side for a short time at the commencement of the opening phase. The total jaw opening, indicated by incisor movement away from the intercuspal position, rarely exceeds the minimum necessary to grasp the food bolus. In Warlpiri people this distance averaged 17.6mm, about the same as recorded in Europeans, but it was slightly greater (18.4mm) in younger subjects than in older (15.4mm).

Because there is no marked resistance to jaw opening, this phase of the masticatory cycle displays the greatest velocity of movement and occupies about 35 per cent of the whole cycle. Jaw velocity decreases as contact is made with the food bolus at the end of the opening phase. The closing phase of the masticatory cycle commences as the food is crushed and the mandible moves further towards the food side. Considerable pressure is generated between the teeth during jaw closure. The pressure, lateral deviation and velocity depend on the size, shape and hardness of food as well as the morphological characteristics of the jaws and teeth. It is interesting that subjects chewing meat display a lateral mandibular shift of about 5.2mm for all age groups, significantly larger than the 3-4mm recorded in Europeans (Hildebrand, 1931). The greatest lateral deviation usually occurs in a more cranial position in Aboriginal people compared with European people, in which a characteristic tear-drop pattern can be recognised with the greatest lateral swing situated below the middle of the masticatory cycle. The crushing phase ends with the teeth near the intercuspal position as final grinding begins.

Tooth contact occurs during the final grinding phase during many, but not all, masticatory cycles. When this occurs, the movement path of the incisors coincides for some distance with the path generated by tooth contact in empty jaw movements. This section of the incisal path is fairly constant in all chewing cycles but occasionally the presence of fine particles between the teeth will give rise to small oscillatory movements during the final grinding phase. The distance over which the masticatory cycle corresponds to the path of contact glide varies in different cycles. At times the two paths coincide at only one point but in many cycles the coincidence occurs for some distance lateral to the intercuspal position and continues until the intercuspal position is reached. This distance averaged 2.8mm in subjects chewing meat and did not vary greatly for different age groups. Because of a flatter cuspal form, the angle of contact glide is fairly shallow in Aboriginal people compared with Europeans and it decreased with age and reduction of cusps by tooth wear.

In summary, the pattern of mastication in the Warlpiri people differed from that commonly observed in European people. Chewing alternates regularly between the right and left sides with a movement path that has a wide, oval form. The lateral excursion of the mandible during chewing is considerably greater in Aboriginal people but the maximum opening does not differ greatly from that in Europeans. Tooth contact occurs in many masticatory cycles usually from a point about 2.8mm lateral to the intercuspal position from which the mandible is guided by cuspal and incisal inclinations back to the intercuspal position.

Development of occlusion

Table 5.3 shows a simplified chart of some of the determinants of occlusal development and function. These determinants are grouped under two main categories, growth-related and function-related, although it must be emphasised that growth and function are not only interdependent but each is subject to overall genetic control that is modified to varying degrees by environmental influences.

Several advantages accrued from studying dental development in the children living at Yuendumu. Intertribal marriages were rare in this Aboriginal society and the population was relatively homogeneous from a genetic point of view compared with most others reported in studies of dental development. Furthermore, the custom of polygyny enabled the genetic aspects of dental morphology to be studied by assembling and analysing records from half-siblings, that is, children with the same father but different mothers.

A further advantage of the Yuendumu population lay in the children's relative freedom from dental decay so that premature loss of deciduous teeth was a rare event. In spite of increasing consumption of refined carbohydrates and other processed foods, Barrett and Williamson (1972) found that 74 per cent of 149 children examined were free of deciduous tooth decay and that less than 4 per cent of all teeth examined were affected. They concluded that the caries experience of young people at Yuendumu ranked among the lowest in the world at that time.

Table 5.3 Determinants of occlusal development and function

A. Growth-related
• Variations in tooth size and shape - genetic and environmental influences • Interactions between developing teeth • Coordination of tooth size during development • Timing and sequence of tooth exfoliation and emergence • Magnitude and direction of jaw rotations during growth • Alveolar development and tooth migrations • Compensatory alveolar development • Changes in dental arch size and shape
B. Function-related
• Development of neuromuscular patterns • Perioral muscle pressures and alveolar development • Premature loss of deciduous teeth • Reduction of tooth size by wear • Tooth loss and migration • Restorative, orthodontic and surgical procedures • Pathological conditions of the teeth, jaws, muscles and joints • Adaptability to changing occlusal conditions

Variations in tooth size

It is thought that tooth size is determined by a polygenic mode of inheritance, that is, the small cumulative effects of a number of genes acting together (Bailit, 1975; Harris, 1975; Townsend and Brown, 1978). However, environmental effects can also be determinants, allowing for the possibility that the continuous variation observed in tooth diameters originates from the superimposed interplay of genes and environment. A developing tooth is exposed to environmental influences from the stage of cellular differentiation until calcification of the crown and roots are complete. Maternal health is important during formation of the deciduous teeth, which is essentially a prenatal process, whereas the permanent teeth are more susceptible to postnatal environment. Tooth size is obviously an important determinant of occlusal morphology and function. In particular, the relative sizes of deciduous teeth and their permanent successors determine, in part, the space available for emergence and subsequent alignment of the permanent teeth within the dental arches. Several studies have aimed to clarify the relative contribution of genes and environment to the control and coordination of tooth size variation.

Table 5.4 Weighted mean estimates of contributions to tooth size variability in Australian Aboriginal people[1]

	Additive genetic %	Common environment %	Within-family environment %
Deciduous			
Mesiodistal	50	19	32
Buccolingual	66	12	23
Combined	58	15	27
Permanent			
Mesiodistal	63	4	33
Buccolingual	66	8	26
Combined	64	6	30

1 Data from Townsend (1980)

Table 5.4 uses data reported by Townsend (1980) to summarise estimates of the genetic and environmental contributions to tooth size in Australian Aboriginal people from Yuendumu. The additive genetic component, which refers to the cumulative effects of genes, accounts for about 60 per cent of tooth size variability in both deciduous and permanent dentitions. It is interesting, however, that the additive genetic component appears to be slightly higher for buccolingual than mesiodistal diameters. Common environment is sometimes termed the maternal effect as it indicates the component of tooth size variability in siblings arising from the common intra-uterine environment of their mother. Common environment explained a much greater proportion of variation in the deciduous dentition, about 15 per cent, compared with about 6 per cent in the permanent. Differences in the timing of tooth calcification, which is predominantly prenatal in the deciduous dentition and postnatal in the permanent, explain this. Space requirements are less likely to be critical for developing deciduous teeth as they reach their full size potential with less interaction than developing permanent teeth. The third component of variability, within family environment, merely indicates the proportion that is due to effects other than additive genetic and common environment. It amounted to about 30 percent in each dentition. This study showed that genetic factors are important in determining tooth size variability but probably not to the extent sometimes suggested.

Like other growth processes, dental development is coordinated with respect to the timing and sequence of tooth calcification, growth of the tooth germs and gingival emergence of the tooth crowns. In addition, there is evidence that the relative sizes of adjacent and opposing teeth are regulated. The mechanisms of coordination operate during the entire development of deciduous and permanent dentitions and they influence not only teeth but also the formation and growth of the jaws and other craniofacial structures.

The nature of tissue interactions during dental morphogenesis is not fully understood but there have been significant advances over recent years in our understanding of interactions that occur between the epithelial and mesenchymal components of developing teeth (Tucker and Sharpe, 2004; Thesleff, 2006; Brook, 2009).

Morphogenetic fields are considered regions in developing tissues under direct genetic control that determines the differentiation, growth and morphology of structures forming within the field. Accordingly, morphogenetic fields are thought to determine the morphological gradients in size or shape of neighbouring structures in a series, for example, phalanges, vertebrae or teeth. Butler (1939, 1963) originally proposed this concept to explain ontogeny and phylogeny of the mammalian dentition, while Dahlberg (1945) expanded it and Osborn (1978) reviewed it. The precise identification of these morphogenetic fields, the extent of genetic control and the complete picture of the biochemical interactions involved are still under investigation, but there is no doubt that the patterns of tooth size variation and correlation point to their existence (Townsend *et al.*, 2009).

According to the *Field Theory*, each tooth class within the mammalian dentition contains a key or polar tooth, which is thought to be more stable in morphology than adjacent teeth in the same field. The maxillary central incisor and the mandibular second incisor are the key teeth within their fields; likewise, the first premolar and first molar are regarded as key teeth within the premolar and molar fields.

The concept of a molar field is well-illustrated by reference to the variabilities of tooth size in the deciduous and permanent molars of Australian Aboriginal people shown in Table 5.5. For both mesiodistal and buccolingual crown diameters in males and females, the variability in size displays an increasing gradient away from the key tooth which is the first molar in the permanent dentition and the second molar in the deciduous. Furthermore, there is a distinct trend for the permanent first molar to be the least variable in the series. These patterns are by no means random and they strongly support the concept of a morphogenetic control over molar teeth that is strongest in the region of the deciduous second and permanent first molars but decreases gradually with distance from the key tooth. This proposal is in keeping with the common clinical observation that the key teeth are more stable or uniform in morphology than their neighbours.

Table 5.5 Coefficients of variation in molar tooth size of Australian Aboriginal people[1*]

	Mesiodistal		Buccolingual	
Tooth	Males	Females	Males	Females
Maxillary				
dm_1	6.9	6.0	6.5	5.4
dm_2	5.9	4.9	5.1	4.3
M1	5.0	4.6	4.5	4.4
M2	5.9	5.7	5.4	5.0
M3	6.5	7.0	6.5	6.3
Mandibular				
dm_1	7.0	5.6	6.5	6.8
dm_2	5.6	4.6	5.0	5.1
M1	5.0	4.4	4.9	4.6
M2	6.0	5.6	5.1	5.0
M3	8.8	6.9	6.1	6.0

1   Data on tooth size from Townsend and Brown (1979) and Margetts and Brown (1978)

*   The coefficient of variation is a measure of the variability of a measurement relative to its arithmetic mean, calculated by expressing the standard deviation as a percentage of the mean.

Further evidence of morphogenetic control appears in the pattern of correlations for size among permanent teeth (Table 5.6). Each tooth is more strongly correlated with a neighbouring tooth of the same tooth class than with a neighbour of different class or more distant teeth. For example, lateral incisors are more highly correlated in size with central incisors than they are with canines; the two premolars display stronger correlations with each other than with their neighbours, the canine and first molar; similarly with the first and second molar. Canines are usually regarded as constituting a single canine field of influence so the patterns of correlation are interesting. In the maxilla, the canines show strongest size association with the first premolars, but in the mandible the correlations with lateral incisors are the strongest. This pattern may be associated with the comparative morphology of the canines, more like the premolars in the maxilla but tending to be incisiform in the mandible. It is interesting that in some herbivores, such as the sheep, lower canines have evolved morphologically to become one of the anterior incisiform teeth.

Table 5.6 Tooth size correlations in the permanent dentition of Australian Aboriginal people – mesiodistal diameters above the diagonal, buccolingual below[1]

	\multicolumn{7}{c}{Maxilla}						
	I1	I2	C	P1	P2	M1	M2
I1	—	**.60**	.52	.55	.46	.56	.37
I2	**.69**	—	.48	.39	.33	.43	.22
C	.57	.54	—	**.62**	.48	.48	.40
P1	.52	.47	**.67**	—	**.73**	.45	.53
P2	.46	.42	.58	**.81**	—	.56	.53
M1	.59	.47	.59	.66	.71	—	**.59**
M2	.52	.41	.59	.63	.71	**.80**	—

	\multicolumn{7}{c}{Mandible}						
	I1	I2	C	P1	P2	M1	M2
I1	—	**.67**	.51	.39	.38	.46	.44
I2	**.82**	—	**.63**	.46	.35	.46	.46
C	.71	.74	—	.56	.46	.44	.49
P1	.58	.60	.65	—	**.68**	.47	.53
P2	.57	.54	.59	**.75**	—	.46	.58
M1	.54	.52	.51	.64	.70	—	**.66**
M2	.63	.57	.59	.66	.72	**.77**	—

1   The highest correlation coefficients between paired tooth diameters are shown in bold type.

Patterns of correlation for tooth diameters in the permanent dentition of Australian Aboriginal people, like the patterns of variability referred to above, are not fortuitous but provide further evidence of overall coordination in tooth size in the developing dentition.

Although our understanding of the molecular interactions occurring during odontogenesis is growing, the concept of morphogenetic fields originally proposed by Butler still provides a useful guideline for the clinician to explain observed variability within the dentition.

Tooth size relationships

Coordinated dental development is also apparent in tooth size relationships between deciduous and permanent teeth and between maxillary and mandibular teeth. These relationships are important in the phases of occlusal development concerned with the emergence and alignment of teeth into optimal aesthetic and functional positions within the dental arches. Positional variations and sub-optimal occlusion may result from discrepancies in the size of permanent teeth relative to deciduous precursors or from alveolar development that is inadequate to accommodate all teeth without crowding.

Table 5.7 shows differences in the mesiodistal crown diameters of permanent teeth and their deciduous precursors for Aboriginal boys and girls. The data derive from longitudinal observations where dental models representing each dentition were available (Brown *et al.*, 1980a). The pattern of size relationships is similar to those reported for other groups, such as North Americans of European ancestry (Moorrees, 1959). All permanent incisors and canines exceeded the deciduous precursors in size, the greatest differences being for the central incisor in the maxilla and the lateral incisor in the mandible. The canines showed least difference in mesiodistal diameter between permanent and deciduous teeth.

For the posterior teeth, however, all deciduous teeth exceeded the permanent successors in size with the exception of the maxillary first premolar, which slightly exceeded the deciduous first molar. The greatest size difference of 3.3mm is in the mandible for the second deciduous molar - second premolar relationship. The mesiodistal diameters of the deciduous teeth relative to the permanent successors increased progressively from anterior to posterior region. Whereas the diameters of deciduous incisors were, on average, about 76 to 80 per cent of the corresponding permanent diameters, the percentage comparison averaged about 85 to 90 per cent for the canines, 99 to 110 per cent for the first deciduous molar and 133 to 144 per cent for the second deciduous molar.

Table 5.7 assesses space requirements and space availability during tooth emergence by the size relationships between combined diameters of corresponding deciduous and permanent tooth groups. In the Aboriginal children, the combined diameters of the permanent incisors exceeded those of the deciduous incisors by about 3mm. However, the combined diameters of the deciduous canine and molars exceeded those of the corresponding permanent teeth by over 1mm in the maxilla and about 3mm in the mandible.

Table 5.7 Differences in mesiodistal diameters of corresponding deciduous and permanent teeth and tooth groups expressed in mm.

Permanent	Deciduous	Maxilla		Mandibular	
		Boys	Girls	Boys	Girls
I_1	di_1	2.1	1.8	1.2	1.4
I_2	di_2	1.6	1.4	1.5	1.5
C	dc	0.9	0.8	1.2	0.8
P_1	dm_1	0.1	0.3	−0.7	−0.8
P_2	dm_2	−2.5	−2.4	−3.3	−3.3
I_1+I_2	di_1+di_2	3.6	3.1	2.8	3.2
P_1+P_2	dm_1+dm_2	−2.3	−2.1	−4.0	−4.0
$C+P_1+P_2$	$dc+dm_1+dm_2$	−1.4	−1.3	−2.8	−3.3
I_1 to P_2	di_1 to dm_2	2.2	1.7	−0.2	−0.2

The larger size excess of the deciduous molars compared with the permanent premolar accounts for this size differential. When researchers compared combined diameters of all teeth, the maxillary permanent teeth from first incisor to second premolar exceeded the deciduous precursors by about 2mm. In the mandible, however, the deciduous teeth were larger by 0.2mm. Tooth size relationships followed similar patterns in boys and girls.

The deciduous teeth are replaced during two phases of development separated by a quiescent period. During Phase 1, which extends from 6.3 to 8.5 years in Aboriginal boys and from 5.1 to 8.1 years in Aboriginal girls, the larger permanent incisors replace the deciduous incisors. In normal development, adequate space is made available by compensating alveolar bone growth, which is evidenced by spacing of the deciduous incisors prior to their exfoliation and replacement.

Table 5.8 Comparison of leeway space expressed in mm in several populations

	Maxilla		Mandible	
Population	Boys	Girls	Boys	Girls
Australian Aboriginal people*[1]	1.4	1.3	2.8	3.3
European North Americans*[2]	1.2	1.5	2.2	2.6
British[3]	0.8	0.7	1.9	2.1
Swedes[4]	1.0	1.3	2.2	2.5
Japanese[5]	1.0	0.9	2.9	2.9
Tristanites[6]	1.0	0.8	1.7	1.5
Pima Indians[5]	0.3	0.8	1.8	2.7

* Leeway space calculated from longitudinal data
1 Brown, Margetts and Townsend (1980a)
2 Moorrees and Chadha (1962)
3 Clinch (1963)
4 Seipel (1946)
5 Hanihara (1976)
6 Thomsen (1955)

Phase 2 extends from about 9.9 to 11.5 years in boys and from 9.1 to 11.1 years in girls and includes emergence of the permanent canines, premolars and second molars. During Phase 2, the relative sizes of the corresponding deciduous and permanent teeth are important determinants of adequate occlusal development. Nance (1947) used the term "leeway space" to describe the size excess of the deciduous canine and molars compared with the permanent canine and premolars. He pointed out that the greater leeway space in the mandible allowed mesial movement of the mandibular first molar relative to the maxillary first molar thus establishing a normal Class 1 molar relationship. In the Aboriginal children the leeway space is quite high compared with many other populations (Table 5.8) and this characteristic is important in the provision of space for unimpaired emergence and alignment of the permanent canines and premolars.

The dental casts of subject 509 shown in Figure 5.4 demonstrate occlusal development in the presence of adequate leeway space. In this Aboriginal girl, the combined diameters of the deciduous canine and molars exceeded those of the permanent successors by over 2mm in the maxilla and over 4mm in the mandible, values that were greater than the averages for the group. Adequate space was available for unimpeded eruption and alignment of the permanent teeth as illustrated by the spacing between the canines, first and second premolars at age 12.7 years. Alignment of the teeth within the dental arches was optimal in this girl with no evidence of crowding.

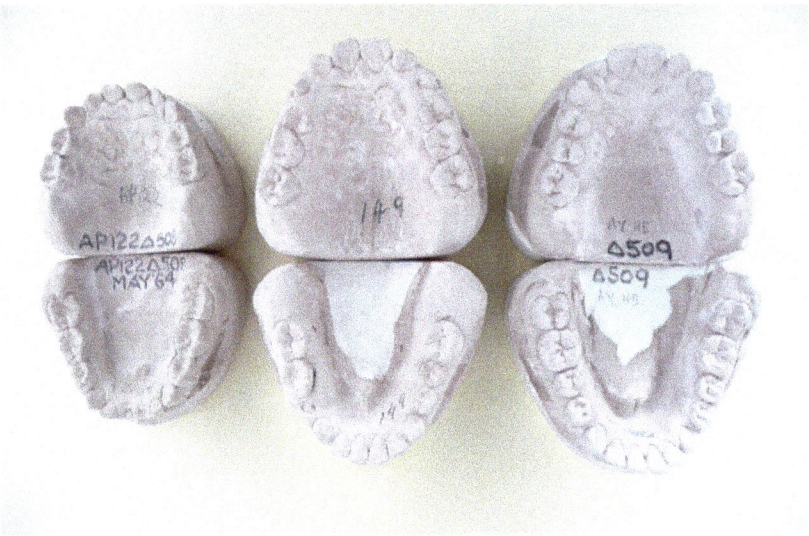

Figure 5.4
Occlusal development in an Aboriginal girl aged 6.7, 11.7 and 12.7 years

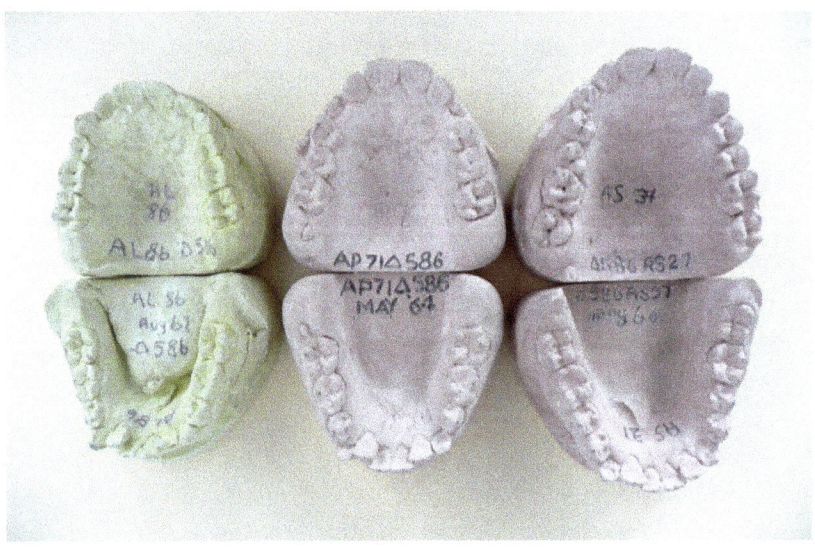

Figure 5.5
Occlusal development in an Aboriginal girl aged 8.6, 10.4 and 12.4 years

In contrast, Aboriginal girl 586, whose dental casts Figure 5.5 shows, had less favourable tooth-size ratios. In this instance the leeway space was well below average for the group; the maxillary canine and premolars exceeded their deciduous precursors in diameter by almost 1mm while in the mandible the size excess of the deciduous teeth was a mere 1.4mm, less than half the average. Maxillary premolar crowding and mandibular anterior crowding was evident at age 10.4 years, although somewhat alleviated two years later. It is interesting that mandibular anterior alignment had improved by age 12.4 years, because of alveolar development, but the right canine remained crowded.

Tooth size correlations

A previous section illustrated the concept of morphogenetic fields exerting control over tooth size with examples relating to the variability of mesiodistal diameters and the correlations between the diameters of adjacent teeth. This section extends the concept by reference to the coordination of tooth size between dentitions and between maxillary and mandibular arches.

Table 5.9 shows the correlation between diameters of corresponding teeth and tooth groups in the deciduous and permanent dentitions of Australian Aboriginal people. The odontometric study of Brown *et al.,* (1980b) reports further details and sample sizes. Although correlations between corresponding single teeth were only moderate, the associations strengthened when the researchers considered combined diameters of groups of teeth. It is particularly interesting that total mesiodistal size, that is, the combined diameters of all teeth, displayed the strongest correlation between deciduous and permanent dentitions. This observation indicates that although the size of individual permanent teeth relative to their deciduous precursors can vary considerably, the developmental process is coordinated so that total tooth size is more rigidly controlled between dentitions. Most correlations between dentitions were higher for buccolingual diameters than for mesiodistal, indicating a tighter coordination between deciduous and permanent tooth size for these dimensions.

Table 5.9 Tooth size correlations between corresponding deciduous and permanent teeth of Australian Aboriginal people[1]

Teeth compared		Maxilla		Mandible	
Permanent	Deciduous	Mesiodistal	Buccolingual	Mesiodistal	Buccolingual
I_1	di_1	0.57	0.56	0.52	0.53
I_2	di_2	0.54	0.31	0.38	0.62
C	dc	0.25	0.41	0.35	0.42
P_1	dm_1	0.36	0.41	0.45	0.47
P_2	dm_2	0.44	0.58	0.42	0.60
I_1+I_2	di_1+di_2	0.54		0.42	
P_1+P_2	dm_1+dm_2	0.47		0.53	
$C+P_1+P_2$	$dc+dm_1+dm_2$	0.49		0.57	
I_1 to P_2	di_1 to dm_2	0.65		0.68	

1   Pooled for boys and girls from Brown *et al.,* (1980b)

Table 5.10 summarises within-dentition associations for tooth size in Aboriginal children. Maxillary and mandibular teeth showed high coordination for size in both the deciduous and permanent dentitions, the level of correlation being considerably higher than for the between-dentition associations reported above. The correlations were even stronger when comparing combined mesiodistal diameters. Coordination for buccolingual tooth size tended to be greater than for mesiodistal.

The tooth size correlations indicate an important aspect of dental development concerned with the establishment of occlusal relationships, namely the existence of coordinating mechanisms that serve to maintain optimal tooth size relationships between and within dentitions. Although there is only moderate coordination between the diameters of single deciduous teeth and their permanent successors, the coordination for total mesiodistal size is much higher. The correlations between maxillary and mandibular teeth in the same dentition were high, particularly for combined diameters, indicating that developmental coordination is stronger for teeth within the same dentition than for corresponding deciduous and permanent teeth.

Table 5.10 Tooth size correlations between corresponding maxillary and mandibular teeth and tooth groups in Australian Aboriginal people[1]

	Deciduous			Permanent	
	Mesiodistal	Buccolingual		Mesiodistal	Buccolingual
di_1	0.77	0.89	I_1	0.67	0.72
di_2	0.71	0.61	I_2	0.58	0.58
dc	0.64	0.77	C	0.72	0.75
dm_1	0.77	0.74	P_1	0.76	0.70
dm_2	0.73	0.84	P_2	0.66	0.78
			M_1	0.66	0.79
			M_2	0.73	0.78
di_1+di_2	0.86		I_1+I_2	0.75	
dm_1+dm_2	0.82		P_1+P_2	0.77	
$c+dm_1+dm_2$	0.86		$C+P_1+P_2$	0.79	
di_1 to dm_2	0.83		I_1 to P_2	0.85	

1   Pooled data for boys and girls from Brown *et al.,* (1980b)

Comparative data for tooth size correlations in other populations, for example North American white children (Moorrees and Reed, 1964), indicate that the coordination for tooth size is particularly strong in Australian Aboriginal people both for between-dentition and within-dentition comparisons. It is likely that this coordination is a significant developmental mechanism in the establishment of optimal occlusal relationships in Aboriginal people.

Dental crown features

Many dental crown features, sometimes referred to as non-metric dental traits, have been described in human populations. These features include extra cusps on specific teeth, altered ridge forms and different groove patterns. Some of the commonly-described characters include Carabelli traits and metaconules (or cusp 5) on maxillary molars, cusp 6 and cusp 7 on mandibular molars, cusp number on molars and mandibular second premolars, groove pattern of molars, protostylids on mandibular molars, and shovel-shaped incisors. Studies of dental morphology in the Yuendumu Aboriginal people showed that their dentitions were characterised by a specific pattern of dental features that tended to distinguish them from other ethnic groups. Metaconules and Carabelli trait were very common on maxillary molars, whereas cusp 7 and protostylids were rare on mandibular molars. It appears that this pattern of expression of dental features represents a characteristic Australian dental complex, distinct from other dental patterns that have been reported previously, such as the Mongoloid or European dental complexes (Hanihara, 1967; Mayhall *et al.*, 1982; Townsend *et al.*, 1990). Figure 5.6 provides examples of some of the dental features observed in the dentitions of Aboriginal people from Yuendumu.

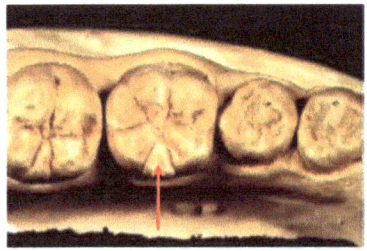 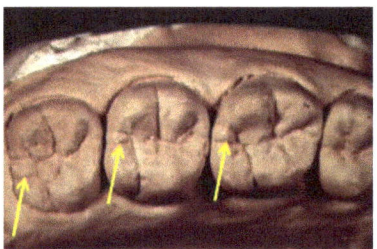
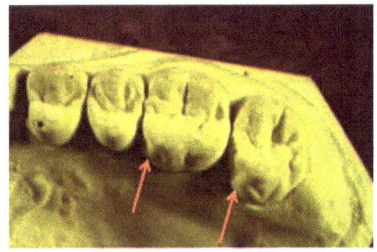 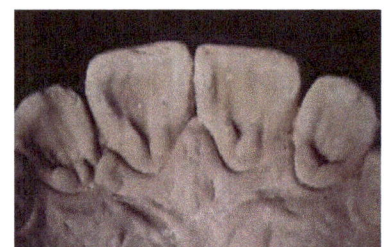

Figure 5.6
Dental features including Cusp 6, Cusp 5, Carabelli trait and shovel-shaped incisors

Tooth exfoliation and emergence

The timing and sequence of tooth formation, progressive calcification and emergence are developmental events that influence dental arch morphology and occlusal relationships. Establishment of occlusal contact occurs towards the end of a complex growth process that commences with the differentiation of tooth germs and progresses through their calcification, migration within the jaw, alveolar penetration gingival emergence and axial alignment. Normal eruption times may be disturbed by local oral conditions. For example, although premature extraction of a deciduous molar tends to accelerate eruption of the permanent premolar, this eruption can be delayed if the loss occurs at certain stages of permanent root formation (Moorrees *et al.*, 1962) or if alveolar bone repair following the extraction hinders the subsequent emergence of the successor (Ando *et al.*, 1965).

Permanent tooth emergence is accompanied by substantial alveolar development and compensatory tooth migrations, which are correlated with the patterns of jaw growth (Björk and Skieller, 1972). Because tooth emergence is an important component of overall craniofacial development, it has been studied in great detail both at the histological level and by clinical comparisons between different populations (Demirjian, 1978).

Developmental timing in the dentition is probably affected more by genetic determinants than by environmental influences (Garn *et al.*, 1965; Hughes *et al.*, 2007). The patterns of tooth emergence vary between different ethnic groups and also between children of the same population, particularly with respect to timing, which is more variable than sequence. Both systemic influences and local oral conditions may affect the process of tooth emergence, causing either acceleration or retardation but the mechanisms involved are not entirely understood. Some agencies affecting tooth emergence may influence the whole dentition while the effect of others, such as conditions predisposing to reduced availability of space, could be limited to individual teeth or groups of teeth.

Socioeconomic environment and nutritional status modify general somatic growth to a considerable extent but the effects of these variables on tooth emergence are probably not great. Evidence concerning the relationships between tooth emergence, socioeconomic class and nutrition is conflicting and no firm conclusions are currently possible. Some authors have reported earlier tooth emergence in children from high socioeconomic classes and in children from urban populations compared with rural but others have refuted these findings (Demirjian, 1978). One of the most detailed clinical studies of tooth emergence was conducted in Chinese children of three socioeconomic groups by Lee *et al.*, (1965), who showed that in the high socioeconomic groups there was a tendency for the anterior teeth to emerge earlier and the posterior teeth later. This observation led to a proposal that emergence of anterior teeth might reflect general physical status, while the later emerging teeth might be influenced, in addition, by oral environment, function and state of preservation of the deciduous precursors.

Several authors have reported positive associations between dental development and general body growth and skeletal maturation but in all instances the correlations were low, indicating that development in the dentition is relatively independent of conditions affecting somatic growth (Tanner, 1962; Garn *et al.*, 1965; Malcolm, 1969; Jenner, 1972). There is some evidence that dental development is more closely associated with morphological growth than with skeletal maturation, particularly during adolescence (Anderson *et al.*, 1975). Earlier tooth emergence was noted in tall and heavy children by Maj *et al.*, (1964), a trend similar to that reported by Garn *et al.*, (1965) who found a low correlation between dental development and caloric balance. In addition, Malcolm and Bue (1970) observed a trend for teeth to emerge later in New Guinea children characterised by slower growth. More recently, Bastos *et al.*, (2007) showed that shorter Brazilian children had fewer emerged teeth.

The premature tooth loss of deciduous precursors has complicated many previous studies of permanent tooth emergence. Unless this is taken into account, comparative studies of tooth emergence may be misleading and difficult to interpret. In the Warlpiri children, premature loss of deciduous teeth because of disease was rare and the patterns of tooth emergence provide useful information on occlusal development. The description that follows is summarised from more detailed accounts published earlier (Barrett, 1957; Barrett *et al.*, 1964; Barrett and Brown, 1966; Brown, 1978; Brown *et al.*, 1979).

Table 5.11 shows the average ages at which the deciduous teeth are exfoliated and the permanent successors emerge in the Aboriginal children. These values were determined from longitudinal observations of dental casts, with the age of a dental event taken as the mid-point of the interval during which the event occurred. This procedure was necessitated by the time interval of one year between successive examinations of the children but, ideally, more frequent observations are necessary for accurate studies of dental development.

Emergence of the permanent teeth followed a pattern similar to that found in other populations, namely a fairly distinct separation of the process into two phases. Phase 1 extends from emergence of the first permanent molar until emergence of the last lateral incisor at which age 12 permanent teeth have emerged. Phase 1 extends from about 6.4 to 8.5 years in the boys and from about 5.1 to 8.1 years in girls. Phase 2 of dental development begins with emergence of the first canine or premolar and continues until completion of the permanent dentition with emergence of the last third molar. This phase extends from about 10.0 to 16.5 years in the boys and from 9.1 to 16.1 years in the girls.

Table 5.11 Average ages of exfoliation and emergence in Australian Aboriginal people: time interval calculated as the age of emergence of a permanent tooth less the age of exfoliation of the deciduous precursor[1]

Teeth Compared		Males			Females		
Deciduous	Permanent	Exfoliation	Emergence	Interval	Exfoliation	Emergence	Interval
			Maxilla				
di_1	I_1	6.9	7.0	0.1	7.2	7.3	0.1
di_2	I_2	8.3	8.5	0.2	8.0	8.1	0.1
dc	C	10.5	10.5	0.0	10.0	10.1	0.1
dm_1	P_1	10.3	10.3	0.0	9.8	9.8	0.0
dm_2	P_2	11.4	11.4	0.0	11.0	11.0	0.0
	M_1		6.4			5.7	
	M_2		11.5			11.0	
	M_3		16.8			16.1	
			Mandible				
di_1	I_1	6.6	6.6	0.0	6.4	6.4	0.0
di_2	I_2	7.2	7.2	0.0	7.2	7.3	0.1
dc	C	9.9	10.0	0.1	9.0	9.1	0.1
dm_1	P_1	10.4	10.5	0.1	9.8	9.9	0.1
dm_2	P_2	11.5	11.5	0.0	11.0	11.0	0.0
	M_1		6.4			5.1	
	M_2		11.2			10.8	
	M_3		16.5			16.1	

1   Data from Brown et al., (1979)

Table 5.11 also shows the time intervals between exfoliation of a deciduous tooth and emergence of the permanent successor. It is interesting that the two events were almost coincidental and that the largest interval was only about 2 months. Although these observations must be interpreted in the light of the limited number of observations available, there is a clear indication that in the Warlpiri children, deciduous teeth are not lost prematurely but are usually retained in place until the permanent successor emerges. Thus, the exfoliation and emergence processes are smoothly integrated events ensuring optimal space within the dental arches for the emergence of permanent teeth.

Compared with Australian children of European ancestry, the Warlpiri children show a tendency for accelerated emergence of teeth during Phase 2 of development. For example, the third molars had emerged, on average, by age 16.1 years in the girls and between 16.5 and 16.8 years in the boys, some years earlier than in many other populations.

Demirjian (1978) summarised studies of tooth emergence and pointed out that the relative timing of emergence in the anterior and posterior segments varies between populations being subject to genetic determination. In an earlier study of the Aboriginal children (Brown, 1978) this aspect of dental development was examined by scoring the ages at which specified numbers of permanent teeth were present.

Table 5.12 compares the ages at which specified numbers of permanent teeth emerged in Australian Aboriginal children and European Western Australian children. The most striking difference between the two populations is evident in the time interval between completion of Phase 1 and commencement of Phase 2. In each population there was a plateau in the emergence process from the time tooth 12 had emerged to the time tooth 13 emerged. In the Aboriginal children, the plateau extended for 1.4 years in boys and 1.0 year in girls but the interval was greater in the children of European ancestry, being 2.0 years in boys and 1.8 years in girls. Aboriginal children were more advanced in dental development than those of European ancestry throughout Phase 2 and all teeth except third molars were present at 11.5 years in Aboriginal boys and 11.1 years in Aboriginal girls. In the European children, however, this stage was not reached until 12.4 years in boys and 11.5 years in girls.

Populations vary considerably in the duration of the quiescent period between Phases 1 and 2 of dental development and in the age at which the plateau stage begins (Hellman, 1943; Lee *et al.*, 1965). Comparative data from several populations showing the relationship between Table 5.13 shows Phase 1 and 2 of dental emergence. The Aboriginal people, compared with many other populations, pass through the quiescent period in a shorter time, indicating that the commencement of the Phase 2 of dental development is accelerated in these children.

It is likely that genetic factors are prominent in determining ethnic differences in the timing of tooth emergence, although local conditions may also play a role. The influences of the general growth pattern, socioeconomic status and nutrition are not entirely clear but these are likely to be low. In the Aboriginal children, dental development appears to be a developmental process that commences rather late with the emergence of primary incisors at about age one year. However, the process accelerates particularly with the emergence of the permanent canine, premolars, second and third molars and is complete with emergence of the third molars at about 16 years. Several factors probably account for these differences.

Table 5.12 Ages of emergence for specified numbers of permanent teeth determined by ranking the mean emergence times of left and right teeth[1]

Number of teeth	Australian Aboriginals		European Australians	
	Boys (yrs)	Girls (yrs)	Boys (yrs)	Girls (yrs)
Phase 1				
1	6.3	5.1	6.3	6.0
4	6.5	6.2	6.4	6.2
8	7.0	7.2	7.6	7.2
12	8.5	8.1	8.3	8.0
Phase 2				
13	9.9	9.1	10.3	9.8
16	10.2	9.8	10.8	10.0
20	10.6	10.0	11.4	10.8
24	11.4	11.0	11.8	11.1
28	11.5	11.1	12.4	11.5
32	16.9	16.2	-	-

1 Data summarised from Brown (1978). Values for European Australians from Halikis (1962).

Table 5.13 Intervals in years between the first and second phases of permanent tooth emergence calculated as the difference between ages at which the last lateral incisor emerges and the first canine or premolar emerges

Group	Boys	Girls	Source
Australian Aboriginal Warlpiri	1.42	0.99	Brown (1978)
European Australians	2.02	1.81	Halikis (1962)
U.S.A. Blacks	2.39	2.04	Garn et al., (1973)
U.S.A. Whites	2.13	1.81	Garn et al., (1973)
England	2.23	1.59	Lee et al., (1965)
New Zealand	2.46	1.88	Lee et al., (1965)
Hawaiian Chinese	0.93	0.91	Lee et al., (1965)
Hong Kong (high socioeconomic)	1.66	1.51	Lee et al., (1965)
Hong Kong (low socioeconomic)	1.03	1.10	Lee et al., (1965)
New Guinea (Kaiapit)	2.60	1.60	Malcolm and Bue (1970)
New Guinea (Lae)	1.90	1.60	Malcolm and Bue (1970)
Uganda	1.70	1.20	Krumholt et al., (1971)

Space availability is no doubt an important determinant of tooth emergence and axial alignment into adequate occlusal relationships. In the Warlpiri children, space availability is optimised by several mechanisms: retention of the deciduous precursors until natural exfoliation; a relative advantage in leeway space, that is, the size difference between deciduous canines and molars and the permanent successors, and a pattern of facial and alveolar growth that is highly coordinated with the processes of tooth migration and emergence.

References

Anderson DL, Thompson GW, Popovich F (1975). Interrelationships of dental maturity, skeletal maturity, height and weight from age 4 to 14 years. *Growth* 39:453–462.

Ando S, Aizawa K, NakashimaT, Shinbo K, SankaY, Kiyokawa K, Oshima S (1965). Studies on the consecutive survey of succedaneous and permanent dentition in the Japanese children. Part I. Eruptive processes of permanent teeth. *J Nihon Univ Sch Dent* 7:141–181.

Bailit HL (1975). Dental variations among populations. *Dent Clin North Am* 19:125–139.

Barrett MJ (1956). Mastication – A Dynamic Process. The University of Adelaide, *Documentary Film*.

Barrett MJ (1957). Dental observations on Australian Aborigines: tooth eruption sequence. *Aust Dent J* 2:217–227.

Barrett MJ, Brown T (1966). Eruption of deciduous teeth in Australian Aborigines. *Aust Dent J* 11:43–50.

Barrett MJ, Williamson JJ (1972). Oral health of Australian Aborigines: survey methods and prevalence of dental caries. *Aust Dent J* 17:266–268.

Barrett MJ, Brown T, Cellier KM. (1964). Tooth eruption sequence in a tribe of Central Australian Aborigines. *Amer J Phys Anthropol* 22:79–89.

Bastos JL, Peres MA, Peres KG, Barros AJD (2007). Infant growth, development and tooth emergence patterns: a longitudinal study from birth to 6 years of age. *Arch Oral Biol* 52:598–606.

Begg PR (1954). Stone age man's dentition. *Amer J Orthodontics* 40:298–312, 373–383, 462–475.

Begg PR, Kesling PC (1977). *Begg Orthodontic Theory and Practice*. 3rd Edition. Philadelphia: Saunders.

Beyron, H. (1964). Occlusal relations and mastication in Australian Aborigines. *Acta Odontol Scand* 22:597–678.

Björk A, Helm S (1969). Need for orthodontic treatment as reflected in the prevalence of malocclusion in various ethnic groups. *Acta Soc Med Scand (Suppl)* 1:209–214.

Björk A, Skieller V (1972). Facial development and tooth eruption. *Amer J Orthodontics* 62:339–383.

Brace CL (1977). Occlusion to the anthropological eye. In: *The Biology of Occlusal Development*. MacNamara JA Jr, editor. Craniofacial Growth Series Monograph 7. Ann Arbor: University of Michigan, pp. 179–209.

Brace CL (1980). Australian tooth size clines and the death of a stereotype. *Current Anthrop* 21:141–153.

Brook AH (2009). Multilevel complex interactions between genetic, epigenetic and environmental factors in the aetiology of anomalies of dental development. *Arch Oral Biol* 54S:S3–S17.

Brown T (1974). Dental decay in Aborigines. In: *Better Health for Aborigines*. Hetzel BS, Dobbin M, Eggleston E, editors. St.Lucia: University of Queensland Press, pp. 97–101.

Brown T (1978). Tooth emergence in Australian Aboriginals. *Ann Hum Biol* 5:41–54.

Brown T, Margetts B, Townsend GC (1980a). Comparison of mesiodistal crown diameters of the deciduous and permanent teeth in Australian Aboriginals. *Aust Dent J* 25:28–33.

Brown T, Margetts B, Townsend GC (1980b). Correlations between crown diameters of the deciduous and permanent teeth of Australian Aboriginals. *Aust Dent J* 25:219–23.

Brown T, Jenner JD, Barrett MJ, Lees GH (1979). *Exfoliation of deciduous teeth and gingival emergence of permanent teeth in Australian Aborigines.* Occasional Papers in Human Biology. Canberra: Australian Institute of Aboriginal Studies, 1:47–70.

Butler PM (1939). Studies of the mammalian dentition. Differentiation of the post-canine dentition. *Proc Zool Soc Lond* 109:1–36.

Butler PM (1963). Tooth morphology and primate evolution. In: *Dental Anthropology.* Brothwell DR, editor. Oxford: Pergamon Press, pp. 1–13

Campbell TD, Barrett MJ (1954). *So They Did Eat.* Documentary Film, The University of Adelaide.

Clinch LM (1963). A longitudinal study of the mesiodistal crown diameters of the deciduous teeth and their permanent successors. *Trans Eur Orthod Soc* 39:202–215.

Coruccini RS (1984). An epidemiologic transition in dental occlusion in world populations. *Amer J Orthodontics* 86:419–426.

Coruccini RS, Townsend GC, Brown T (1990). Occlusal variation in Australian aborigines. *Am J Phys Anthropol* 82:257–265.

Dahlberg AA (1945). The changing dentition of man. *J Amer Dent Assoc* 32:676–690.

Demirjian A (1978). Dentition. In: *Human Growth. Vol. 2. Postnatal Growth.* Falkner F, Tanner JM, editors. New York: Plenum Press, pp. 413–444.

Garn SM, Lewis, AB, Kerewsky RS (1965). Genetic, nutritional and maturational correlates of dental development. *J Dent Res* 44:228–242.

Garn SM, Sandusky ST, Nagy JM, Trowbridge FL (1973). Negro-Caucasoid differences in permanent tooth emergence at a constant income level. *Arch Oral Biol* 18:609–615.

Halikis SE (1962). The variation in eruption of permanent teeth and loss of deciduous teeth in Western Australian children, IV, Sequence of permanent tooth eruption and deciduous tooth loss. *Aust Dent J* 7:400–408.

Hanihara K (1967). Racial characteristics in the dentition. *J Dent Res (Suppl)* 46:923–926

Hanihara K (1976). *Statistical and comparative studies of the Australian Aboriginal dentition.* Bulletin No 11, Tokyo: The University of Tokyo.

Harris JE (1975). Genetic factors in the growth of the head. *Dent Clin North Am* 19:151–160.

Hellman M (1943). The phase of development concerned with erupting the permanent teeth. *Am J Orthod Oral Surg* 29:507–526.

Helm S (1979). Etiology and treatment need of malocclusion. *J Can Dent Ass* 45:673–676.

Hildebrand GY (1931). Studies in the masticatory movements of the human lower jaw. *Scand Arch Physiol Suppl* 61.

Hughes TE, Bockmann MR, Seow K, Gotjamanos T, Gully N, Richards LC, Townsend GC (2007). Strong genetic control of emergence of human primary incisors. *J Dent Res* 86:1160–1165.

Jenner JD (1972). *Dental Development in Australian Aborigines. A Study of Relations with Growth and Skeletal Maturity around Adolescence.* MDS Thesis: The University of Adelaide.

Krumholt L, Roed-Petersen B, Pindborg JJ (1971). Eruption times of the permanent teeth in

622 Ugandan children. *Arch Oral Biol* 16:1281–1288.

Lee MMC, Chan ST, Low WD, Chang KSF (1965). Eruption of the permanent dentition of Southern Chinese children in Hong Kong. *Arch Oral Biol* 10:849–861.

Maj G, Bassini S, Menini G, Zannini O (1964). Studies on the eruption of permanent teeth in children with normal occlusion and malocclusion. *Trans Eur Orthod Soc* 40:107–130.

Malcolm LA (1969). Growth and development of the Kaiapit children of the Markham Valley, New Guinea. *Am J Phys Anthropol* 31:39–51.

Malcolm LA, Bue B (1970) Eruption times of permanent teeth and the determination of age in New Guinean children. *Trop Geog Med* 22:307–312.

Margetts B, Brown T (1978). Crown diameters of the deciduous teeth in Australian Aboriginals. *Am J Phys Anthropol* 48:493–502.

Mayhall JT, Saunders SR, Belier PL (1982). The dental morphology of North American Whites: a reappraisal. In: *Teeth: form, function and evolution*. Kurten B, editor. New York: Columbia University Press, pp.245–258.

Moorrees CFA (1959). *The Dentition of the Growing Child. A Longitudinal Study of Dental Development Between 3 and 18 Years of Age*. Cambridge: Harvard University Press.

Moorrees CFA, Chadha JM (1962). Crown diameters of corresponding tooth groups in the deciduous and permanent dentitions. *J Dent Res* 41:466–470.

Moorrees CFA, Reed RB (1964). Correlations among crown diameters of human teeth. *Arch Oral Biol* 9:685–697.

Moorrees CFA, Fanning EA, Grøn AM, Lebret L (1962). The timing of orthodontic treatment in relation to tooth formation. *Trans Eur Orthod Soc* 38:87–101.

Nance HN (1947). The limitations of orthodontic treatment. I. Mixed dentition diagnosis and treatment. *Am J Orthod Oral Surg* 33:177–223.

Osborn JW (1978). Morphogenetic gradients: fields versus clones. In: *Development, Function and Evolution of Teeth*. Butler PM, Joysey KA, editors. London: Academic Press, pp. 171–201.

Saunders SR, Mayhall JT (1982). Developmental patterns of human dental morphological traits. *Arch Oral Biol* 27:45–49.

Seipel CM (1946). Variation of Tooth Position. *Svensk Tand Tidsk* 39:Suppl.

Smith P, Brown T, Wood WB (1981). Tooth size and morphology in a recent Australian Aboriginal population from Broadbeach South East Queensland. *Am J Phys Anthropol* 55:423–32.

Tanner JM (1962). *Growth at Adolescence*. 2nd Edition. Oxford: Blackwell Scientific Publications.

Thesleff I (2006). The genetic basis of tooth development and dental defects. *Am J Med Genet*, Part A,140:2530–2535.

Thomsen S (1955). *Dental morphology and occlusion in the people of Tristan Da Cunha. Results of the Norwegian Scientific Expedition to Tristan Da Cunha, 1937–1938*. No. 25. Oslo, Det Norske Videnskaps-Akademi.

Townsend GC (1980). Heritability of deciduous teeth in Australian Aboriginals. *Am J Phys Anthropol* 53:297–300.

Townsend GC, Brown T (1978). Inheritance of tooth size in Australian Aboriginals. *Am J Phys Anthropol* 48:305–314.

Townsend GC, Brown T (1979). Tooth size characteristics of Australian Aboriginals. *Occasional*

Papers in Hum Biol 1:17–38.

Townsend G, Yamada H, Smith P (1990). Expression of the entoconulid (sixth cusp) on mandibular molar teeth of an Australian Aboriginal population. *Am J Phys Anthropol* 82:267–274.

Townsend GC, Harris EF, Lesot H, Clauss F, Brook A (2009). Morphogenetic fields within the human dentition: a new, clinically relevant synthesis of an old concept. *Arch Oral Biol* 54S:S34–S44

Tucker AS, Sharpe PT (2004). The cutting-edge of mammalian development: how the embryo makes teeth. *Nat Rev Genet* 5:499–508.

6
Facial Growth Patterns in the Warlpiri

Dental development, including the establishment of occlusal relationships between opposing teeth, occurs as part of the progressive growth of the facial structures occurring from early childhood through the adolescent period to adulthood. During this time, there is extensive growth of the alveolar bone around the teeth, remodelling of the jaws, rotation of the face in relation to the cranial base, and migration of teeth until they come into occlusion (Brown *et al.*, 1990).

Björk and Skieller (1972) described the characteristic patterns of facial growth and tooth eruption in Danish children. In this study, metallic implants inserted into the maxilla and mandible served as stable reference markers on which serial cephalometric roentgenograms were superimposed to trace the extent and direction of growth changes in the jaw and tooth migrations during emergence. In the Danish children, facial development was marked by a general tendency for the face to rotate forwards with age in relation to the anterior cranial base. On average, the forward rotation was greater in the mandible than the maxilla and it was strongly associated with growth at the mandibular condyle. Forward rotations of the jaws were accompanied by extensive remodelling processes that were particularly evident along the lower mandibular body, the posterior border of the ramus and the nasal floor. The paths of tooth emergence were determined by a combination of active eruption within the jaws and bodily rotation of the jaws. Thus, the observed patterns of tooth emergence illustrate a form of compensatory adaptation to the rotations of the jaws during growth.

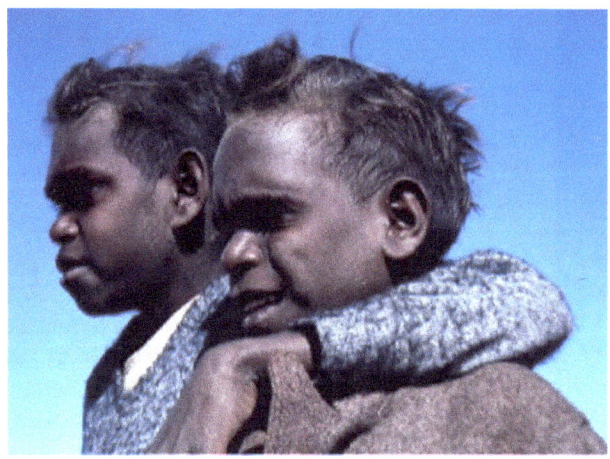

Figure 6.1
Max Jungarrayi and friend displaying mid-facial prognathism

Mid-facial prognathism

A striking morphological feature of the face in Australian Aboriginal people is the relative protrusion of the mid-facial region compared with many other groups (Figure 6.1). The prognathism is most marked in the alveolar regions of each jaw but, in contrast, the basal areas as indicated by the anterior nasal spine in the maxilla and the chin point in the mandible are not unduly prominent in relation to the anterior cranial base. From our studies of the dentition of the Warlpiri we have noted that alveolar prognathism results from the relatively large tooth diameters and a marked migration of the entire dental arches in an anterior and occlusal direction during growth. This progressive relocation of the dentition during its emergence is an important feature of occlusal development in this group.

The longitudinal growth records of an Aboriginal boy observed between the ages of 6.9 and 16.3 years illustrate these aspects of dental development. This analysis integrates data from cephalometric roentgenograms with measurements of dental casts and observations of tooth emergence. The boy is representative of his group and although his growth pattern indicates interesting principles of occlusal development, additional analyses would allow for a fuller appreciation of variations in facial growth within this population.

Figure 6.2 illustrates the general pattern of growth changes in the craniofacial structures between 6.9 and 16.3 years. Serial radiographs were superimposed according to stable reference structures in the cranial base, which have been described in implant studies (Björk, 1969, 1980; Björk and Skieller, 1972, 1974, 1976). The initial stage of the procedure consists of placing a sheet of cellophane printed with cross lines on the first radiograph of the series so that the horizontal line passes through point nasion and the centre of sella turcica where it is intersected by the vertical reference line. Subsequent films in the series are superimposed according to anatomical reference structures and the cross lines are transferred onto these from the first film. Structures used for superimposition include the trabecular regions of the cribriform plate, the anterior wall of the sella turcica and, from the end of the juvenile period, the anterior contour of the middle cranial fossa.

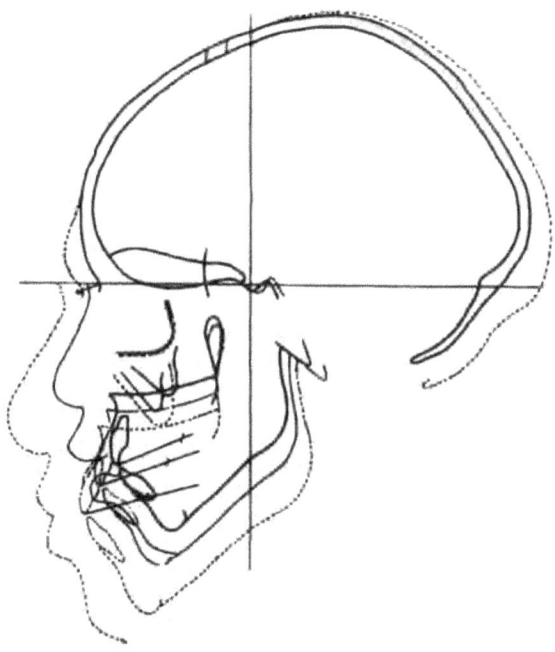

Figure 6.2
General craniofacial growth pattern - boy aged 6.9 to 16.3 years

These structures are known to be reasonably stable in morphology during the growth period likely to be of most interest to the orthodontist. In the Aboriginal boy examined, growth changes in the cranial vault included a downward and forward displacement of the nasion point from its initial position, a gradual expansion of the sella turcica with resorption along the posterior wall and floor, pronounced expansion of the frontal bone with separation of outer and inner tables as the frontal sinus developed and the progressive expansion and lowering of the occipital region of the vault.

With continuing facial growth, the maxilla and mandible were displaced downwards away from the cranial base, but the inclinations of the nasal floor, the lower border of the mandible and the mandibular ramus to the original nasion-sella line did not change greatly during this period. Progressive relocation of the mandibular condyles downwards and backwards, away from the cranial base, occurred because of growth processes in the condyles and the lateral cranial base. The development of mid-facial prognathism is also obvious in cephalometric tracings.

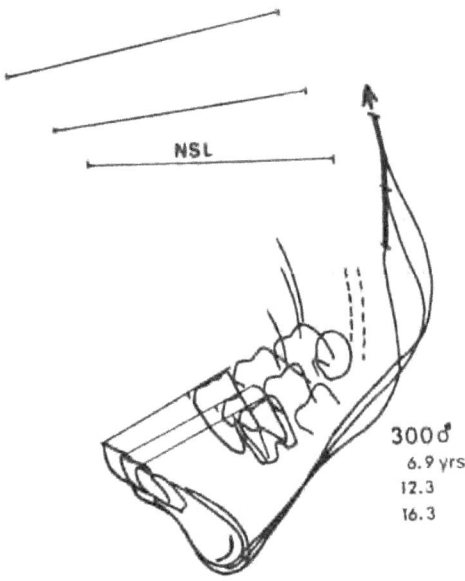

Figure 6.3
Mandibular remodelling and tooth emergence shown by superimposition of growth records on stable reference structures

Figure 6.3 shows mandibular growth and remodelling where tracings of successive radiographs have been superimposed according to the structural method (Björk 1969; Björk *et al.*, 1984). Natural reference structures used for mandibular superimposition included the anterior border of the chin, trabecular structures related to the mandibular canal, inner cortical structures at the lower symphyseal border and the lower contour of a tooth germ prior to root formation. These anatomical references have been shown to be relatively stable during growth by the implant studies referred to above.

Superimposition by this method demonstrates the direction of condylar growth and the extent and sites of remodelling processes. Between the ages of 6.9 and 16.3 years there was a gradual forward rotation of the entire mandible away from the cranial base as indicated by the change in inclination of the nasion-sella reference from first to last records. The forward rotation of the mandible amounted to 11.5 degrees, somewhat greater than the average of 6.0 degrees reported for Danish children by Björk and Skieller (1972). Remodelling of the mandible consisted of marked deposition along the posterior border of the ramus, resorption along the anterior border of the ramus, deposition below the symphysis and anterior part of the lower mandibular border, and resorption along the posterior segment of the lower border. Because of this remodelling, the orientation of the mandible within the face remained fairly stable as evidenced by minimal change in the inclinations between the anterior cranial base, mandibular border and ramus.

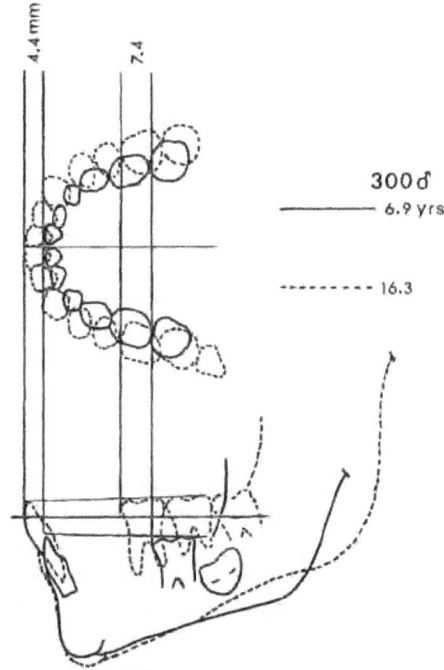

Figure 6.4
Mandibular growth and dental arch development

Figure 6.4 shows tooth movements and alveolar development in the Aboriginal boy in which dental arch tracings have been integrated with the mandibular growth analyses. As the primary teeth were being replaced, there was a marked upward and forward displacement of the entire dental arch. However, the displacement was not uniform in all regions of the dental arch. Whereas the first permanent molars migrated 7.4mm forwards during the growth period, the anterior movement of incisors was only 4.4mm.

Thus, the depth of the dental arch measured anterior to the first molars decreased by about 3mm. This decrease was probably associated partly with the closure of spaces as the deciduous molars were replaced by the smaller premolars and partly with an increase in bimolar breadth of about 4mm during the observation period.

Growth rotation, remodelling and alveolar development in the maxilla are shown in Figure 6.5 with superimposition along the anterior border of the zygomatic process which may be used as a natural reference structure in the absence of implants provided it can be visualised clearly on serial films. Björk and Skieller (1976) have described the method for maxillary superimposition by the structural technique.

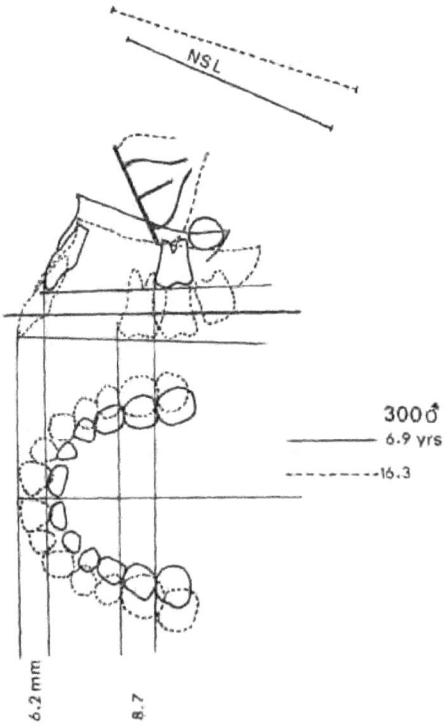

Figure 6.5
Maxillary growth and dental arch development

Forward rotation of the maxilla, indicated by the changing inclination of the nasion-sella reference line, amounted to 5.5 degrees, about half the forward rotation of the mandible but somewhat greater than the average anterior rotation of 2.5 degrees reported for Danish children (Björk and Skieller, 1972). The anterior rotation of the maxilla was accompanied by lowering of the nasal floor by remodelling and by lengthening of the maxilla in a posterior direction. Alveolar development was also pronounced in the maxilla with the entire dental arch migrating downwards and forwards away from the stable reference structures. The anterior displacement of the first molars was 8.7mm in the maxilla, slightly more than the forward migration of the mandibular first molars. The incisors moved forwards 6.2mm so that the depth of the maxillary arch anterior to the first molars decreased with age. In relation to the stable reference structures, the occlusal line rotated anteriorly with growth by about 3 degrees in both the maxilla and mandible. This is the expected pattern with forward growth rotations of the jaws where occlusal movement of the molars exceeds that of the incisors with a consequent change in occlusal line inclination (Björk and Skieller, 1972).

Table 6.1 Dimensional changes in the dental arches of an Australian Aboriginal boy[1]

Age in years	Arch breadth		Difference in arch breadth	Arch length		Difference in arch length
	Maxilla	Mandible		Maxilla	Mandible	
5.5	–	32.2		29.1	26.4	2.7
6.9	35.3	33.0	2.3	28.3	27.1	1.2
8.5	36.1	33.3	2.8	29.8	27.5	2.3
10.3	37.2	34.5	2.7	29.8	27.1	2.7
11.3	38.0	34.9	3.1	28.7	26.0	2.7
12.3	38.4	36.1	2.3	27.5	26.0	1.5
13.3	38.8	36.1	2.7	27.9	24.4	3.5
14.3	39.5	36.4	3.1	27.1	24.4	2.7
15.3	39.9	36.8	3.1	26.7	24.0	2.7
16.3	40.3	37.2	3.1	26.0	23.3	2.7
Dimensional change						
6.9-16.3 years	5.0	4.2		-2.3	-3.8	

1 Arch breadth and arch length defined in text (in mm).

Dimensional changes in the dental arches during the observation period of almost 10 years are summarised in Table 6.1 and illustrated in Figures 6.6 and 6.7. For this analysis, a tangent to the most anterior points on the right and left first permanent molars was constructed on tracings of standardised photographs of the maxillary and mandibular arches. Arch length was measured as the perpendicular distance from the tangent to the labial surface of the most prominent central incisors; arch breadth was recorded as the distance between the most palatal points of the molars projected onto the tangent. These arch dimensions, expressed in actual size, refer only to the arch segment anterior to the first molars.

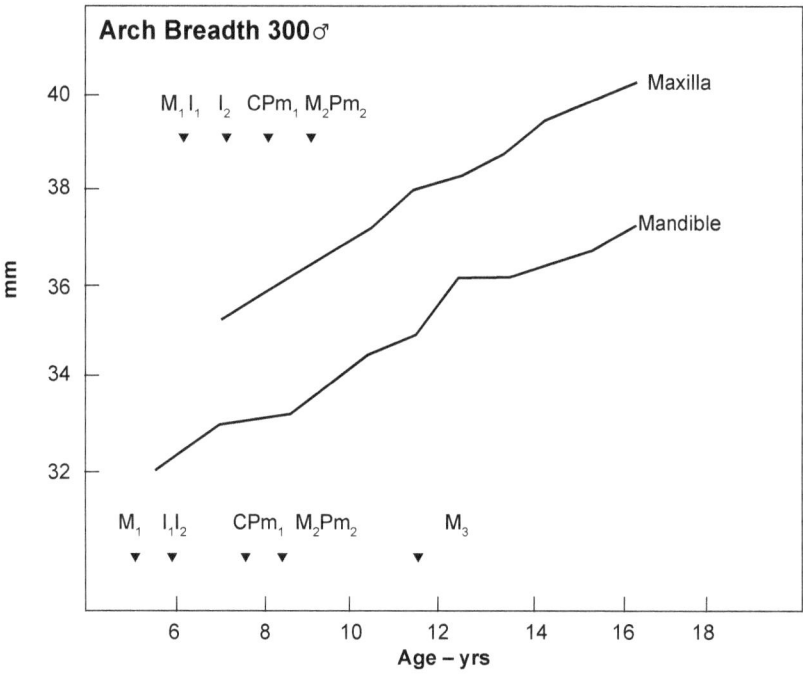

Figure 6.6
Changes in dental arch breadths with times of tooth emergence indicated.

The changes in dental arch dimensions followed the pattern reported in several studies of other populations and summarised by Riedel (1977), namely an increase in arch breadth and a decrease in arch length both in the maxilla and the mandible. Dental arch breadths increased steadily over the examination period by about 5mm in each arch thus keeping the difference between maxillary and mandibular breadths at about 2mm to 3mm.

Lengths of the dental arches showed an initial increase, more marked in the maxilla, during emergence of the permanent incisors, canine and first premolar. Thereafter the lengths decreased with emergence of the second premolar and second molar. The overall decrease amounted to about 2mm in the maxilla and 4mm in the mandible. In the Aboriginal subject, occlusal development was marked by a substantial forward migration of the entire dental arch relative to the supporting basal bone. This was accompanied by substantial alveolar development leading to mid-facial prognathism. During the same period, the dental arches displayed dimensional changes, an increase in breadth and a reduction in length, as the deciduous teeth were replaced by their permanent successors. As a consequence of the marked forward migration of the teeth, the reduction in arch lengths, resorption along the anterior border of the ramus, and the lengthening of the maxilla posteriorly, adequate space was provided for unimpeded emergence and alignment of the posterior permanent teeth.

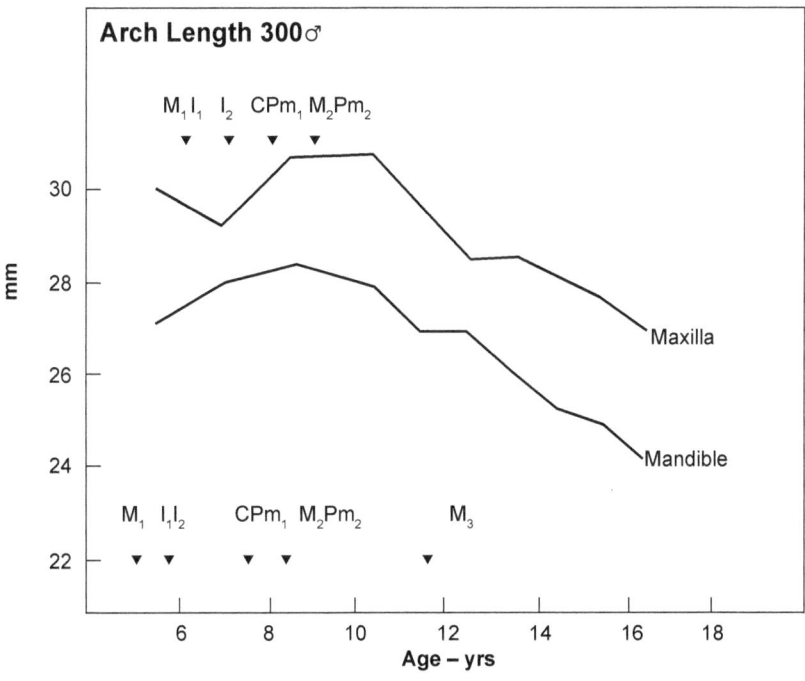

Figure 6.7
Changes in dental arch depths with times of tooth emergence indicated.

Although not all of the third molars had emerged by age 16 years in this subject, there appeared to be adequate space for these teeth in the dental arches.

Agenesis and impaction of third molars are rare in Aboriginal people compared with other populations, where tooth-crowding problems are frequent. For example, Macintosh and Barker (1978) reported an incidence of only 1.5 per cent for mandibular third molar agenesis in Aboriginal people - among the lowest of all populations.

Figures 6.8, 6.9 and 6.10 show occlusal photographs of the Aboriginal boy used to demonstrate dental development and facial growth. The age span represented is from 5.5 years to 16.3 years. Interesting features to note are:

1. Age 5.5 years. Well-formed dental arches with spacing in the anterior region particularly between the deciduous second incisors and canines. The mandibular first molars have already emerged at this stage.

2. Age 6.9 years. In the maxilla, the central incisors have emerged and the deciduous lateral incisors have moved distally to approximate the deciduous canines. The first permanent molars are also in position. All mandibular permanent incisors have emerged with some crowding and axial rotation or the lateral incisors.

3. Ages 10.3 to 13.3 years. During this three-year period, the deciduous canines and molars were replaced by the permanent successors and the permanent second molars emerged. This transitional stage was marked by the provision of adequate space for the emergence of the premolars, particularly in the mandible (Age 11.3). The permanent canines have also emerged into an adequate position and alignment with no crowding.

4. Age 16.3 years. In the final stage, the mandibular left third molar has emerged and the entire dental arch is well-formed with no evidence of any significant crowding. Note that the mandibular incisor crowding, evident at about 6.9 years, is now considerably improved. It would be expected to reduce even further during later development, particularly if interproximal tooth wear reduced the mesiodistal diameters of these teeth.

The analyses of facial growth and occlusal development in the Aboriginal boy demonstrate several important biological processes that are coordinated during the maturation of the masticatory structures. The general pattern of facial growth did not vary greatly from that described in European populations, namely a forward rotation of each jaw away from the cranial base. In this boy, the rotation continued throughout the growth period and was particularly marked during the adolescent growth cycle that was judged from observations of body height to commence at about 10 years and peak at 13 years. Although the forward rotation of the maxilla and mandible was above average by European standards, the inclinations of the occlusal plane, mandibular border, mandibular ramus and nasal floor remained fairly constant throughout growth. This was accomplished by substantial remodelling of the mandible and maxilla, which served to maintain a stable relationship between the jaws and the other cranio-cervical structures. Remodelling, described in more detail by Björk and Skieller (1972) and Björk (1980), appears to be a general growth mechanism to compensate for the jaw rotations.

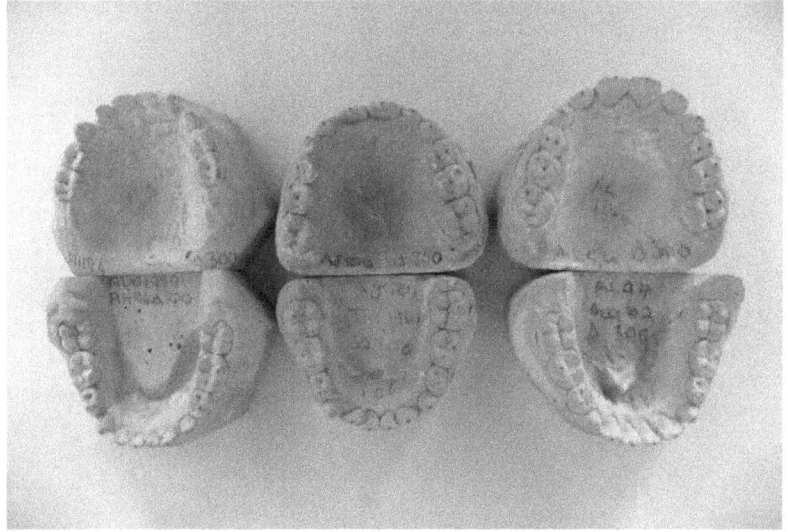

Figure 6.8
Occlusal development in an Aboriginal boy aged 5.5, 6.9 and 8.5 years

Alveolar development was more marked in the Aboriginal boy than in Europeans, leading to the characteristic mid-facial prognathism. The jaw rotations were accompanied by a substantial occlusal and anterior migration of the entire dental arches. At the same time, replacement of the deciduous molars by the smaller permanent premolars provided additional space for unimpeded eruption of the posterior permanent teeth. The establishment of well-formed dental arches with the teeth in good axial alignment was the result of favourable size relationships between the deciduous and permanent teeth and a high degree of coordination between the basic growth processes, compensatory remodelling of the jaws and alveolar development during emergence of the permanent teeth.

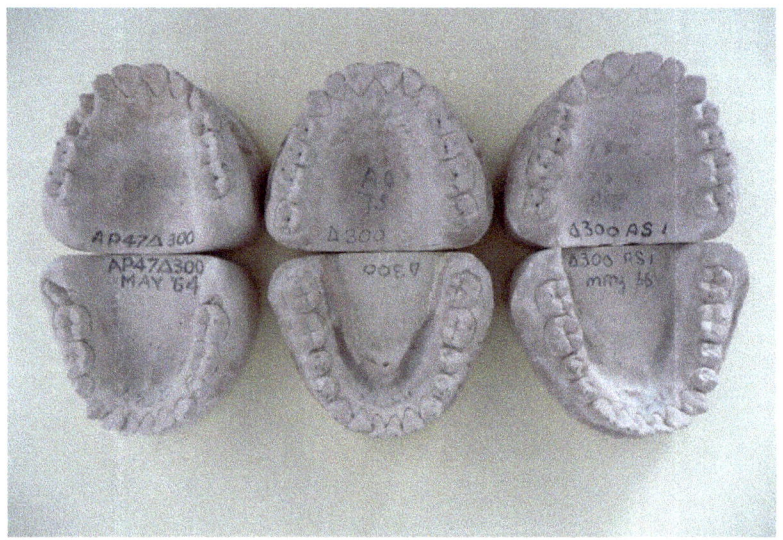

Figure 6.9
Occlusal development in an Aboriginal boy aged 10.3, 11.3 and 13.3 years

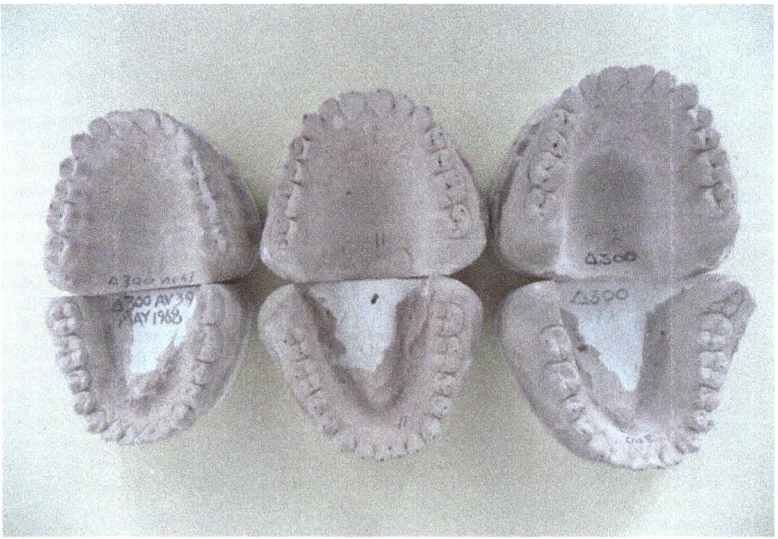

Figure 6.10
Occlusal development in an Aboriginal boy aged 14.3, 15.3 and 16.3 years

Lip and tongue pressures in relation to occlusion

Before leaving the subject of occlusal development, we will briefly discuss the relationships between dental arch form and tongue and lip pressures in Australian Aboriginal people. There is a general belief that the teeth occupy positions of stability between the muscular forces exerted by the tongue from the inside and the lips and cheeks from the outside. This concept arises from the view that the resultant of forces acting on the teeth must be balanced if the teeth remain stable. The views and results reported here are summarised from the work of Proffit *et al.*, (1975) and Proffit (1978), who examined lip and tongue pressures in Warlpiri people from Yuendumu. Proffit's observations allowed interesting comparisons between Aboriginal people, with large well-developed dental arches, and North American Whites with smaller and relatively constricted arches. Proffit measured muscle pressures in 18 subjects by the use of intra-oral pressure transducers coupled with a multichannel strain gauge amplifier with analogue tape output. He assessed pressures exerted on the labial and lingual aspects of the maxillary and mandibular arches during swallowing, speaking and at rest.

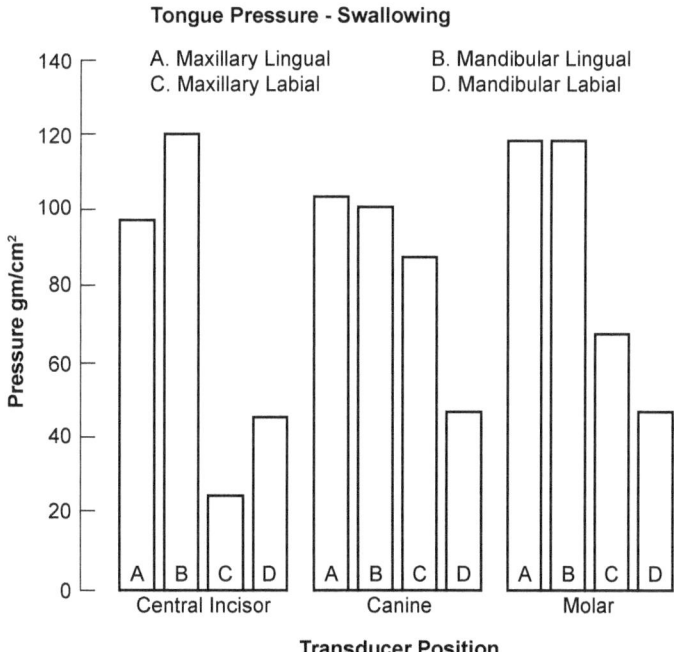

Figure 6.11
Labial and lingual tongue pressures during swallowing in Australian Aboriginal people

Figure 6.11 charts the average labial and lingual pressures during swallowing in Aboriginal peoples. Proffit noted that the maximum tongue pressures during swallowing greatly exceeded those generated by the lip, indicating a distinct lack of equilibrium, a situation also noted in North American subjects. Figure 6.12 shows comparisons of tongue pressures during swallowing between the two groups. It is interesting to note that tongue pressures in the Warlpiri people were considerably smaller than those in the North American Whites. Proffit interpreted these observations to indicate that the simplistic expectation from equilibrium theory that dental arch size related directly to tongue pressure was not sustainable. In fact the opposite appeared to be true, both within each group and for the between group comparisons, so that there was no evidence that arch dimensions were directly related to pressures generated by the tongue during swallowing.

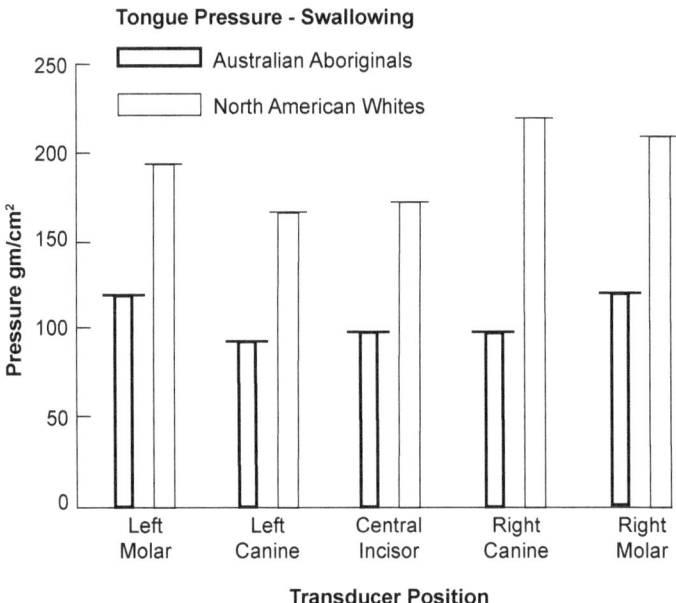

Figure 6.12
Comparison of tongue pressures during swallowing in Australian Aboriginal people and North American whites

These observations refer to comparisons of arch dimensions and soft tissue pressures between two populations that vary considerably, both morphologically and functionally. The comparison should not be taken to infer that arch dimensions are unaffected by soft tissue pressures during a child's development. The association of diminished arch dimensions and microglossia is a well-known clinical observation that establishes a developmental relationship.

Figure 6.13 compares resting muscle pressures in the two groups for the tongue while Figure 6.14 does so for the lip and cheek. Although the two groups did not differ for resting tongue pressures as much as they did for swallowing pressures, the Aboriginal group still displayed smaller pressures in the incisor, canine and molar regions. Thus, there was no evidence for any direct relationship between dental arch size and resting tongue pressure, so far as group comparisons were concerned. In contrast, resting lip and cheek pressures were similar in the two groups, a finding that Proffit interpreted as support for the concept that dental arch circumference might be limited by resting pressures of the lips and cheeks.

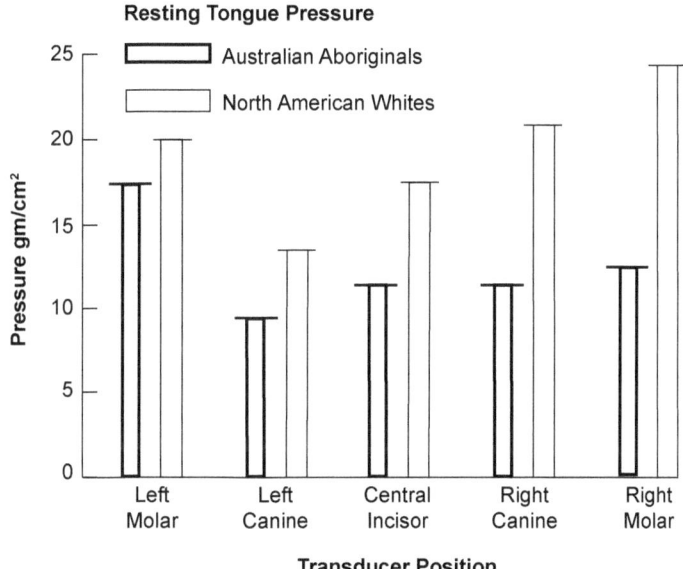

Figure 6.13
Comparison of resting tongue pressures in Australian Aboriginal people and North American whites

In his discussion of equilibrium theory, Proffit drew attention to the relationship between incisor inclination and the relative positions of the upper and lower jaws. The incisors tend to be proclined when the mandible is retrognathic in relation to the maxilla and retroclined with the reverse situation. Brown (1965) noted this relationship in an earlier study of Australian Aboriginal adults. He reported that a combination of high maxillary prognathism and relatively low mandibular prognathism was compensated to some extent by a decrease in upper alveolar development and an increase in the chin angle, both of which would tend to decrease the effect of jaw base discrepancies in incisal relationships. In a similar way, a discrepancy in the sagittal jaw relationship produced by relatively high mandibular prognathism was compensated by a reduction in the chin angle and a reduction in both overbite and overjet of the incisors, making for more harmonious tooth relationships. Björk (1963, 1964) discussed similar modifications of a compensatory nature that occurred during normal development of occlusion in Danish children. He suggested that this form of modification was mediated by lip and tongue musculature and by forces involved in intercuspation.

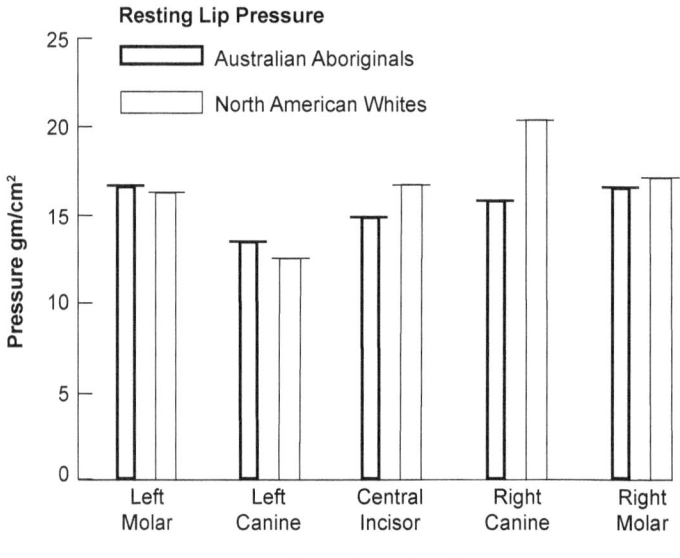

Figure 6.14
Comparison of resting tongue pressures in Australian Aboriginal people and North American whites

It has been known for some time that Australian Aboriginal people have a noticeably shorter neck than Europeans. Solow *et al.*, (1981) explored this characteristic further, producing evidence that the cranio-cervical angulation, that is, the angular relationship between head and cervical vertebrae, also differed in Aboriginal people. Solow and Tallgren (1971a, 1971b, 1976, 1977) demonstrated a strong relationship between cranio-cervical angulation and facial morphology and it is plausible that population differences in this feature may be related to the observed differences in facial build and even arch form. Proffit (1978) noted that, because of their shorter necks, Aboriginal people tend to have a smaller pharyngeal cavity than Europeans, and consequently the tongue is carried in a higher and more forward position. He concluded that the different resting posture of the tongue might well be related to the different dental arch form.

In summary, Proffit's work on equilibrium theory using evidence from Aboriginal people indicates that resting soft tissue pressures are significant in establishing the vertical positioning of teeth, while the lip and tongue pressures during activity are not. Certainly, the topic of muscle pressures and equilibrium is far from complete clarification and it is likely that other factors such as forces generated during tooth intercuspation and metabolic activity of the periodontal structures may be involved.

Tooth wear and continuously changing occlusion

This section further discusses wear of the natural dentition with particular reference to changing occlusal relations and masticatory function. Tooth wear can occur during mastication by vigorous chewing activity and the inclusion of abrasive particles in food. However, tooth wear may also result from other causes, such as the non-masticatory use of teeth as tools or the empty tooth grinding of bruxism. Wear produced by food or other exogenous factors is commonly referred to as abrasion, whereas wear produced by tooth-to-tooth contact, such as tooth grinding, is usually referred to as attrition.

Barrett (1977) described several non-masticatory uses of teeth in Australian Aboriginal people, such as grasping, grinding, biting, piercing, cutting, tearing, shredding and crushing. For example, when living under hunter-gatherer conditions, Aboriginal people would frequently use their teeth as substitutes for tools in stripping bark from a freshly cut small branch that they worked into a spear, digging stick or other wooden object. Also, they often used teeth as a vice or clamp to grip various materials during manufacture or even to sharpen the pointed sticks used in tooth evulsion ceremonies. They often chewed dried animal sinews for softening prior to use as binding materials. Molnar (1972) and Barrett (1977) describe these and other non-masticatory uses of teeth caused wear. However, it is sometimes difficult to distinguish between masticatory and non-masticatory wear on tooth surfaces. Attention is also warranted to tooth wear resulting from grinding and clenching as performed during the empty movements of bruxism. This condition, well known in modern populations, may be associated with pathogenic sequelae, including muscle fatigue and pain, periodontal involvement and temporomandibular joint problems.

Even a cursory examination of the dentitions of earlier humans or many present-day groups who have not adopted western food habits indicates that abrasive wear was a normal dental characteristic that progressed with age during the lifetime of the individual. This is in sharp contrast to the situation found in modern industrialised societies where abrasion of teeth tends to be comparatively light even in later life. In modern humans, it is rare to find total elimination of posterior tooth cusps through physiological tooth wear, although this was a common feature of earlier dentitions.

Coarse foods, often with the inclusion of abrasive substances, formed the usual diet of humans for most of history, probably until the 18th century when the industrial age saw the advent of new food technologies culminating in the softer pre-processed diets which are characteristic of today's urban dweller. Under conditions of continuing physiological tooth wear, occlusal relations were not static but gradually changed throughout life. Masticatory efficiency was by no means impaired by tooth wear and, providing the rate and extent of tooth wear were within the ability of the individual to adapt, the process served to establish and maintain optimal occlusal relationships. It is rather paradoxical that clinical dentistry today bases itself on concepts of occlusion derived from observations of non-worn dentitions with tooth-to-tooth relationships that did not exist until relatively recent times.

Various dental researchers have studied the processes involved in wear and their effects on dental occlusion in many earlier populations. In Australian Aboriginal people, tooth wear was a normal characteristic of dentitions that functioned in a natural manner. Wear was continuous throughout life and it commenced when the first deciduous teeth emerged into occlusal function. Wear occurred on both the occlusal and the proximal tooth surfaces, leading to substantial changes in the size and shape of tooth crowns with age. As a result, dental morphology and occlusal relationships were continually modified and the pattern observed in a subject on one examination represents only a single phase in a complex series of progressive events.

With tooth wear, occlusal relationships tended to pass through three distinct phases, which have been termed by Barrett (1969) as wear-in, wear-out and last-stage. The wear-in phase commenced early and had the effect of eliminating cuspal interferences and other occlusal irregularities that would persist in the modern dentition in the absence of substantial abrasion. As wear continued, cusps were gradually reduced in height and the opposing tooth surfaces became flatter and broader in area leading to greater efficiency in the masticatory cycles. Furthermore, mandibular closure during grinding strokes became freed from the guiding influence of cusps and the intrusive masticatory stroke gradually widened in response to flatter occlusal surfaces. Incisor relations and therefore the biting function were also modified with the gradual acquisition of an edge-to-edge occlusion in the anterior region. Other effects on occlusion, which a later section describes, also took place during the wear-in phase (Figure 6.15).

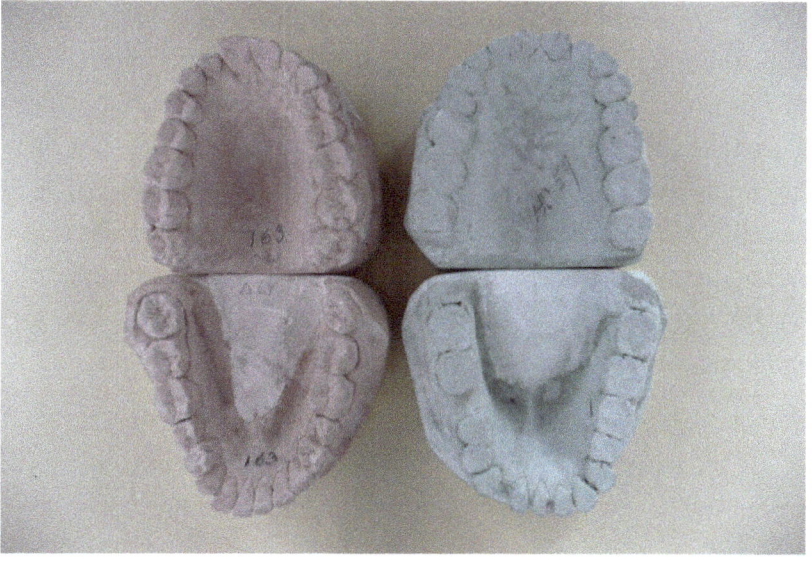

Figure 6.15
Dental casts of Aboriginal adults from Yuendumu, Central Australia (left)
and Kalumburu, Northwest Australia (right),
showing different degrees of tooth wear

With continued vigorous use of the dentition, wear progressed, first with dentine exposure and eventually total elimination of cusps and, in many instances, substantial reduction of crown height down to gum level. With multi-rooted teeth, wear often extended even further, past the root furcation, so that only root fragments remained, which in turn were sometimes tipped laterally to provide new occlusal surfaces. There is no doubt that these changes represent the wear-out phase. Nevertheless, biological compensatory mechanisms operated to enable many individuals to retain their complete dentitions, even though considerably worn, in a state of functional efficiency with little evidence of detrimental pathology.

In many subjects, mostly older individuals, the rate and extent of tooth wear exceeded the ability of the masticatory system to adapt, and in these instances it could no longer be considered physiological but was distinctly pathological. The dentition had entered its last-stage. Because of extensive tooth wear, dental pulps were often exposed and infected with subsequent periapical and alveolar sequelae. Moreover, excessive occlusal loads sometimes led to degeneration of the temporomandibular joint structures and the advent of progressive arthritic changes on the articular surfaces.

Occlusal Wear

Barrett (1958) examined serial dental casts to describe occlusal wear in the deciduous dentition of Aboriginal subjects, noting that the process commenced as the teeth first made functional contact. By the time the first permanent molars emerged at about 6 years of age, the deciduous molars showed extensive wear, often with dentine exposure. Campbell (1925) also noticed deciduous teeth of Aboriginal people living a traditional lifestyle had considerable occlusal wear. It is interesting that although Aboriginal children participating in the growth study were breast-fed until relatively late (about 3-5 years) they were also given solid food that requires vigorous chewing from an early age.

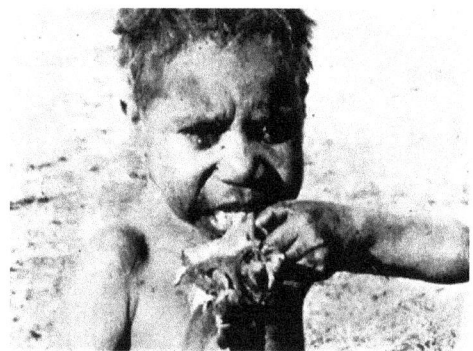

Figure 6.16
Unidentified Warlpiri boy, from the film *So they did eat*.
(if online click HERE to link to an extract from the film)

Figure 6.17 shows the pattern of occlusal wear on opposing deciduous molars. A similar process occurs on permanent first molars. Typically, wear progresses most rapidly on the buccal cusps of the lower molar and the lingual cusps of the upper molar because both the external and central slopes of these cusps are involved in the grinding phase of mastication. This process eventually leads to an oblique occlusal plane directed towards the palate in the upper first molar - the so-called ad-palatum wear, which is the opposite to the type of occlusal curvature in the coronal plane described as normal in most texts on tooth occlusion.

This pattern of wear resulted in a gradual reduction in cusp height, particularly the lower buccal cusps and upper lingual cusps with the result that areas of tooth surface opposed during mastication increased. Barrett (1958) also described minor positional changes in the upper and lower molars as they reached a state of optimal working equilibrium with each other. With increasing wear, there is a tendency for the maxillary arch to become broader relative to the mandibular, probably due to a combination of growth at the palatal suture and compensatory adjustments in alveolar remodelling. The oblique occlusal plane may indeed act in a similar way to bite planes in modifying the direction and magnitude of growth processes, although no longitudinal evidence is available to support this.

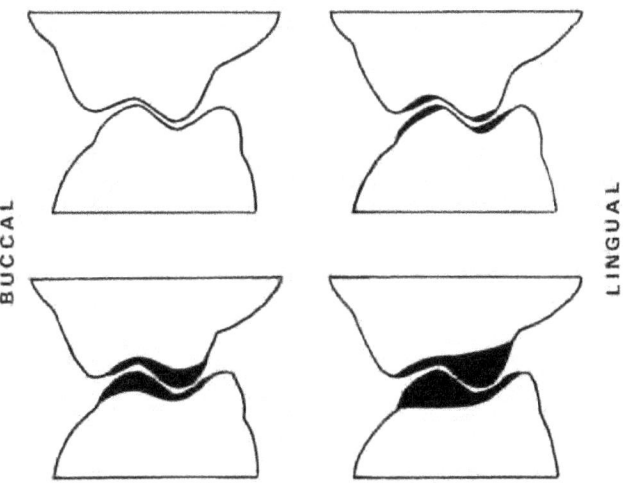

Figure 6.17
Stages in occlusal wear of deciduous molars
(after Barrett, 1958)

With emergence and articulation of the permanent first molars, these teeth assume a major occlusal load during food grinding, particularly if there is heavy wear to the deciduous molars (Molnar and Ward, 1977). It is not until the second molars and premolars come into occlusion, some six years later, that additional surface area is added to reduce the load carried by the already heavily worn first molars. It is not unusual, then, to find evidence of rapid and marked wear on first permanent molars while wear on the other permanent posterior teeth is considerably less.

The ad-palatum wear on deciduous molars referred to above occurs also on the maxillary permanent premolars and first molars. However, in many subjects the plane of wear changes progressively in regions posterior to the first molars. The pitch of the occlusal plane may be almost horizontal on the upper second molars and it may slope upward and buccally on the third molars. Usually the wear planes on the opposing lower teeth closely reciprocate those on the upper. The compound occlusal plane, which many observers of heavily worn dentitions have noted, is usually described as being helicoidal (Figure 6.18).

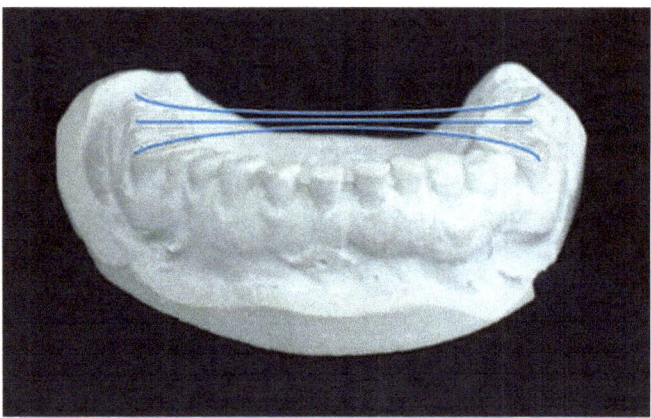

Figure 6.18
Photograph of dental model showing presence of helicoidal plane associated with varying amounts and direction of wear on the lower molar teeth

Campbell (1925) described the helicoidal plane in Australian Aboriginal people and suggested that it resulted from differences in breadth between the upper and lower dental arches. In the first molar region, maxillary arch breadth is greater and the masticatory grinding phase results in greater wear on buccal cusps of lower molars and lingual cusps of upper molars. However, mandibular arch breadth is sometimes greater in the region of the third molars, and in these instances, the reverse wear pattern takes place. As Campbell summarises:

in the Australian specimens this compound attritional curve is always present when the arch width at the third molars is greater in the lower than in the upper. When the arch widths at this region are the same or the upper the greater, then the attritional curve alters accordingly.

Campbell's explanation of the helicoidal occlusal plane appears to have wider acceptance than alternative theories and, furthermore, this characteristic type of occlusal wear probably has evolutionary significance. For example, Tobias (1980) noted that the helicoidal plane is absent in every specimen of Australopithecus but it appears in Homo habilis, where it is associated with posterior dental arch reduction. Tobias regards the appearance of helicoidal planes as a conspicuous indication of the gradual transition from Australopithecus to Homo habilis, whereas Richards and Brown (1986) believed that a helicoidal plane could be expected in most heavily worn dentitions and that it had no taxonomic significance.

In Australian Aboriginal people living a traditional lifestyle, occlusal wear was continuous and often extensive. Beyron (1964) reported less wear in present-day Aboriginal people from Yuendumu, with about 8 per cent of subjects aged 45 years or older showing Broca Grade IV wear. The transition to Broca Grade II occurred at about 20 years of age and in the majority of subjects the incisors and first molars displayed most wear and the third molars the least.

The extent and rate of tooth wear are governed by several factors including the thickness and hardness of enamel, the magnitude of forces applied during mastication, the consistency of food, the inclusion of abrasive particles, and the nature of the final grinding phase of the masticatory cycle. We do not completely understand the interaction and relative importance of these factors but without doubt, vigorous mastication and the inclusion of abrasive material in food were important determinants of tooth wear in Australian Aboriginal people.

Compensatory processes accompanied tooth wear with varying effectiveness in different subjects. When wear progressed at a tolerable rate or extent, the compensatory mechanisms were usually adequate. However, with excessive wear, the ability to adapt was sometimes exceeded and pathological changes resulted. Three main compensatory processes will be briefly mentioned, secondary dentine production, alveolar remodelling and temporomandibular joint remodelling. The laying down of secondary dentine was an effective barrier to advancing tooth wear and in most instances this mechanism served to prevent pulpal exposure with periapical sequelae. At times, wear progressed until no clinical crowns remained and yet pulps were still not involved. However, this was not always the case.

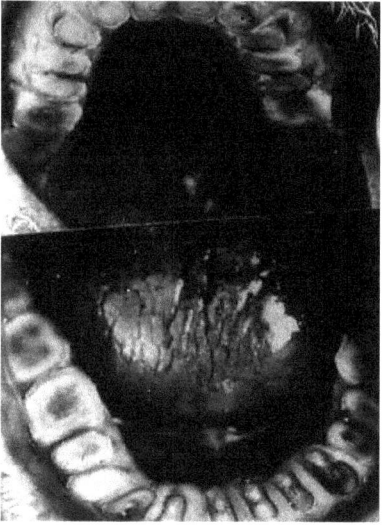

Figure 6.19
Severe tooth wear in an Aboriginal male from Kalumburu, Northwest Australia, aged about 70 years, showing loss of adjacent tooth contacts, deposition of secondary dentine, helicoidal occlusal plane and alveolar development

It was once thought that continual eruption of teeth in their sockets was the sole compensatory adjustment for tooth wear but Figure 6.19 demonstrates that this is unlikely. It shows an Aboriginal subject with wear down to gum level but with no noticeable over-eruption of the teeth. A more likely mechanism is continual alveolar growth and remodelling, as discussed by Ainamo and Talari (1976) and Berry (1976). The subject shown in Figure 6.19 also demonstrates that alveolar development accompanied the tooth wear. During progressive wear, it is also probable that tooth movements and alveolar remodelling take place to ensure optimal occlusal relationships, as described by Barrett (1958) and referred to above. Continual alveolar development appears to be one mechanism by which loss of occlusal tooth substance is compensated, and it is interesting that increases in facial heights through adult life have been reported in some populations where occlusal wear is minimal. The third compensatory mechanism is remodelling of the articular surfaces of the temporomandibular joint in response to changing occlusal relationships and, with advanced wear, increasing occlusal stress.

Interproximal wear, sometimes referred to as proximal or approximal wear, is the wearing away of adjacent tooth surfaces with a gradual reduction of the mesiodistal diameters and dental arch perimeters. This type of tooth wear invariably accompanied occlusal wear and it is due to the rubbing together of adjacent tooth surfaces during vigorous mastication.

Loss of tooth substance by interproximal wear can be quite extensive. For example, Campbell (1925) reported differences between unworn and worn teeth of Australian Aboriginal people of 1.6mm and 2.4mm in the maxilla and mandible respectively for the combined mesiodistal diameters of premolars and molars. Begg and Kesling (1977) reported a reduction of 10.56mm in lower dental arch perimeter due to interproximal wear prior to the emergence of the third molars. These authors believed that interproximal wear is an important process in occlusal development of the naturally functioning dentition by providing adequate space for emergence and alignment of teeth. While this is undoubtedly true, other factors also operate during occlusal development in Aboriginal people.

With progressive interproximal wear, the areas of contact between adjacent teeth became broadened so that contact occurred over extensive flattened areas rather than at limited point contacts between convex surfaces as described in the modern non-worn dentition. While this was taking place, tooth contact was preserved by mesial movement so that dental arch form became more stabilised by the increasing areas of tooth contact. However, when tooth crowns were substantially reduced in old age, adjacent tooth contacts were lost.

The pattern of interproximal tooth wear was not always consistent and wear facets could occur on the mesial or distal or on both surfaces, the size of the facet varying according to enamel density, duration of the wear and degree of lateral masticatory stress (Campbell, 1925). At times, a convex surface would rub into the flattened or concave surface of the adjacent tooth. This has led some authors to conclude that the relative hardness of the enamel of adjacent teeth determined which tooth was worn and which did the wearing. Some authors state that earlier erupting teeth underwent surface hardening and thus the harder surface would wear into the softer enamel of a later emerging tooth (Beyron, 1964). Campbell (1925), however, illustrated interproximal wear with the later emerging tooth wearing into the surface of the older tooth, which led him to suggest that the unworn tooth might have slightly greater hardness. Although relative surface hardness may indeed determine the patterns of interproximal wear to some extent, other factors such as relative movement between adjacent teeth and the direction and magnitude of forces generated during the grinding phase or mastication are probably of equal importance. There does not appear to be any consistent pattern of interproximal tooth wear that offers a simple explanation.

Occlusal function in the worn dentition

Continual occlusal and interproximal wear in the Aboriginal dentition resulted in modifications to tooth size and shape and progressive changes to the occlusal relationship between upper and lower teeth. As the wear-in phase of occlusal development continued, the pre-eruptive forms or cusps and incisal edges were lost and cuspal interdigitation and incisor overbite were not retained as they are in the dentition of modern industrialised humans.

Cuspal interdigitation was replaced by contact over broad surfaces that conformed to a helicoidal plane. Continuing wear increased both the area of opposing tooth surfaces and eventually the number of teeth contacting in lateral mandibular positions. With advancing tooth wear, changes also occurred in maxillo-mandibular relationships, of which the most noticeable was the development of an edge-to-edge incisor relationship. The neuromuscular and temporomandibular joint systems adapted to these occlusal changes and efficient trouble-free mastication was preserved.

Beyron (1964) analysed tooth contacts in a limited number of males from Yuendumu. Although based on only 46 subjects ranging in age from 15 to 45 years, his study provides one of the few detailed accounts of tooth relationships in dentitions subject to wear. In spite of the loss of cuspal morphology, the inclined planes of maxillary and mandibular cusps usually enabled the observer to articulate the dentition in a position of maximum tooth contact corresponding to the intercuspal position or centric occlusion of the non-worn dentition. In this intercuspal position, 75 per cent of Aboriginal subjects, aged 24 years or younger, displayed tooth contacts from second molars to the premolars with no contact between canines and incisors. Only 13 per cent of these younger subjects showed contact as far anteriorly as the canines.

With increasing age, however, more teeth were brought into contact in this position so that 44 per cent of the adult group (aged 25-44 years) and 62 per cent of the mature group (over 45 years) showed contact from second molars to canines. Beyron observed contact from second molars to incisors in 23 per cent of the mature group whereas in only 15 per cent contact was limited to the first premolars. Beyron found a similar situation when examining positions of right and left lateral cuspal contacts. Working side contacts from second molars to incisors were displayed by 38 per cent of younger subjects, 56 per cent of adults and 69 per cent of mature subjects. Beyron also reported no contacts on the non-working side in any subject. Occlusal relationships in the Aboriginal subjects departed markedly from those described as normal in currently held views of dental occlusion in at least three ways.

First, contact between incisors in the intercuspal position is not common even in older subjects. Second, lateral contact movements involve at least premolars and molars and in older subjects the canines and incisors are also included. Third, the number of teeth contacting in lateral positions increases with age as a result of wear and the wear-in process.

During the grinding phase of the masticatory stroke, initial tooth contact usually occurs 2-3mm lateral to the position of maximum intercuspation. In the Aboriginal subjects, contact between maxillary and mandibular teeth during intrusive movements tends to shift from one group of teeth to another. As the intercuspal position is approached, the greatest number of teeth come into contact, usually the same teeth that contact in the intercuspal position.

This type of group function is termed segmental occlusion, which Barrett (1969) described in Aboriginal people as follows:

> maximum contact of opposing tooth surfaces did not occur simultaneously all the way round the arches in one position of the mandible relative to the maxilla but could only be effected segmentally. That is, molar teeth on one side could be brought into most intimate functional contact only at slightly eccentric relations of the mandible, the premolars and canines in another position, incisors in another position, and so on around the arch. Intimate functioning occlusion was limited to a particular segment at anyone time and occlusal contact elsewhere was absent or minimal.

Another interesting consequence of tooth wear is the gradual elimination of incisor overbite and the development of the edge-to-edge relationship so characteristic of the adult and mature Aboriginal dentition. Most observers of the naturally functioning dentition have reported this phenomenon. Beyron (1964), for example, reported a decrease in incisor overbite from 1.06mm in young subjects to 0.0mm in subjects aged 45 years or older. It is interesting, however, that incisor overjet was reduced by only a small amount during the same age span.

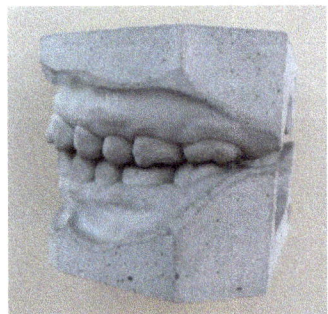 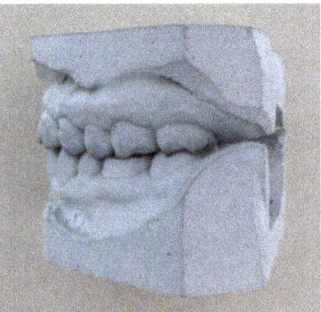 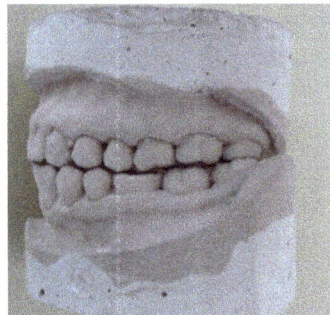

Figure 6.20
Dental casts of a Warlpiri girl aged 12.9, 15.9 and 29.9 years showing changing incisor relationships

There is little doubt that in Aboriginal people the elimination of incisor overbite with age is consequent upon the wear process. However, edge-to-edge incisor relationships sometimes appear in younger Aboriginal people with little tooth wear and in some European children living in urban environments. In the Navajos of Tuba City, Arizona, edge-to-edge incisor relationships appear to be the general rule even in the unworn dentition (Brace, 1977).

Various researchers have proposed a number of causative factors to explain the change in incisor relationships with advancing wear. Begg and Kesling (1977) attribute the elimination of overbite to anterior migration of the mandibular dentition relative to the maxillary, proclination of lower incisors and retroclination of the upper incisors. Mesial migration of mandibular teeth relative to the mandibular body certainly occurs with interproximal wear, as evidenced by the changing relation between the mental foramen and the posterior teeth. However, without longitudinal observations and stable reference markers it is impossible to determine if the tooth migration is greater in the mandibular arch. On the other hand, remodelling changes on the mandibular condyle and articular eminence associated with heavy wear suggests a progressive anterior shift of the entire mandible with continuing tooth wear.

Similar repositioning of the mandible into an anterior functioning position is a common clinical finding in patients with posterior tooth loss and patients wearing complete dentures with worn occlusal surfaces. Brace (1977) prefers to debate the question from an alternative approach, namely that overbite in the present day dentition results from the continual eruption of the incisors when they are not used in natural opposition to each other as they were in pre-industrial humans.

A particularly interesting variety of occlusal relationship, observed in some Aboriginal subjects, is alternate intercuspation. Chapter 3 (see Figure 3.6) discusses this type of occlusion.

Although Barrett was probably the first to describe the functional significance of alternate intercuspation, Turner (1871) reported it, referring to the disparity in widths of the upper and lower dental arches. This form of occlusal relationship is by no means unique to human populations. It is analogous to the morphology displayed by animals such as herbivores that employ wide grinding strokes during mastication. In these, the disparity between upper and lower dental arch breadths is very marked.

Alternate intercuspation is sometimes present in the deciduous dentition as well as the permanent, and it may either intensify or diminish as occlusal development proceeds. One of the present authors has noticed the occlusal feature in dental casts and skeletal material from other pre-industrialised groups, such as Bedouins of Israel, South African Bantus, North American Indians and Greenland Eskimos (Brown, personal observations). Telfer (1978) also described alternate intercuspation, and analysed metric data from the dental casts of Yuendumu people. The phylogenetic and ontogenetic significance of alternate intercuspation is not yet fully understood, nor is it known whether it has a strong genetic basis.

The impression is gained when studying alternate intercuspation that the disparity in arch breadths permits a wider range of lateral jaw movement with perhaps an increase in opposing tooth contacts as the jaw moves medially during the final phase of the masticatory stroke. Masticatory efficiency is by no means impaired by a lack of any position resembling the respected intercuspal position of modern occlusion concepts.

In the preceding section, we gave an account of the constantly changing occlusal relationships in the natural functioning dentition of Australian Aboriginal people. Continuing tooth wear had the effect of bringing a greater area of occlusal surface into activity during the grinding phase of mastication. This occlusal change, accompanied by the broad flat masticatory stroke, enabled food to be milled between flat tooth surfaces rather than comminuted between sharp cusps and fossae - much in the manner of a pestle and mortar.

Progressive occlusal wear was accompanied by compensatory changes, which served to maintain equilibrium in the masticatory components for optimal function. Loss of tooth enamel and dentine were compensated by the deposition of secondary dentine and a reduction in face height was minimised by alveolar development, which tended to carry the teeth occlusally. There was also an anterior displacement of the mandibular arch relative to the maxillary with establishment of edge-to-edge incisor relationships. This changing arch relationship probably involves movement of the mandibular teeth relative to maxillary as well as a bodily repositioning of the mandible but current knowledge does not completely explain the mechanisms involved.

The temporomandibular joints are considered to be load-bearing during part of the masticatory cycle and they have the ability to compensate for altered functional demands, such as those resulting from progressive occlusal wear. Adaptation to occlusal stress is effected by remodelling processes that are evident on the articular surfaces of many specimens showing tooth wear. Under normal circumstances, joint remodelling serves to maintain equilibrium between structures and function in the joint tissues, an important correlate of optimal function. Some authors hold the view that tooth wear was always physiological and beneficial and that compensatory mechanisms were always effective. However, this is not the case and in many instances tooth wear under harsh environmental conditions progressed to a stage where the individual's adaptive potential was exceeded, equilibrium was lost and degenerative changes occurred in the teeth, jaws and temporomandibular joints, as described in more detail by Richards and Brown (1981).

Functions of tooth cusps

The conventional view usually regards tooth cusps as important features of occlusal morphology, essential for efficient mastication and serving to stabilise maxillo-mandibular arch relations in a position of centric occlusion or maximum intercuspation. The restoration of their form and manner of interdigitation is a significant function of modern dental practice. And yet, even a cursory examination of the dentitions of Australian Aboriginal people and other populations characterised by tooth wear leads to the inescapable conclusion that tooth cusps are not very important for either mastication or jaw positioning. As described earlier, cuspal form was retained for only a transitory period of occlusal development and, with continuing wear, cusps were lost so that mastication was effected between broad and flat occlusal surfaces with sharp enamel rims. Provided there were no pathological sequelae in later life, arising from pulpal involvement or joint degeneration, the loss of cusps did not impair masticatory function.

Some authors, including Mills (1976) and Berry (1976), hold the view that tooth wear in the higher primates, including humans, is not only physiologically correct but also highly desirable. According to this view the reduction of tooth wear in modern industrialised humans has been accompanied by an increase in dental decay, periodontal disease and malocclusion. What then are the functions of tooth cusps if they are not required for mastication?

Notwithstanding the evolutionary significance of tooth cusps, Campbell (1946, 1956) considered that the modern civilised dentition represented an "entirely unnatural state of occlusal configuration" that was in reality retention of an immature occlusal condition quite unsuitable for adult masticatory function. Campbell therefore proposed that tooth cusps served an important developmental role in the biomechanics of tooth eruption and dental arch formation.

According to Campbell, the cusps and fossae serve to guide opposing teeth into correct position so that arch alignment is established and maintained. He also pointed out that development of tooth roots and alveolar bone is not complete when teeth first meet in occlusion. Cuspal interdigitation maintains tooth position and stability until firm and effective implantation is achieved following completion of root form and alveolar support. As tooth usage becomes more vigorous, alveolar compactness increases. At about this stage, intercuspation is no longer essential in the naturally functioning dentition and tooth wear is already changing cuspal morphology.

From more recent knowledge of masticatory physiology, other functions of tooth cusps can be proposed apart from the role in tooth eruption and arch formation. For example, it is well established that jaw movements are effected by a complex system of neuromuscular pathways controlled by sensory inputs from the oral tissues, muscles and joints. An important part of this neural control comprises the proprioceptive impulses originating in the periodontal ligaments. It is highly likely that masticatory reflexes are initiated, learned and reinforced through sensory inputs to the central nervous system generated when the newly emerged teeth meet in occlusal contact during masticatory function. In view of the high occlusal sensitivity of teeth, cusps probably play an important part in the establishment of neural reflexes concerned with jaw positions and movements. Once these patterns are established they are reinforced and refined by tooth contact during mastication and swallowing but the original cuspal morphology is no longer so important.

Tooth cusps may also be involved in the fine adjustments of growth rates and directions during development of the facial skeleton but this role must remain speculative for the present. The experimental work of Petrovic and colleagues, summarised by Petrovic and Stutzmann (1977), supports this concept. These authors proposed an interesting servosystem in which the maxillary dental arch acts as a constantly changing reference input. The lower dental arch responds to the reference input and is adjusted, by growth of the mandible, to a position of optimal occlusal relationship.

This adjustment, the authors suggest, is mediated by activity in the lateral pterygoid and masseter muscles effecting variations in the rate and direction of growth at the mandibular condyles. Petrovic and colleagues have also suggested ways by which the servosystem operates in conjunction with hormonal influence but further experimental work is required to refine their hypothesis. This research, so far, supports the view that clinical devices fitted to vary the antero-posterior position of the mandible may affect jaw growth through altered activity of the associated muscles.

In the light of the work by Petrovic and colleagues, it seems reasonable to suggest that maxillo-mandibular relationships are established during growth by complex mechanisms, as yet unknown, that involve neural inputs from the teeth, muscles and joints. These inputs may control fine adjustments to the rates and directions of jaw growth so that occlusal relationships are optimised. The work of Björk and Skieller (1972) indeed indicates the feasibility of this hypothesis by demonstrating the strong coordination between the patterns of jaw growth and tooth emergence. It is perhaps not coincidental that in the naturally functioning dentition tooth cusps are well on the way towards elimination by the time facial growth nears completion in early adulthood.

To conclude, this chapter takes the view that many concepts of dental occlusion are based on observations of dentitions that no longer function in a natural and physiological way. It could be argued that many clinical procedures used in dentistry today arose empirically out of "urgent practical endeavours to keep pace with the dental troubles and disasters which have been so prevalent in the degenerate dentition of modern civilised man" (Campbell, 1956).

Our studies of occlusal development and function in Australian Aboriginal people illustrate the extent of changes in the jaws and dentition subsequent to the gradual transition to a way of life largely free from the environmental harshness experienced by earlier populations. In many industrialised populations, masticatory function is not as vigorous as we observed in the Aboriginal people at Yuendumu, resulting in less stimulation for growth of the mid-facial region and development of the alveolar processes. Consequently, there is often inadequate space within the dental arches to enable optimal occlusal development, leading to varying degrees of dental crowding, malocclusion, and third molar impaction (Brown *et al.*, 1990).

Orthodontists are particularly concerned with occlusal irregularities ranging in severity from minor degrees of crowding or rotation to the gross anomalies associated with some genetically determined craniofacial abnormalities. Occlusal disorders are often accompanied by a heightened susceptibility to dental decay and periodontal disease, conditions that have increased in prevalence in many populations with the adoption of lifestyles that are less dependent on the naturally functioning dentitions.

The studies of Aboriginal people at Yuendumu have demonstrated some important biological processes involved in the development of functionally efficient dentitions. In the first instance, a high degree of coordination between the sizes of corresponding deciduous and permanent teeth sets the scene for orderly development. Similarly, maxillary and mandibular teeth are highly correlated in size, thus minimising the chances of occlusal disorders arising from tooth size discrepancies. Although genes predominantly control tooth size, there is no doubt that local environmental conditions, such as the space available for calcifying tooth crowns, are also important. Morphogenetic fields probably maintain an overall control over tooth development but we do not yet fully understand the mechanisms involved.

In Aboriginal children, the size excess of deciduous molars compared with the permanent premolars is usually favourable. In spite of large permanent teeth, an Aboriginal person usually has little difficulty in accommodating them without significant crowding. Consequently, the dental arches tend to be well formed and less prone to the crowding irregularities often found in other contemporary dentitions.

Of equal importance in occlusal development are the patterns of tooth emergence and craniofacial growth. In this respect, note that the Aboriginal children who were involved in the Yuendumu Growth Study seldom lost their deciduous teeth prematurely through decay. Furthermore, facial growth was characterised by a prominent occlusal and anterior movement of the dental arches, resulting in marked alveolar development and mid-facial prognathism. This anterior drift of the dentition together with remodelling of the mandibular ramus provided adequate space for unimpeded emergence of the later teeth.

Apart from morphological differences in the dento-facial structures, there are also striking differences in masticatory function between Aboriginal people living in their traditional way and many modern groups. The dentition of Aboriginal people living a traditional lifestyle continually changes with age as a result of vigorous function and wear. Tooth cusps, for example, are not very important for efficient mastication as they gradually wear away with no evidence of impaired function. Flattened occlusal surfaces and a broad masticatory stroke cope with coarse food far better than cusps and short chopping movements. Up to a point, we may consider tooth wear physiological and beneficial, particularly as it provides a wear-in process that optimises occlusal relationships for vigorous mastication without the hindrance of cuspal interferences (Kaifu *et al.*, 2003). In the modern non-worn dentition, however, masticatory strokes are usually limited in extent and power and they are often conditioned by cuspal morphology.

In instances of extreme wear on teeth, leading to worn-out dentitions, degenerative arthritis of the temporomandibular joints is a likely outcome together with pulpal and periapical pathology in many cases. Nonetheless, it is patently obvious that, generally, the dentition of the Australian Aboriginal person living a traditional lifestyle functioned in a healthy and physiological way until late in life, free of many of the disorders and diseases that are the penalty of so-called civilisation.

References

Ainamo J, Talari A (1976). Eruptive movements of teeth in human adults. In: *The Eruption and Occlusion of Teeth.* Poole DFG and Stack MV, editors. London: Butterworths, pp. 97–107.

Barrett MJ (1958). Dental observations on Australian Aborigines: Continuously changing occlusion. *Aust Dent J* 3:39–52.

Barrett MJ (1969). Functioning occlusion. *Ann Aust Coll Dent Surg* 2:68:80.

Barrett MJ (1977). Masticatory and non-masticatory use of teeth. In: *Stone Tools as Culture Markers: Change, Evolution and Complexity.* Wright RVS, editor. Canberra: Australian Institute of Aboriginal Studies, pp. 18–23.

Begg PR, Kesling PC (1977). *Begg Orthodontic Theory and Practice.* 3rd Edition. Philadelphia: Saunders.

Berry DC (1976). Excessive attrition. In: *The Eruption and Occlusion of Teeth.* Poole DFG, Stack MV, editors. London: Butterworths pp.146–155.

Beyron H (1964). Occlusal relations and mastication in Australian Aborigines. *Acta Odontol Scand* 22:597–678.

Björk A (1963). Variation in the growth pattern of the human mandible: longitudinal radiographic study by the implant method. *J Dent Res* 42:400–411.

Björk A (1964). Sutural growth of the upper face studied by the implant method. *Trans Europ Orthod Soc* 40:49–65.

Björk A (1969). Prediction of mandibular growth rotation. *Am J Orthod* 55:585–599.

Björk A (1980). Mandibular growth rotations. Paper presented 55th Congress of the European Orthodontic Society, May 15–19th, 1979, Barcelona, Spain. *Eur J Orthod* 2:59–61.

Björk A, Brown T, Skieller V (1984). Comparison of craniofacial growth in an Australian Aboriginal and Danes, illustrated by longitudinal cephalometric analysis. *Eur Orthod J* 6:1-14.

Björk A, Skieller V (1972). Facial development and tooth eruption. *Am J Orthod* 62:339–383.

Björk A, Skieller V (1974). Growth in width of the maxilla studied by the implant method. *Scand J Plast Reconstr Surg Hand Surg* 8:26–33.

Björk A, Skieller V (1976). Postnatal growth and development of the maxillary complex. In: *Factors Affecting the Growth of the Midface.* MacNamara JA Jr, editor. Craniofacial Growth Series Monograph 6. Ann Arbor: University of Michigan, pp. 61–99.

Brace CL (1977). Occlusion to the anthropological eye. In: *The Biology of Occlusal Development.* MacNamara JA Jr, editor. Craniofacial Growth Series Monograph 7. Ann Arbor: University of Michigan, pp. 179–209.

Brown T (1965). *Craniofacial Variations in a Central Australian Tribe: A Radiographic Investigation of Young Adult males and Females.* Adelaide: Libraries Board of South Australia.

Brown T, Townsend GC, Richards LC, Burgess VB (1990) Concepts of occlusion: Australian evidence. *Am J Phys Anthropol* 82:247–256.

Campbell TD (1925). *Dentition and Palate of the Australian Aboriginal.* Adelaide: The Hassell Press.

Campbell TD (1946). Tooth cusps. *Aust Dent J* 50:305–307.

Campbell TD (1956). Comparative human odontology. *Aust Dent J* 1:26–32.

Kaifu Y, Kasai K, Townsend G, Richards L (2003). Tooth wear and the "design" of the human dentition: a perspective from evolutionary medicine. *Yearb Phys Anthropol* 46:47–61.

Macintosh NWG, Barker BCW (1978). The Tabon Cave mandible. *Arch Phys Anthrop Oceania* 13:143–166.

Mills JRE (1976). Attrition in animals. In: *The Eruption and Occlusion of Teeth*. Poole DFG, Stack MV, editors. London: Butterworths, pp. 133–145.

Molnar S (1972). Tooth wear and culture: a survey of tooth functions among some prehistoric populations. *Curr Anthropol* 13:511–526.

Molnar S, Ward SC (1977). On the hominid masticatory complex: biochemical and evolutionary perspectives. *J Hum Evol* 6:557–568.

Petrovic AG, Stutzmann JJ (1977). Further investigations into the functioning of the peripheral "comparator" of the servosystem (respective positions of the upper and lower dental arches) in the control of the condylar cartilage growth rate and of the lengthening of the jaw. In: *The Biology of Occlusal Development*. McNamara JA Jr, editor. Craniofacial Growth Series Monograph 7, Ann Arbor: University of Michigan, pp. 255–291.

Proffit WR (1978). Equilibrium theory re-examined: To what extent do tongue and lip pressures influence tooth position and thereby the occlusion? In: *Oral Physiology and Occlusion*, Perryman JH, editor. London: Pergamon Press, pp. 55–77.

Proffit WR, McGlone RE, Barrett MJ (1975). Lip and tongue pressures related to dental arch and oral cavity size in Australian Aborigines. *J Dent Res* 54:1161–1172.

Richards LC, Brown T (1981). Dental attrition and degenerative arthritis of the temporomandibular joint. *J Oral Rehab* 8:293–307.

Riedel RA (1977). Post-pubertal occlusal changes. In: *The Biology of Occlusal Development*. McNamara JA Jr, editor. Craniofacial Growth Series Monograph 7. Ann Arbor: University of Michigan, pp. 113–140.

Solow B, Tallgren A (1971a). Natural head position in standing subjects. *Acta Odontol Scand* 29:591–607.

Solow B, Tallgren A (1971b). Postural changes in craniocervical relationships. *Tandlaegebladet* 75:1247–1257.

Solow B, Tallgren A (1976). Head posture and craniofacial morphology. *Am J Phys Anthropol* 44:417–436.

Solow B, Tallgren A (1977). Dentoalveolar morphology in relation to craniocervical posture. *Angle Orthod* 47:157–164.

Solow B, Barrett MJ, Brown T (1981). Head posture and craniofacial morphology in Australian Aboriginals. *J Dent Res* 60:473. Abstract.

Telfer PJ (1978). *Comparative Study of Dental Arch Morphology and Occlusion*. MDS Thesis, University of Adelaide.

Tobias PV (1980). The natural history of the helicoidal occlusal plane and its evolution in early Homo. *Am J Phys Anthropol* 53:173–187.

Turner W (1891). The relations of the dentary arcades in the crania of Australian Aboriginals. *J Anat Physiol* 25:461–471.

7
People and Personalities Involved with the Project

The International Researchers

Henry Lennart Beyron 1909–1992

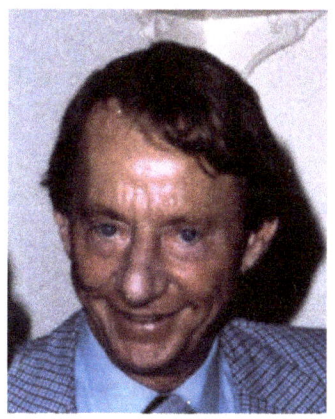

Figure 7.1
Henry Lennart Beyron

Henry Lennart Beyron was born at Norrmalmstorg 1, Stockholm, Sweden, on 5 August 1909. He attended the Royal Dental School and the Royal Caroline Medico-Chirurgical Institute in Stockholm from 1928–1932. He graduated as a Doctor of Dental Surgery in 1931 and achieved a Master of Science in Dentistry from the Northwestern University, Chicago, Illinois, USA, in 1938. He became an Associate Professor in the Prosthetic Department of the Royal Dental School, Stockholm, in 1942. His advancement continued when he was appointed as the Principal Dental Surgeon to Kings Gustaf V and VI of Sweden.

Henry Beyron was widely known in the world of dental research as an expert in the field of dental occlusion. Murray Barrett and Beyron first met each other in the 1950s when Barrett was on study leave in Scandinavia. Beyron's association with the research at Yuendumu began in January 1957 when he wrote a letter to Barrett outlining his intention to present a series of lectures in the United States on the subject of "Functional Analysis of Occlusion". In this letter, he stated that he would be interested in presenting these lectures in Australia. Barrett replied to Beyron's enquiries with an offer of co-operation should he decide to come to Adelaide and work on Aboriginal data. From an analysis of this correspondence, it appears that Beyron was encouraged to come to Adelaide with the possibility of being able to study occlusion involving Aboriginal subjects in the field. In September 1957, the Australian Dental Association considered the proposal that Beyron visit Yuendumu. A letter from Mr John Wark, the Honorary Secretary of the Association, gave tentative approval to both his lecture tour and his visit to Yuendumu. Much of this letter concerned the financial arrangements, such as honorarium, travelling and accommodation expenses.

Correspondence continued throughout the year, confirming arrangements for Beyron to come to Adelaide after a series of lectures he was to give in Hobart, Melbourne, Sydney and Brisbane. In October 1957, Beyron accepted an offer from the Federal Office of the Australian Dental Association that outlined the terms and conditions of his Australian lecture tour and of his visit to the Yuendumu Settlement (Barrett, 1953-1957).

Beyron arrived in Adelaide in late December 1957 and left Adelaide with Draper Campbell and Murray Barrett for Yuendumu on 7 January 1958. The prime purpose of this trip to Yuendumu was for Beyron to learn more about the Aboriginal dentition. Barrett and Campbell initially provided Beyron with assistance in both obtaining data and providing suggestions and editorial input to a paper Beyron was preparing regarding his trip. An example of the depth and commitment Barrett and his co-researchers made toward the manuscript can be gained by viewing papers stored in the Murray Barrett Laboratory on the 6th floor of the Adelaide Dental School. The folder contains 44 pages of Beyron's manuscript with Murray Barrett's corrections made in red crayon. Attached to each page is another typed page with all the corrections inserted in their correct places (Barrett, 1953-1973). In the acknowledgements, Beyron writes:

To Dr Barrett I am especially indebted for his assistance in collecting the material observations, casts, articulator records, photographs and cine films, and for his aid in editing the manuscript (Beyron, 1964).

The collaboration between Beyron and Barrett illustrates not only the trust Beyron had in Barrett's ability to modify the paper, but also that international researchers were recognising the importance of the research being undertaken at Yuendumu. Nonetheless, Barrett was greatly disappointed that Beyron would not agree to his request for co-authorship, particularly in view of both his and his colleagues' substantial input into Beyron's paper. It was specially upsetting given that the paper dealt with occlusal relations, a topic that was central to Barrett's research endeavours, and the fact that Barrett made many years of research material and experience with Aboriginal people freely available to Henry Beyron.

Despite this disappointment over the authorship of the paper, relations between Barrett and Beyron continued amicably until Barrett's death in 1975. Beyron died in Stockholm in 1992.

Arne Björk 1911–1996

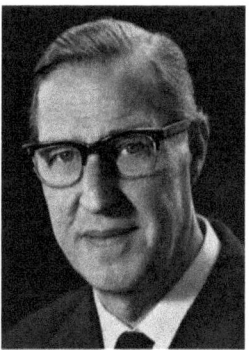

Figure 7.2
Arne Björk

Arne Björk was born in 1911, in the Dalarna district of Sweden, a beautiful region of lakes and forests, to which he regularly returned for summer vacations. After qualifying in dentistry, he practised in Västerås from 1937 until 1951. He also served as Professor of Orthodontics at the Malmö School of Dentistry between 1949 and 1950. In 1951 he was appointed to the Professorship of Orthodontics at the Royal Dental College, Copenhagen, a position he held until his retirement in 1981.

His thesis *The Face in Profile* (Björk, 1947) set new standards for the application of the emerging technique of radiographic cephalometry for the study of craniofacial morphology. It served as a model text in this discipline. His best-known work, however, was the series of publications from the 1950s until his retirement based on his pioneering studies in which he used tantalum implants to analyse facial growth patterns (Björk, 1955, 1968). Björk was able to describe jaw rotations, alveolar bone growth, bone remodelling and tooth emergence in ways that provided a clearer understanding of the complex patterns of facial growth and the development of malocclusions. Although at variance with contemporary concepts of facial growth, Björk's work gained immediate international attention. Thereafter, many international researchers were privileged to work and study with Björk and many Danish scholars used his research records for their dissertations.

Björk published extensively in his lifetime and received many prestigious awards and invitations to lecture overseas. On his 60th birthday he was presented with a volume of essays written by local and overseas researchers who had worked with him. One of these essays was by Adelaide authors (Brown *et al.*, 1971). The volume was also printed in the Tandlægebladet (Danish Dental Journal 1971; 75: 1143-1340). On the occasion of his 80th birthday, the Danish Dental Journal published a special issue of 10 articles written by Arne Björk's Danish colleagues and ex-students.

A close working relationship between Arne Björk, his colleagues and the Adelaide dental researchers was established after Murray Barrett's first visit to Sweden and Denmark. The relationship firmed when Sven Helm, a member of Björk's staff, visited Yuendumu and spent time in Adelaide in 1965 for epidemiological studies of malocclusion in different ethnic groups (Björk and Helm, 1969; Helm, 1979). The following year Tasman Brown spent most of his first sabbatical leave in Arne Björk's department. The purpose of the extended stay was to absorb the Björk philosophy of craniofacial growth, to observe the use of implants and to meet staff and postgraduate students working with the implant material. Of special significance during this period was the liaison Brown established with Beni Solow, who, like Brown, was pioneering the application of multivariate factor analysis to craniofacial growth studies.

The relationship between the Danish and Adelaide research groups continued. In subsequent years, Brown spent parts of two other sabbaticals in Copenhagen, Solow carried out research at Yuendumu, and Arne Björk and his research associate Vibeke Skieller visited Adelaide in 1975 for an extended stay that included lectures to Adelaide orthodontists.

Without doubt Arne Björk had a very significant influence on the establishment of the extended phase of the Yuendumu study and the methodology and analytical procedures used by the Adelaide group and their students. He died in 1996.

Beni Solow 1934–2000

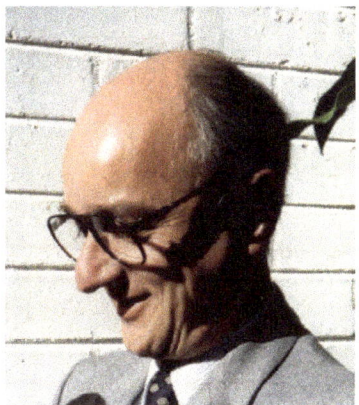

Figure 7.3
Beni Solow

Beni Solow was born in Copenhagen, Denmark, in 1934. He attended the Metropolitan High School and qualified as a dentist at the Royal College, Copenhagen, in 1957. He obtained the degree of Doctor of Orthodontics (dr.odont) in 1966. The title of his doctorate thesis was *The pattern of craniofacial associations. A morphological correlation and factor analysis study on young male adults* (Solow, 1966). The study of cephalometric measurement, craniofacial growth patterns, and factors that influenced the control mechanisms governing craniofacial development became the main themes of his research.

In 1966 when Brown spent several months at the Royal Dental College, Denmark, he and Beni Solow spent many hours discussing cephalometric analysis, automatic data analysis and the application of factor analysis to research projects in which they were involved. Through this liaison Beni Solow became very familiar with the Adelaide project and a few years later he notified Murray Barrett of his intention to attend an Australian and New Zealand Association for the Advancement of Science (ANZAAS) conference in Adelaide in August 1969 (Barrett, 1953-1957). In this letter, Solow mentioned that he was interested in studying computerised cephalometrics. He also mentioned that in a previous discussion with Tasman

Brown he had became aware of a planned trip to Yuendumu from 23 August to 4 September 1969, and asked whether he could join the research group. In further communications, Solow described both the project and the methodology he planned to use during this visit. Solow noted that the name of his project was "Head Balance" and that it was a multivariate correlation study relating natural head position to facial morphology. He planned to compare cephalometric data of Warlpiri subjects with data previously obtained from Danish male and Finnish female subjects.

The problems experienced in setting up the necessary equipment and participants were formidable. Initially, Solow had hoped to acquire data from 100 males and 100 females. He thought this was the minimum number that he could use in conjunction with the data obtained in Scandinavia. In reality, he examined about 24 participants of either sex each working day, giving a total of about 120 for the duration of the visit. The age of the participants ranged from 19 to 40 years in males and 19 to 40 years in females. Solow published the results of his research at Yuendumu in a joint paper that focussed on head posture and craniofacial morphology in Australian Aboriginal people (Solow *et al.*, 1982).

In 1982 Solow became the Professor of Orthodontics in the Department of Orthodontics, The Royal Dental College, Copenhagen, taking over as head of the department following the retirement of Professor Arne Björk. Professor Beni Solow died on 11 August 2000 during an exploratory surgical procedure.

Sven Helm 1927–

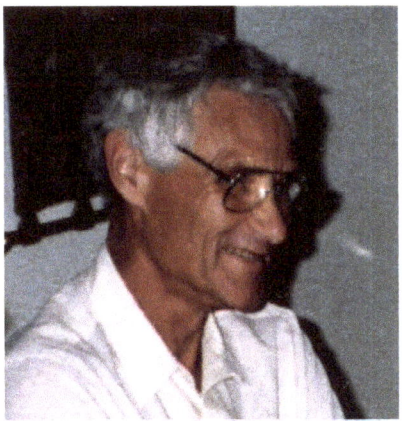

Figure 7.4
Sven Helm

Sven Helm was born in 1927 and graduated in dentistry from the Royal Dental College, Copenhagen, in 1951. He served in the Danish Armed Service Dental Corps, after which he worked in the Public Health Service in Northern Sweden for a further two years. On his return to Denmark, he organised the Public Dental School Service, in which he developed an orthodontic section. Having received a research grant from the Royal Dental College, Copenhagen, he elected to remain in academia, working with Arne Björk.

His purpose in accepting an offer to visit Yuendumu was to carry out an epidemiological survey of malocclusion in children and young adults, to record examples of malocclusion in the dental casts, and to obtain measurements, where possible, of asymmetry in the skull. He visited Yuendumu in August 1965 and whilst at the Settlement he examined 205 Aboriginal participants and obtained intra-oral radiographs of approximately 75 participants.

A report written after this visit noted that the results of Helm's survey of malocclusion would provide a valuable basis for comparisons to be made between the Aboriginal data and those obtained from other ethnic groups, notably Danish, Bantu, Indian and Chinese schoolchildren (Barrett, 1953-1957).

Helm, being an orthodontist, was interested in understanding malocclusion but also in treating the condition. In a joint publication with Arne Björk, he outlined the need for treatment as reflected in the prevalence of malocclusion in different ethnic groups, which included the data he had collected at Yuendumu (Björk and Helm, 1969).

Tadashi Ozaki 1924–

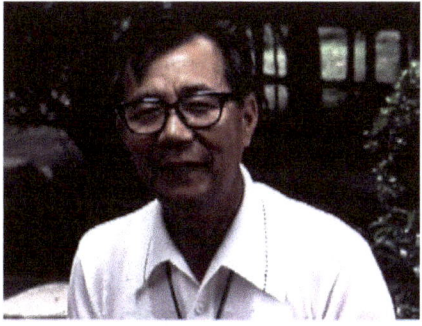

Figure 7.5
Tadashi Ozaki

In November 1965, Murray Barrett wrote a letter to Professor Shin-ichi Kato of the Department of Anatomy, Nihon University, Tokyo, Japan. In this letter, Barrett requested permission to visit Professor Kato's department to study craniofacial characteristics. In a reply to this enquiry, Professor Kato took advantage of Barrett's communication and requested that a member of his staff, Dr Tadashi Ozaki, visit The University of Adelaide to conduct research in anatomy. From this communication, a strong research base developed between Barrett and Tasman Brown from Adelaide and Dr Ozaki and his colleagues from Japan.

Tadashi Ozaki was born on 4 August 1924. He entered Nihon University in 1946 and graduated as a Doctor of Dental Surgery (DDSc) in 1953. He acquired a Doctor of Medical Science degree (DMSc) at the Tokyo University School of Medicine in 1960, and in the same year became Lecturer in Anatomy at the Nihon University. He became an Associate Professor in 1962 and Professor of Anatomy at the School of Dentistry, Nihon University, in 1968.

He arrived in Adelaide in mid-November 1968 after much correspondence between the Australian and Japanese university departments. The intention was for Ozaki to remain in Australia for two years. A problem that faced both the Adelaide research team and Ozaki was to find ways of assisting him financially during his time in Australia. One method was for him to apply for a Leverhulme Visiting Fellowship. Unfortunately, his application did not meet the requirements for a fellowship but, subsequently, Nihon University agreed to finance his visit.

Ozaki's areas of interest concerned correlations between measurements of the dental arches of Australian Aboriginal people, and comparing dental arch size, tooth size and facial morphology between Aboriginal and Japanese subjects. With these interests in mind, Ozaki visited Yuendumu from 20 May to 7 June 1969.

During his visit to Yuendumu, Ozaki was involved in obtaining growth data, with particular reference to hand and wrist measurements. Inspection of the field trip registers reveals that Ozaki was the only Japanese academic to visit Yuendumu as a member of a dental team. Subsequently, many other Japanese academics have visited Adelaide to study the material acquired at Yuendumu and to publish their findings in research papers.

Ozaki also worked with Eisaku Kanazawa, Mitsuo Sekikawa and Kazu Kasai producing papers relating to intercuspal distances of both upper and lower molar teeth and making comparisons between Australian Aboriginal and Japanese populations (Ozaki *et al.*, 1987; Sekikawa *et al.*, 1986, 1988; Kanazawa *et al.*, 1988, 1991; Kasai *et al.*, 1993). In many of these papers, it is apparent that the aim was to compare observed dental traits in the Aboriginal population at Yuendumu with other ethnic groups, including Indians, early settler Americans and Pacific Island populations.

Another Japanese researcher to visit Adelaide was Kazuro Hanihara who published numerous papers between the years 1970–1979 concerning crown size, tooth measurement, sexual dimorphism and dental traits in Australian Aboriginal people (Hanihara, 1970, 1974, 1976, 1977, 1978, 1979).

William Robert Proffit 1936–

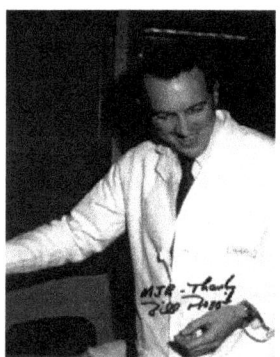

Figure 7.6
William R Proffit

In December 1969, Tasman Brown received a letter from Alton W Moore who, at that time was the Associate Dean of The School of Dentistry, University of Washington, Seattle, USA. This letter introduced William R Proffit as a colleague who wished to spend a sabbatical leave in Australia.

William Robert Proffit was born on 19 April 1936 at Erwin, North Carolina, USA. He obtained his BSDent degree in 1956 and his DDSc doctorate in 1959 from the University of Carolina. He also obtained a PhD degree (Physiology) from the Medical College of Virginia in 1962, and a MSDent degree (Orthodontics) in 1963 from the University of Washington, Seattle, USA.

Replying to a communication from Tasman Brown, Proffit outlined his research interests in dentistry in general and his interest in orthodontics in particular. As correspondence between Proffit and Brown continued, a research program developed that became dependent on the involvement of Murray Barrett. In the late 1960s and early 1970s, a study was designed to examine tongue pressures and positions within the oral cavity. Proffit had observed that amongst the non-European populations there were no data on lingual pressures. As the dental arch dimensions in the Aboriginal population differed noticeably from Europeans, primarily in width and depth, it was considered important to determine whether these physical differences might be associated with differences in lip and tongue pressures.

In May 1972 a team comprising Murray Barrett, his Adelaide colleagues David Parker and Leslie Reynolds, together with William Proffit, commenced a study of tongue and lip pressures of 18 Aboriginal teenagers at Yuendumu aged between 13 and 17 years. These teenagers had participated in examinations during earlier visits, and the team had available records from dental casts, radiographs and body measurements. The researchers placed pressure sensitive transducer devices at various locations in the mouth and recorded pressure waves on magnetic tape while the participants drank water, swallowed, and repeated certain Warlpiri words. (see Chapter 6.)

The research resulted in the publication of three papers. Proffit wrote one for an orthodontic audience using the Aboriginal data to increase knowledge of muscle pressures and tooth position (Proffit, 1975). He and his co-authors designed the second paper for a research audience and compared muscle pressure and tooth position between North American whites and Australian Aboriginal people (Proffit *et al.*, 1975). The third paper focussed on speech production. The intention of this paper was to differentiate physiologically certain sounds made between Australian Aboriginal and North American subjects (Proffit and McGlone, 1975).

Stephen Molnar 1931–

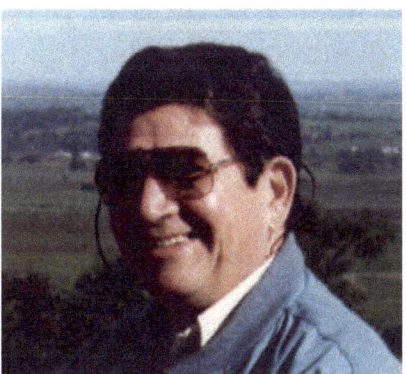

Figure 7.7
Stephen Molnar

Stephen Molnar, who was a PhD student of Loring Brace, became interested in tooth wear in relation to culture in early human populations. His descriptive publication, *Tooth wear and culture: A survey of tooth functions among some prehistoric populations* (Molnar, 1972), was described by Barrett as "a valuable review of tooth wear and culture which should stimulate further studies of tooth wear in relation to masticatory physiology and dental anthropology" (Barrett, 1972). In commenting on Molnar's paper, Barrett drew attention to his own studies and those of others that described the progress of tooth wear in Australian Aboriginal people from the stage of the deciduous dentition through adulthood to the eventual breakdown of the dental mechanism including the teeth and the temporomandibular joints, with consequential periapical and alveolar pathology.

The interest shown in his paper by Barrett and the expansive comments obviously encouraged Molnar to study tooth wear in Aboriginal people to expand his data from other groups. With this in mind, he corresponded with Barrett seeking permission to visit Adelaide and examine the cast collection and other available material. He received this permission and Molnar commenced the lengthy task of attracting research funding to enable his visit. It was unfortunate that delays in appropriate funding and other commitments prevented Molnar from making his visit to Adelaide until after Barrett's death in 1975. He eventually secured his research funding and arrived in Adelaide with his wife Iva in 1979 for an extended stay to study Aboriginal tooth wear rates, tooth wear variability and dental arch shape.

He compared data obtained from the skeletal material of the Murray River Valley (Swanport) region (then held by the South Australian Museum and since reburied), and data from the contemporary Aboriginal population at Yuendumu. The purpose of this research was to consider tooth wear and explain how it could contribute to dental disease and be a contributory factor to problems with dental occlusion. As time passed these comparisons became important when addressing questions about alterations in the dentition with changes from a nomadic subsistence-based lifestyle to a less demanding settlement lifestyle.

Molnar completed his observations in Adelaide and returned to Missouri and Washington University with further data and photographs from the Adelaide cast collection to provide material for ongoing studies with his PhD student, Jeff McKee, who completed his thesis on tooth wear and craniofacial shape a few years later (McKee, 1985). The St Louis group published several papers on these topics in the 1980s and 1990s (Molnar *et al.*, 1983a, 1983b; McKee and Molnar, 1988a, 1988b; Molnar *et al.*, 1989; Molnar and Molnar, 1990, 1992).

Subsequently Steve and Iva Molnar returned to Adelaide to help set up the chewing simulating machine that was to be used by the Adelaide group to study aspects of tooth wear and jaw movements (see Chapter 8).

Other interest from the USA

Documentary evidence of interest by Americans in the research work at Yuendumu can be traced back as far as 1963. **Coenraad Moorrees** from the Forsyth Dental Infirmary, Boston, Massachusetts, sent a letter to Murray Barrett asking to be kept informed of the research being conducted at Yuendumu, and to be sent reprints of work already published. Moorrees was particularly interested in the development of longitudinal growth studies.

Another American dentist who was interested in longitudinal growth studies was **Edward C McNulty**, who arrived in Adelaide in September 1966 as the recipient of a Special Research Fellowship awarded by the National Institute of Dental Research for one year. After the year had expired, he applied for, and received, a six-month extension. During his stay in Adelaide, he joined the field expedition to Yuendumu in May 1967. His proposed research project was accepted for candidature in the Master of Dental Surgery Degree programme at the University of Adelaide. He was interested in computer-based craniofacial measurement and analysis. His MDSc thesis investigated growth changes in the faces of Aboriginal people using a co-ordinate system to analyse cephalometric radiographs (McNulty, 1968). This study built on a technique pioneered by Thompson (1917) and applied by Moorrees (1953) that was based on the deformation of mesh grids. Two papers resulted from his analyses of the Yuendumu cephalometric material (Barrett *et al.*, 1968; McNulty *et al.*, 1968).

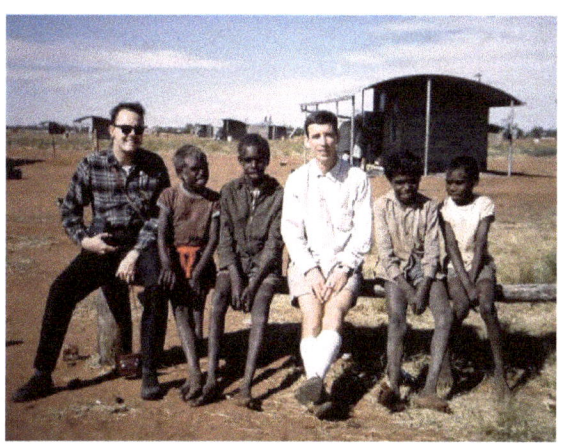

Figure 7.8
Edward McNulty (left) and R McClean with unidentified Warlpiri boys at Yuendumu, 1967

McNulty returned to the United States and eventually became the Professor and Chairman of the Department of Orthodontics, New York College of Dentistry. He died in early April 2001.

It should be noted that access to the records acquired during visits to Yuendumu was not restricted to dental graduates. They were also available to those whose interest was of a broader anthropological nature. One American anthropologist to study the Yuendumu dental models was **Charles Loring Brace**, who was interested in tooth size and its relation to the development of cooking technology and food habits. His description of tooth size clines explained variation in the indigenous population of Australia, using data from the Warlpiri and other geographical and temporal populations (Brace, 1980). His theory that migration and contact with Western foods and technology could influence Aboriginal people's tooth size has stimulated much interest and debate.

Robert Corruccini was another anthropologist whose interest concerned physical changes in the dentition. The essence of his research was dental occlusion and how occlusion could change over time. Looking at similar pre-contact Aboriginal specimens to those that Molnar had studied, Corruccini noted distinguishable changes in the occlusion between the skeletal material and the Yuendumu dental models. In a paper that considered measurable occlusal characteristics in Aboriginals, Corruccini noted that there were small but significant changes in features such as overbite, overjet, tooth rotations and tooth displacements over a generation. The essence of Corruccini's work was to describe and explain the noticeable physical characteristics of the dentition that occurred with transition from a hunter-gatherer lifestyle to a western-influenced settlement lifestyle (Corruccini *et al.*, 1990).

The Adelaide Researchers

Murray James Barrett 1916–1975

Murray James Barrett was born and educated in Adelaide, South Australia. He graduated with a Bachelor of Dental Surgery degree in 1939 from The University of Adelaide, and obtained a Master of Dental Surgery degree in 1949 after completing the requirements in the physical sciences and his chosen clinical field of prosthodontics. It is noteworthy that Barrett was the second person to obtain the MDSc degree at The University of Adelaide, opportunities for postgraduate study and research in fields of dentistry being scarce at that time. He was an undergraduate and postgraduate dental student under Campbell's Deanship and subsequently formed a working relationship with him after joining the teaching staff in 1947. In common with other dental students in Campbell's time, Barrett was influenced by Campbell's knowledge of Aboriginal life and customs and by his enthusiasm for exploring the relationships between diet, food habits and dental disease. After his graduation with the BDS degree, he served during the Second World War as a dental officer in the Royal Australian Air Force, with part of his service spent in Papua New Guinea. Besides gaining experience in clinical dentistry, the war provided Barrett with the opportunity to develop organisational skills and the necessary self-discipline for his future career.

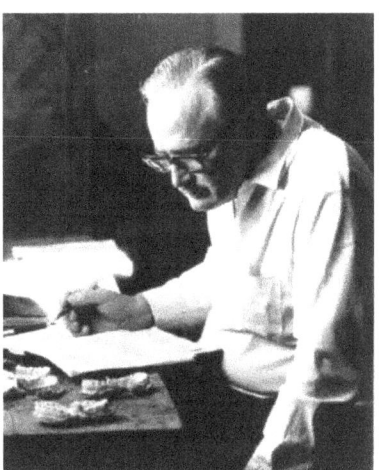

Figure 7.9
Murray James Barrett

He was a meticulous planner and organiser and, to a large extent, a perfectionist. In his later academic career it was not unusual for Barrett to amend draft after draft of a research paper, sometimes as many as ten times, before he felt it ready for publication. It was said of him that he acquired his talents for planning and organising from his time in the Air Force, and his mastery of the English language and devotion to anthropological research from Campbell (Rogers *et al.*, 2009). It is difficult to estimate the influence Campbell had over Barrett, but it would seem it was enough to persuade Barrett to devote his working life to academia as opposed to pursuing a career as a private dental practitioner.

When the Second World War ended in 1945, Barrett joined a general dental practice operated by Roger G Willoughby on North Terrace, Adelaide. Willoughby was a highly respected dental clinician and also a part-time tutor at the Dental School. It was probably on Willoughby's advice that Barrett undertook the Master of Dental Surgery course specialising in a clinical discipline. After obtaining this degree, a teaching career in the Dental School of The University of Adelaide appealed to Barrett and the University appointed him as a Demonstrator in Prosthetic Dentistry in 1947, Senior Demonstrator in 1949, and Reader (now Associate Professor) in 1951. An academic's two key roles are teaching and research, and Barrett's appointment as Reader elevated him to a senior position on the staff of the Dental School. After appointment his research direction was fostered by Campbell, and like

Campbell before him, Barrett had to balance his research interests with the teaching and administrative demands of a busy academic career.

In July 1957, Barrett submitted a thesis entitled "Dental Observations on Australian Aborigines" to the University of Adelaide's Education Committee to be considered for a doctorate degree award (DDSc). He based the thesis on observations made at Yuendumu during the field expeditions of the early 1950s. After consideration by the appointed external examiners, it was decided that the degree would not to be awarded. The examiners' reports, which are filed in The University of Adelaide archives, make it apparent that the main criticisms related to Barrett's inability to conform to either the conventional anthropological norms of the day or to the examiners' views of how such material should be presented. They may have confused the requirements for the Adelaide DDSc degree with those for the PhD degree in their own universities (Melbourne and Sydney). The DDSc regulations required a significant contribution to dental science in the form of a specially written thesis or a collection of papers. In the early 1960s, the Faculty of Dentistry decided to create a second chair alongside that of Professor AM Horsnell. The selected discipline was Restorative Dentistry and, as a senior staff member in this discipline, Murray Barrett was an obvious candidate. However, a change of Faculty objectives led to them establishing the proposed chair in the emerging field of Oral Biology, with Professor John Thonard being the successful candidate.

In 1973, Murray Barrett was nominated for a Personal Chair in Restorative Dentistry. This nomination and the letters supporting it emphasise the high level of support for Barrett by his colleagues. Letters of support came from Professors Profitt, Strehlow, Horsnell, de la Lande, Birdsell, Doctors Makinson and Beasley, as well as from Professors A Dahlberg, SJ Kreshover and G Davis (Barrett, 1953-1957). The nomination documents referred to the significance of Barrett's 50 research papers. In a letter of recommendation, the Head of the Adelaide Dental School, Professor AM Horsnell, drew attention to the $60,000 grant awarded to Barrett and Brown by the National Institutes of Health, USA, to support the Yuendumu study.

The Personal Chair Committee, which at the time was a sub-committee of the Council of the University, did not recommend Barrett's appointment to a Chair. No evidence exists in the University's archives as to the reasons for this decision. However, four candidates for Chairs within the University were nominated in the same year (1973) and presumably the academic standing of the other three candidates was considered to be greater than Murray Barrett's. At this time, the appointment of personal Chairs was a relatively recent innovation in The University of Adelaide. It was also a general rule of the University at that time to appoint only three academic staff to personal Chairs per year.

These decisions in no way lessened the magnitude of Barrett's academic achievements. While they were disappointing to Barrett from a personal point of view, if anything they strengthened his resolve to pursue and promote both his teaching and research endeavours.

Although research was a major factor in Murray Barrett's academic life, it did not consume every minute of his time. He was heavily involved in the management of the Adelaide Dental School, sat on various boards and committees within and outside the university, taught and supervised undergraduate and postgraduate students, and contributed to curriculum development.

For both the Faculty of Dentistry and the Dental School, the decade between 1960 and 1970 was a very active one in both departmental restructuring and building development. From these phases of re-structuring and development, Murray Barrett's abilities as both an administrator and committeeman become clear. He was prepared to argue strenuously for what he believed to be right and was meticulous in recording and storing all correspondence (both incoming and outgoing), no matter how insignificant.

Murray Barrett's invitation to be a member of the planning committee created to design the new dental hospital and school highlights another aspect of his administrative skills. This project began in 1958 and was completed in 1969. The demolition and construction comprised two stages, with Barrett having considerable input into the second stage (1964-1969). This stage was concerned with erection of a six-storey building designed to unite to the first stage construction's north wing (1962) and south wing (1964). The second-stage building committee comprised of Professors Horsnell and Thonard, and Doctors Barrett, Cran, Makinson, Sims and Scollin.

During this period (1964), Murray Barrett became Dean of the Faculty of Dentistry, succeeding Professor AM Horsnell, who was on sabbatical leave. The members of the Faculty elected him and he held the position of Dean for one year.

Despite his involvement in matters relating to university life, Barrett did not neglect his responsibilities to the profession. He was appointed Chairman of the Australian Dental Association (South Australian Branch) 1954 and Federal Councillor of the Australian Dental Association 1953, 1954. He also devoted time to serving on allied research boards. He was elected Chairman of the Board for Anthropological Research in 1968, and in the same year he was elected as a Member of the Australian Institute of Aboriginal Studies.

Yuendumu held a very special place in both the heart and mind of Murray Barrett, and it was shortly after his last sabbatical leave spent at Yuendumu that he died after major cancer surgery on 24 February 1975, aged 59 years.

Tasman Brown 1929–

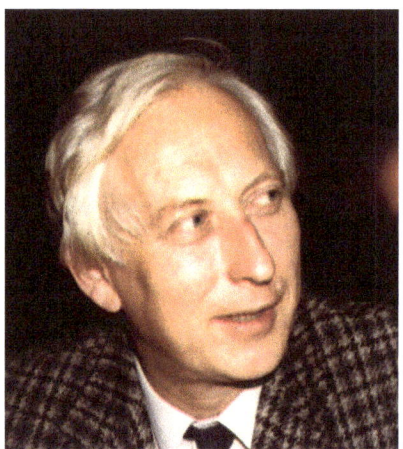

Figure 7.10
Tasman Brown

Tasman Brown graduated in dentistry from The University of Adelaide in 1950. Many of his teachers were prominent scientists of the mid-20th century. They included anatomists Andrew Abbie and Ross Adey, botanist/pathologist John Cleland, and dentist/anthropologist Draper Campbell. Murray Barrett was one of his clinical teachers. All had an important influence on Brown's future career, fostering his interest in basic sciences, particularly Campbell who regularly drew upon his profound knowledge of Aboriginal people to illustrate lectures in dental anatomy. All these teachers were members of the team to visit Yuendumu in 1951 under Campbell's leadership.

After graduation, Brown worked in a country dental practice for nine years, all but six months as the sole practitioner. His experience as a clinician served as an important foundation for a later academic career. Few opportunities for further study were available at that time but in 1958 he commenced a programme of coursework and research for a Master's degree. The inclusion of biological sciences in the programme convinced him that he should follow a career in academia rather than in private dental practice. The outcome of this decision was his appointment in 1960 as Lecturer in Dental Anatomy at the Dental School, The University of Adelaide, to take over the teaching duties of the recently retired Draper Campbell.

His location in the Anatomy Department brought him into closer association with Professor Abbie, who was later appointed his supervisor for the research component of the Master's degree. As part of his duties, Brown presented lectures in topographical anatomy, dental anatomy and comparative anatomy as well as tutoring in histology and clinical dental practice. Thus, he became fully committed to basic science teaching and research. At the time, Abbie was conducting his anthropometric survey of Australian Aboriginal communities and publishing extensively in the fields of anatomy and physical anthropology. It was an exciting environment in which to work.

Brown's future research direction was decided when Murray Barrett invited him to join his long-term dental study at Yuendumu. Barrett wished to take the Yuendumu project to another level by augmenting his observations of the dentition with a parallel study of general and craniofacial growth, somatometry and skeletal maturation. The first field trip incorporating this new approach was in 1961, with Brown undertaking the additional observations. After the 1961 trip, Brown completed his Master's degree in 1963 with a thesis on craniofacial variations that the Libraries Board of South Australia later published (Brown, 1965). As his supervisor for this research, Abbie introduced Brown to the wider anthropological literature, including classical texts in foreign languages. At the same time, Brown immersed himself in the scientific writings of dental anthropologists including Campbell, Moorrees, Pedersen, Seipel and Lundström. The medical and anthropological literature relating to Australian Aboriginal people was also essential reading.

During the following years, Murray Barrett and Tasman Brown co-authored a series of papers dealing with tooth morphology, tooth eruption and craniofacial growth. At times, they shared authorship with postgraduate students or other collaborators. This Yuendumu research was facilitated by a generous research grant to Barrett and Brown from the Institute of Dental Research, National Institutes of

Health, Bethesda, Maryland. In 1962, the installation of computing facilities for general use in the university was a significant event for Brown. Barrett and Brown now had the means to process their accumulating data from Yuendumu speedily and accurately. They attended courses to achieve competency in computer programming, a skill they retained and used extensively.

It soon became apparent to Brown that he should apply multivariate analysis to his Yuendumu cephalometric and somatometric data to examine the interactions between multiple variables. The pioneer work by Professor William Howells and his students at Harvard University's Department of Anthropology provided a useful model. After developing and testing appropriate computer programmes against published examples, Brown felt ready to apply the methodology of factor analysis to a series of craniometric variables obtained from skeletal material.

During a sabbatical leave taken in 1966 at the Royal Dental College, Denmark, Brown studied the concepts and methodology of Professor Arne Björk, who pioneered the use of metallic implants to analyse facial growth. Brown also met Beni Solow, the Department Leader, who was also applying multivariate analysis to cephalometric data. The two enjoyed many vigorous and beneficial discussions on their experience with the method. Later that year Beni Solow published his doctoral dissertation (Solow, 1966). Brown received his DDSc degree in 1968, and the Australian Institute of Aboriginal Studies, Canberra, later published his thesis, with minor revisions (Brown, 1973). Apart from his work with Björk and Solow, Brown renewed acquaintance with Sven Helm, a dental epidemiologist who had spent time in the Adelaide laboratory the previous year.

Before returning to Adelaide, Brown travelled to the United States to establish contact with several researchers involved in anthropology or growth studies, including C Moorrees, E Hunt Jr and W Howells in Boston, WM Krogman in Philadelphia, S Garn in Yellow Springs and R Moyers in Michigan. The last visit on this trip was to Tokyo, where he met Tadashi Ozaki ahead of Ozaki's forthcoming extended stay in Adelaide.

Brown joined Barrett and others on annual field trips to Yuendumu until 1971 when the data-gathering phase of the study concluded. After Murray Barrett's death in 1975, Brown was determined to build upon his colleague's heritage by taking the study in new directions. Honours and postgraduate students continued to work in what was known at the time as the Anthropology and Genetics Research

Laboratory. Of special importance and relevance to the new directions were the projects of his three PhD students. Grant Townsend specialised in dental morphology and genetics and used the accumulated family data from Yuendumu to produce one of the first detailed analyses of genetic and environmental determinants of tooth size (Townsend, 1976). Lindsay Richards directed his research to the study of masticatory function, leading to a definitive account of adaptation to heavy occlusal loading and excessive tooth wear (Richards, 1983). Amanda Abbott initiated a new phase of the research. With Brown, she developed methods for the acquisition of cephalometric data in three dimensions. She also explored the use of finite element analysis to these types of data (Abbott, 1988).

The 1970s and 1980s were busy years for Brown. Further sabbaticals brought him back to Denmark in 1973 and 1979, when he collaborated with Arne Björk and assistant Vibeke Skieller in a study of facial growth (Björk *et al.*, 1984). Discussions with Beni Solow led to him adopting his unique method for producing growth charts from semi-longitudinal data. Brown later programmed this for the analysis of the Yuendumu somatometric data (Appendix B). During these decades, he also visited Tanner and Whitehouse in London, studying the methods they used in the acquisition and analysis of growth data. Here, Brown also discussed the curve-fitting methods of Preece and Baines and later applied them to the Yuendumu height measurements (Brown and Townsend, 1982). Two scientists from the United States spent extended visits to the Adelaide laboratory around this time and each worked with the Adelaide team to develop new research concepts and methodology. Stephen Molnar from St Louis, Missouri, was an expert in tooth wear, and Bhim Savara from Portland, Oregon, introduced his technique for three-dimensional photography and measurement. Brown and Abbott later expanded this and applied it to biplanar cephalometric radiographs at the Australian Craniofacial Unit.

After a period as Visiting Professor at the School of Dentistry at Matsudo, Japan, with Professor Tadashi Ozaki, and a further month as Visiting Professor at the Dental School, Dunedin University, New Zealand, with Professor Martin Kean, Tasman Brown retired from his full-time post at the university in 1991. He continued to supervise students and participate in research and accepted a part-time appointment as Research Director at the Australian Craniofacial Unit, Adelaide. In this role, Brown applied his experience in computer technology and cephalometric research to assist in the development of three-dimensional data acquisition and, for the Unit's orthodontist, a comprehensive semi-automatic system for cephalometric analysis. The Unit used these systems for the analysis and diagnosis of craniofacial abnormalities. He retired from the Unit in 1998.

During his academic career, Tasman Brown served on many local and national committees, was Dean of the Dental Faculty for a term and in 1978 received the inaugural Alan Docking Prize for research awarded by the International Association for Research (Australian and New Zealand Division). In 1994, he was made a Member of the Order of Australia for his contributions to dental research and postgraduate dental education.

Other staff on the project

Several staff members of the Adelaide Dental School visited Yuendumu or other Aboriginal communities on one or more occasions, either to follow their own line of research or to assist the principal investigators in their work schedules.

Alexander Cran, an oral pathologist, travelled to Yuendumu in the years 1956, 1957 and 1958 with Campbell and Barrett to investigate the teeth and gingivae of Central Australian Aboriginal people. From this initial research, he published papers concerning diet and dental caries (Cran, 1959, 1960).

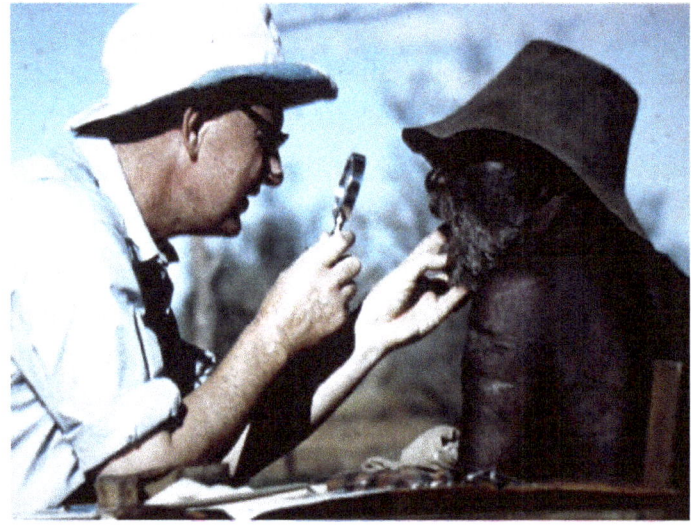

Figure 7.11
Alec Cran examines an unidentified Warlpiri man, 1955 (courtesy of PG Dellow)

Geoffrey Heithersay, an Adelaide dentist, did not visit Yuendumu, but spent time at Haast's Bluff in 1956 as a member of a team led by Professor Andrew Abbie of The University of Adelaide. Heithersay conducted a dental survey that led to the publication of observations on the Haast's Bluff community (Heithersay, 1959, 1960, 1961). **Elizabeth Fanning**, who was the Reader in Dental Health, joined the Yuendumu research team in 1962 to assist in the radiological examinations. She was co-author with Barrett and Brown in a paper describing the long-term objectives of the Yuendumu study (Barrett *et al.*, 1965) and she later co-authored papers on tooth formation in Australian Aboriginal people and Australians of European ancestry (Fanning and Moorrees, 1969; Fanning and Brown, 1971).

Peter Reade, a specialist in immunology and dental medicine, visited Yuendumu in 1961 and again in 1966. After an earlier field visit to Koonibba in South Australia, he published a report on his dental observations of the Aboriginal population (Reade, 1965). In 1970, **John Williamson**, an oral surgeon, was a member of the Yuendumu team when he studied the oral health of young children and adults. **Grant Townsend**, who was an undergraduate dental student at the time, also travelled to Yuendumu and acted as a recorder in this study. The aim of the investigation was to establish guidelines related to the levels of oral mucosal and periodontal health, as well as the prevalence of dental caries and other observable pathological conditions. Associated with this study was an assessment of the prevalence and severity of fluorosis in the Yuendumu children. The results of this work appeared in two papers (Barrett and Williamson, 1972; Williamson and Barrett, 1972).

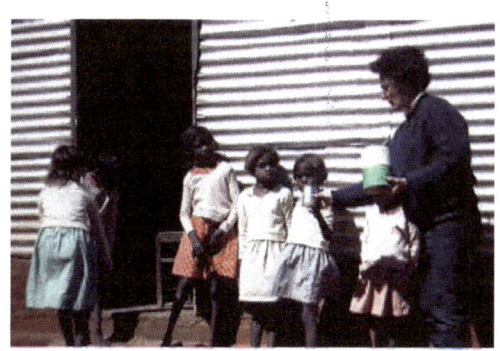 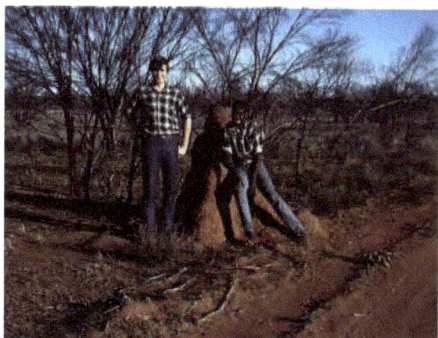

Figure 7.12
Left, Elizabeth Fanning with a group of school girls in 1962, and right, Grant Townsend and an unidentified Warlpiri man in 1970

The Adelaide researchers and those who came from overseas to study at Yuendumu always received substantial support from numerous members of The University of Adelaide professional staff. **Leslie Reynolds**, **Norman Harrison** and **Thomas Rollings** provided the dental technical requirements. **Sandra Pinkerton**, **Marie Cummings**, **Geraldine Kuusk, Wendy Schwerdt** and others provided secretarial expertise and laboratory assistance to both Murray Barrett and Tasman Brown. More recently, **Michelle Bockmann** has become the Manager of the Murray Barrett Research Laboratory and **Karen Squires** has provided administrative assistance to members of the Craniofacial Biology Research Group.

At Yuendumu

The Warlpiri men **Harry Nelson Jakamarra**, **Jimmy Jungarrayi** and **Sandy Japaljarri** were always at hand to find participants and to help fulfil requests that were difficult to meet without a detailed knowledge of the local community and their customs. These men and many other local Warlpiri were ever helpful in enlisting community participation and approval. The local teachers were always co-operative

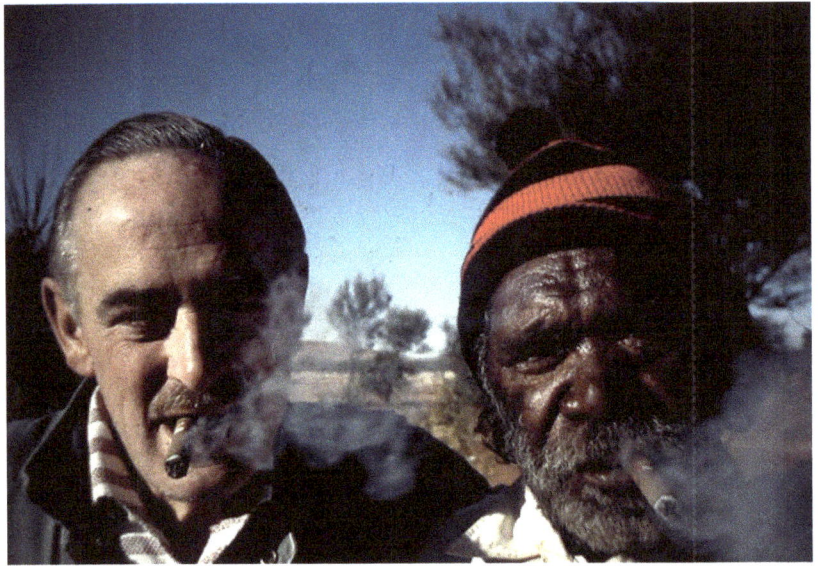

Figure 7.13
Murray Barrett and Jimmy Jungarrayi Spencer

and willingly assisted the researchers when school children were scheduled for examination.

The Missionaries: Tom Fleming (1909–1990) and Pat Fleming (1914–1995)

Tom Fleming and his wife Pat were Baptist missionaries at Yuendumu for 25 years. Not only did they host the dental teams during many periods of fieldwork, but also they played an integral and very essential role in the dental study itself. Without their freely given hospitality, assistance and knowledge of the Warlpiri, the long-term study would hardly have been established let alone continued for many years.

After theological training in Melbourne, Tom Fleming worked with the Baptist Home Mission and then when war intervened in 1939, he enlisted in the Second A.I.F., eventually transferring to the Y.M.C.A. He served with the Eighth Division, first in Malaya and then as a prisoner of war in Singapore. From there, the Japanese sent him to the Sandakan prison camp in British North Borneo (now Sabah) and then to Kuching.

Although his time in the Japanese prison camps left him in ill health for some months after the war, he became interested in inland missions, Yuendumu in particular. He applied for and was accepted for the position of Baptist missionary at Yuendumu, where Tom and Pat arrived in April 1950. They remained there until Tom's retirement to Alice Springs in July 1975.

The Flemings were well known and respected throughout the Northern Territory for their work at Yuendumu. Their achievement at Yuendumu is the church with its stained glass windows.

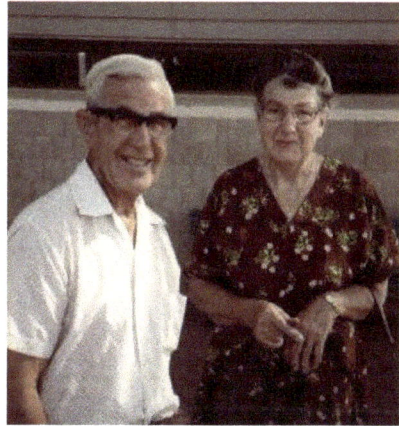

Figure 7.14
Tom and Pat Fleming (courtesy of Jolyon Fleming)

After Tom Fleming's death in 1990, his widow Pat received many written tributes that express the esteem in which Tom was held. Extracts from three of these tributes follow.

The Flemings and the Dental Teams

By Tasman Brown, The University of Adelaide, written in September 1992

The association between the Flemings and the dentists from Adelaide commenced in 1951 when the first team of scientists from Adelaide visited Yuendumu Settlement, the year after Pat and Tom had arrived at the recently established Baptist Mission. As a consequence of this visit the team leader Draper Campbell and Murray Barrett became good friends of the Flemings who took a close interest in the studies being conducted.

In the 1950s, Draper Campbell produced a series of documentary films on the life and crafts of the Warlpiri people. Barrett was the camera man. In addition Barrett commenced a longitudinal growth study involving dental examinations and dental models of young children. Tom was a fruitful source of information on numerous occasions during these years. His knowledge of the Aboriginal people was encyclopedic when it came to customs, beliefs, kinships and many other aspects of Warlpiri life. His input into a paper regarding the Warlpiri practice of removing an anterior tooth was significant (Barrett *et al.,* 1978).

The hospitality and kindness afforded all guests by Tom and Pat was given generously without thought of the personal inconvenience that the never-ending stream of visitors caused. Even a casual glimpse at the Flemings' Visitors' Book from Yuendumu conjures up visions of the many people descending on these kind people in their own home - clergy, dentists, doctors, psychiatrists, politicians, writers, dancers, curators, anthropologists, anatomists, to name a few. The annual visits of the dental teams were marked by fairly continuous scientific work during the day, tempered by times of relaxation when Tom would take us with him on one of his pastoral visits to a neighbouring cattle station. During our visits to Yuendumu, Pat provided most evening meals although I might add there was always some assistance with the washing-up on these occasions. Tom generously made his first church building available for our work area, provided we tidied the room prior to the Sunday services.

The success of the research work is indicated by the publication of numerous papers over the years and by the esteem in which the Yuendumu material is held by scientists worldwide. Tom was a quiet and continuing contributor to the success of this scientific work. One example could be singled out. Since the earliest days of the ministry at Yuendumu, Tom and Pat had maintained detailed records of births, deaths and marriages in the Warlpiri community. Without any doubt, these records were the most complete of their kind for any Aboriginal community. With the assistance of Murray Barrett, these records were computerised and constantly checked and re-checked by informants every year. Pat amended the records regularly and these amendments were forwarded to Adelaide to be computerised. The records have been used on numerous occasions for a variety of purposes. Many years ago, Doctor Nicholas Peterson made extensive use of them during legal consideration of the land claims in Central Australia. The Yuendumu council of elders also makes considerable use of them as they contain the only documented records of former generations for many Aboriginal families.

From a scientific point of view, the family records have proved to be extremely valuable because genealogies can be constructed from them. These genealogies, which define mother-father-son-daughter relationships within families as well as cross-family relationships, have been verified by blood analysis to be substantially correct. The great advantage of access to accurate genealogies for genetic research is that they allow the scientist to estimate the influence of genes and environment on the natural variation observed in populations. A dental scientist from Adelaide, Grant Townsend (*now Professor*), used the Yuendumu genealogies and dental models to show that inheritance accounted for only about 60% to 70% of variation in the size of teeth. The study was one of the first in the world to demonstrate this and the findings changed our thinking about dental development and helped to explain the way in which environmental conditions affect our dental appearance and function. Several other genetic studies using these genealogies have followed. By assisting in the compilation of Warlpiri genealogies Tom and Pat Fleming had a very substantial input into a piece of work that became quite significant in the scientific world (Fleming *et al.*, 1971).

[…]

Films were also shown regularly at Yuendumu, the feature of the week being eagerly awaited. These were always a source of enjoyment, particularly Westerns which were great favourites. On special occasions, usually when the Adelaide dental team was in residence, one of the documentary films produced by Campbell and Barrett and illustrating Warlpiri crafts would be shown. A capacity audience would attend, usually with Tom presiding over proceedings. Howls of sheer delight would follow the appearance on the screen of one of the film's performers who, of course would be known to every member of the audience and related to many. Usually the *star* would be present for the screening.

[…]

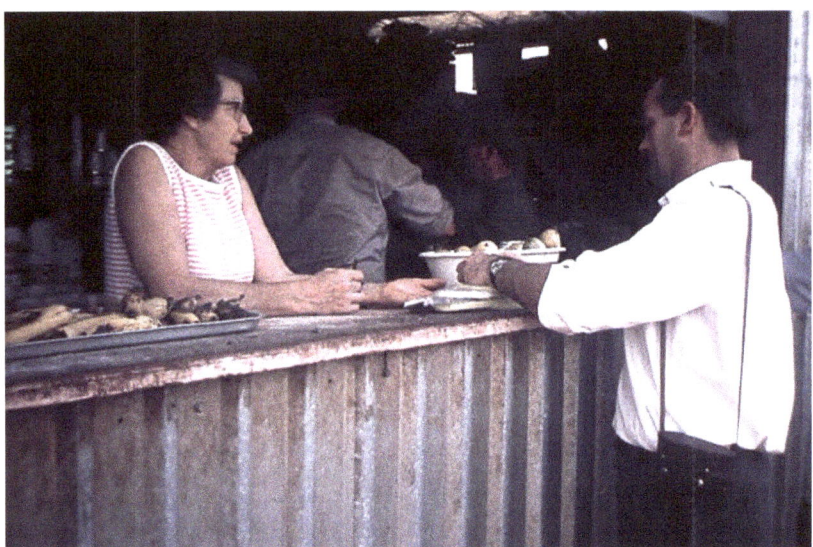

Figure 7.15
Pat Fleming serving team member Michael Nugent at the Yuendumu store, 1969

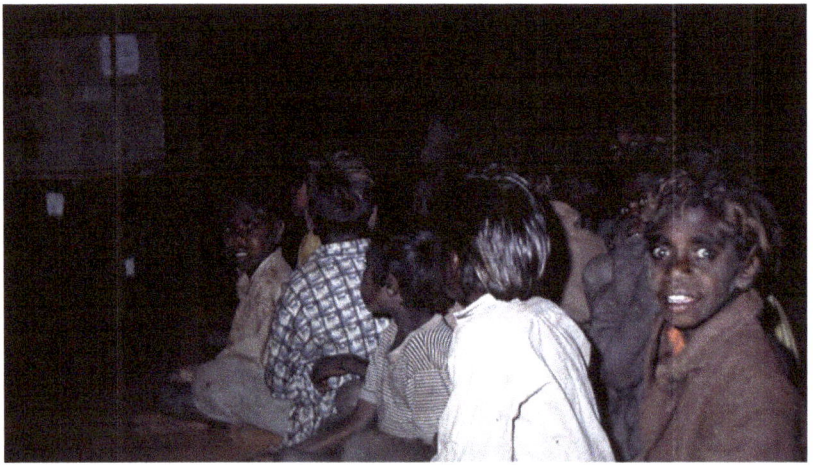

Figure 7.16
Benjamin Japangadi and friends at a movie evening at Yuendumu

By Ted Egan, Superintendent at Yuendumu 1958–62, Administrator of The Northern Territory 2003–07

It's not surprising that a benign man like Tom Fleming would end up being called "Tom Father". His hair was prematurely white, no doubt one of the health-shattering results of years in a Japanese POW camp. But it was more his gentle, wise, reliable presence that gave him the father figure stature.

You always felt that here was a well of knowledge and wisdom that you could always draw from. His intelligent eyes would focus his undivided attention on you, and he made you feel you were the most important person in the world, and that your beliefs and attitudes were eminently worth his time. He had a wry sense of humour, and the sort of tolerance you would expect from a man who was truly Christ-like.

He was obviously a deeply religious man, yet I never once discussed religion with him. I feel sure his thesis on religion was that it was something you displayed by your own lifestyle and code of ethics, rather than something you tried to impose on people by rigid precepts. I met Tom, his dear wife Pat, and their boys Adrian and Jolyon at Yuendumu, where Tom was the Baptist Minister for many years, and I was the Superintendent of the Aboriginal Reserve for four of those years 1958–62. Tom and Pat were wonderful support for me in what were often difficult times, and we developed a lifelong friendship therefrom. We shared a lot of dramas, and some parental laughs for I had young children of my own, and they and the Fleming boys mixed freely, as friends and playmates, with the local Aboriginal kids. One day we all raised our eyebrows as five-year olds Greg Egan and Jolyon Fleming got into a dust-up and began to use language that Tom said "took him back to the war years".

Among the Aboriginal people and the station people of Central Australia, the Reverend Tom Fleming was much-loved and deeply respected. He went slowly about the work of spreading the Christian message, for he did not seek miracles, or too forcefully proselytise, or create "rice Christians' through gifts or coercion. His own demeanour, and his unabashed love of his fellow human-beings, unsoured by his horrible war experiences, were the attributes which caused him to have such a profound influence on everybody he met.

While as a friend I mourn his passing, I know that men such as "Tom Father' never really die. One of the cleverest catch-lines of advertising I have ever seen was the bye-line used to promote the film Crocodile Dundee. Above the poster of the laconic Paul Hogan was the statement "There's a little bit of him in all of us". Well, there's a bit of Tom Fleming in all the people who ever met him, for he gave you all he had, and asked nothing in return.

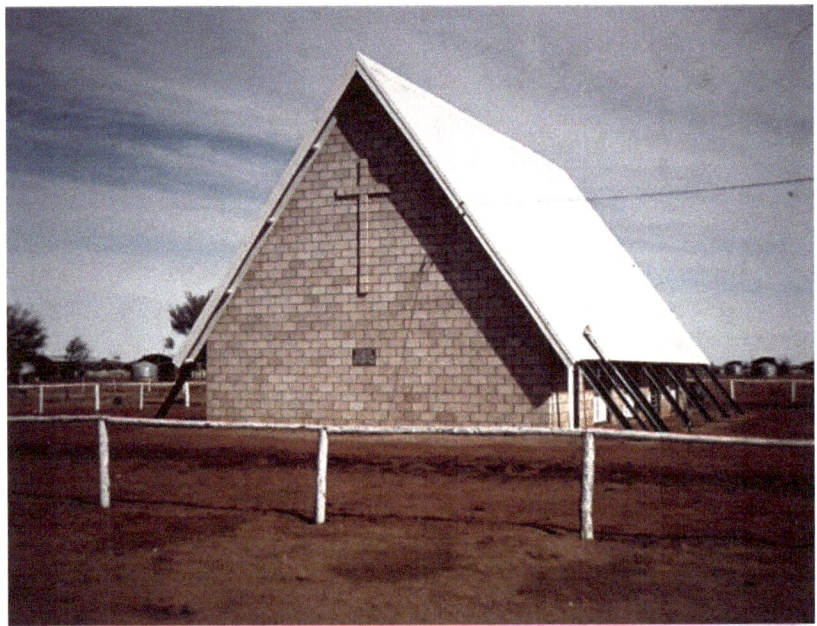

Figure 7.17
The "new" church at Yuendumu

By James Marshall, Warlpiri man from Yuendumu

We will never forget old Fleming.

He was like a father for us. He helped and guided us, and was always thinking of the future and taught and trained us for the future.

In the early days when there was no policeman, when there was trouble and fighting he would go and help sort it out.

Jungarrayi started everything here - the Social Club, the sports weekend, the museum. He had a lot of feeling for yapa[1]. He wanted to help them go the right way.

---

1   Yapa - the term for Warlpiri people. (TB)

He was always there in trouble. He helped me when I was in trouble and they were going to spear me. He went and talked to them in the camp for me and helped sort things out.

He was always with the old people - always helping them. He knew them. He was always in the sorry camps with the people.

He wasn't in a hurry to make people Christians. He didn't force people. He thought about Christianity yapa way.

He never tried to throw our culture away. He was a man of God but he was always thinking of supporting the culture.

Today there are a lot of people in this community who have been trained to do different things because of Jungarrayi.

He loved Yuendumu and Central Australia and died close to here.

He knew everything about Warlpiri people. The paintings in the church window show that.

When he died and they had a service for him, all the people came. People came from other places too. That is what they all thought of him.

References

Abbott AH (1988). *The Acquisition and Analysis of Craniofacial Data in Three Dimensions.* PhD Thesis, The University of Adelaide.

Barrett MJ (1953–1957). *Correspondence and personal notes.* Murray James Barrett Laboratory, School of Dentistry, The University of Adelaide.

Barrett MJ (1957). *Dental Observations on Australian Aborigines.* Thesis presented for the Degree of Doctor of Dental Science. Murray James Barrett Laboratory, Dental School, The University of Adelaide.

Barrett MJ (1972). Tooth wear and culture: a survey of tooth functions among some prehistoric populations. Molnar S, editor. Comment in: *Curr Anthropol* 13:516.

Barrett MJ, Fleming TJ, Djagamara NA (1978). *Tooth evulsion in the Walbiri area.* Canberra: Australian Institute of Aboriginal Studies. (Restricted Access Publication.)

Barrett MJ, Brown T, Fanning EA (1965). A long-term study of the dental and craniofacial characteristics of a tribe of Central Australian Aborigines. *Aust Dent J* 10:63–68.

Barrett MJ, Brown T, McNulty EC (1968). A computer-based system of dental and craniofacial measurement and analysis. *Aust Dent J* 13:207–212.

Barrett MJ, Williamson JJ (1972). Oral health of Australian Aborigines: survey methods and prevalence of dental caries. *Aust Dent J* 17:37–50.

Beyron H (1964). Occlusal relations and mastication in Australian Aborigines. *Acta Odontol Scand* 22:597–678.

Björk A (1947). The Face in Profile. An anthropological x-ray investigation on Swedish children and conscripts. *Svensk Tandläkare-Tidskrift* (40 Suppl).

Björk A (1955). Facial growth in man, studied with the aid of metallic implants. *Acta Odontol Scand* 13:9–34.

Björk A (1968). The use of metallic implants in the study of facial growth in children: Method and application. *Am J Phys Anthropol* 29: 243–254.

Björk A, Helm S (1969). Need for orthodontic treatment as reflected in the prevalence of malocclusion in various ethnic groups. *Acta Socio-Med Scand* (1 Suppl):209S–214S.

Björk A, Brown T, Skieller V (1984). Comparison of craniofacial growth in an Australian Aboriginal and Danes, illustrated by longitudinal cephalometric analysis. *Eur J Orthod* 6:1–14.

Brace CL (1980). Australian tooth-size clines and the death of a stereotype. *Curr Anthropol* 21:141–164.

Brown T (1965). *Craniofacial Variations in a Central Australian Tribe: A Radiographic Investigation of Young Adult Males and Females.* Adelaide: Libraries Board of South Australia.

Brown T (1973). *Morphology of the Australian Skull Studied by Multivariate Analysis.* Canberra: Australian Institute of Aboriginal Studies. Australian Aboriginal Studies No. 49.

Brown T, Townsend GC (1982). Adolescent growth in height of Australian Aboriginals analysed by the Preece-Baines function: a longitudinal study. *Ann Hum Biol* 9:495–505.

Brown T, Barrett MJ, Grave KC (1971). Facial growth and skeletal maturation at adolescence. *Tandlaegebladet* 75:1221–1222.

Corruccini RS, Townsend GC, Brown T (1990). Occlusal variation in Australian Aboriginals. *Am J Phys Anthropol* 82:257–265.

Cran JA (1959). Relationship of diet to dental caries. *Aust Dent J* 4:182–190.

Cran JA (1960). Histological structure of the teeth of Central Australian Aborigines and the relationship to dental caries incidence. *Aust Dent J* 5:100–104.

Fanning EA, Moorrees CFA (1969). A comparison of permanent mandibular molar formation in Australian Aborigines and Caucasoids. *Arch Oral Biol* 14:999–1006.

Fanning EA, Brown T (1971). Primary and permanent tooth development. *Aust Dent J* 16:41–43.

Fleming DA, Barrett MJ, Fleming TJ (1971). Family records of an Australian Aboriginal community. *Abor Stud News* 3:15.

Hanihara K (1970). Preliminary reports on dental anthropology of the Australian Aborigines. (in Japanese) *J Anthrop Soc Nippon* 78:75–76.

Hanihara K (1974). Factors controlling crown size of the deciduous dentition. (in English). *J Anthrop Soc Nippon* 82:128–134.

Hanihara K (1976). *Statistical and comparative studies of the Australian Aboriginal dentition*. Bulletin, No.11. The University Museum, The University of Tokyo, Tokyo.

Hanihara K (1977). Distance between Australian Aborigines and certain other populations based on dental measurements. *J Hum Evol* 6:403–418.

Hanihara K (1978). Difference in sexual dimorphism in dental morphology among several human populations In: *Development, Function and Evolution of Teeth*. Butler PM, Joysey KA, editors. London: Academic Press, pp. 127–133.

Hanihara K (1979). Dental traits in Ainu, Australian Aborigines, and New World populations. In: *The First Americans: Origins, Affinities and Adaptions*. Laughlin WS, Harper AB, editors. New York: Gustav Fischer, pp. 125–134.

Heithersay GS (1959). A dental survey of the Aborigines at Haast's Bluff, Central Australia. *Med J Aust* 1:721–729.

Heithersay GS (1960). Attritional values for Australian Aborigines, Haast's Bluff. *Aust Dent J* 5:84–88.

Heithersay GS (1961). Further observations on the dentition of the Australian aborigines at Haast's Bluff. *Aust Dent J* 6:18–28.

Helm S (1979). Etiology and treatment need of malocclusion. *J Can Dent Assoc* 45:673–676.

Kanazawa E, Morris DH, Sekikawa M, Ozaki T (1988). Comparative study of the upper molar occlusal table morphology among seven human populations. *Am J Phys Anthropol* 77:271–278

Kasai K, Richards LC, Brown T (1993). Comparative study of craniofacial morphology in Japanese and Australian Aboriginal populations. *Hum Biol* 65:821–834.

McKee JK (1985). *Patterns of Dental Attrition and Craniofacial Shape Among Australian Aborigines*. PhD Thesis, The Washington University, St. Louis.

McKee JK, Molnar S (1988a). Measurements of tooth wear among Australian Aborigines: II Intrapopulational variation in patterns of dental attrition. *Am J Phys Anthropol* 76:125–136.

McKee JK, Molnar S (1988b). Mathematical and descriptive classification of variations in dental arch shape in an Australian Aboriginal population. *Arch Oral Biol* 33:901–906.

McNulty EC (1968). *Growth Changes in the Face. A semi-longitudinal Cephalometric Study of the Australian Aboriginal by Means of a Coordinate Analysis*. MDSc Thesis, The University of Adelaide.

McNulty EC, Barrett MJ, Brown T (1968). Mesh diagram analysis of facial morphology in young adult Australian Aborigines. *Aust Dent J* 13:440–446.

Molnar S (1972). Tooth wear and culture: A survey of tooth functions among some prehistoric populations. *Curr Anthropol* 13:511–515.

Molnar S, McKee JK, Molnar I, Przybeck TR (1983a). Tooth wear rates among contemporary Australian Aborigines. *J Dent Res* 62:562–564.

Molnar S, McKee JK, Molnar I (1983b). Measurements of tooth wear among Australian Aborigines: I. Serial loss of the enamel crown. *Am J Phys Anthropol* 61:51–65.

Molnar S, Richards LC, McKee JK, Molnar I (1989). Tooth wear in Australian Aboriginal populations from the River Murray Valley. *Am J Phys Anthropol* 79:185–196.

Molnar S, Molnar IM (1990). Dental arch shape and tooth wear variability. *Am J Phys Anthropol* 82:385–395.

Molnar S, Molnar I (1992). Dental arch shape and tooth wear among the prehistoric populations of the Murray River valley. In: *Craniofacial Variation in Pacific Populations*. Brown T, Molnar S, editors. Adelaide, South Australia: Anthropology and Genetics Laboratory, The University of Adelaide, pp. 99–112.

Moorrees CFA (1953). Normal variation and its bearing on the use of cephalometric radiographs in orthodontic diagnosis. *Am J Orthod* 39:942–950.

Ozaki T, Kanazawa E, Sekikawa M, Akai J (1987). Three-dimensional measurement of occlusal surface of upper first molars in Australian Aboriginals. *Aust Dent J* 32:263–269.

Proffit WR (1975). Muscle pressure and tooth position: North American Whites and Australian Aborigines. *Angle Orthod* 45:1–11.

Proffit WR, McGlone RE (1975). Tongue-lip pressure during speech of Australian Aborigines. *Phonetica* 32:200–220.

Proffit WR, McGlone RE, Barrett MJ (1975). Lip and tongue pressure related to dental arch and oral cavity size in Australian Aborigines. *J Dent Res* 54:1161–1172.

Reade PC (1965). Dental observations on Australian Aborigines, Koonibba, South Australia. *Aust Dent J* 10:361–370.

Richards LC (1983). *Adaptation in the Masticatory System: Descriptive and Correlative Studies of a Pre-Contemporary Australian Population*. PhD Thesis, The University of Adelaide.

Rogers J, Townsend G, Brown T (2009). Murray James Barrett dental anthropologist: Yuendumu and beyond. *HOMO J Comp Hum Biol* 60:295–306.

Sekikawa M, Akai J, Kanazawa E, Ozaki T (1986). Three-dimensional measurement of the occlusal surfaces of lower first molars of Australian Aboriginals. *Am J Phys Anthropol* 71:25–32.

Sekikawa M, Kanazawa E, Ozaki T, Brown T (1988). Principal component analysis of intercusp distances on the lower first molars of three human populations. *Arch Oral Biol* 33:535–541.

Solow B (1966). The Pattern of Craniofacial Associations. A Morphological and Methodological correlation and Factor Analysis Study of Young Adult Males. *Acta Odontol Scand* 24 (Suppl 46).

Solow B, Barrett MJ, Brown T (1982). Craniocervical morphology and posture in Australian Aboriginals. *Am J Phys Anthropol* 59:33–45.

Thompson, DW (1917). *On Growth and Form*. London: Cambridge University Press.

Townsend GC (1976). *Tooth Size Variability in Australian Aboriginals: A Descriptive and Genetic Study.* PhD Thesis, The University of Adelaide.

Williamson JJ, Barrett MJ (1972). Oral health of Australian Aborigines: endemic dental fluorosis. *Aust Dent J* 17:266–268.

8
The Past, the Present and the Future

The end of field trips to Yuendumu and the post-1970 years

The early stages of the Yuendumu Growth Study received research funding from The University of Adelaide. From April 1964, the project received substantial support for a further seven years until March 1971 from a Public Health Service Grant of the United States Department of Health, Education and Welfare. The National Institute of Dental Research, Bethesda, Maryland, approved this grant.

Towards the end of the 1960s it was becoming apparent to Barrett and Brown that a decision was needed about whether to continue the yearly visits to Yuendumu after the grant expired or to stop and concentrate more on data analysis. Time was always a precious commodity, and so much of it was required to make the field trips worthwhile. The extensive organisation needed to plan the trips and the costs involved made it increasingly difficult to justify further visits to Yuendumu after the 1971 expedition. They reached the decision to stop the field trips after considering several factors. First and foremost was the vast accumulation of field records awaiting further analysis: 1,717 sets of dental casts representing 446 participants, 1169 sets of radiographs representing 288 individuals, as well as somatometric observations, family histories, photographs, and film and sound recordings.

Table 8.1 indicates the "longitudinality" of the records obtained between 1961 and 1971. For example, the third row shows that 31 children were 6 years of age at first examination. Only one of these children was examined on 10 occasions, but 10 were examined on 9 occasions, 14 on 8 occasions and so on. The oldest of these participants in 1971 was 15 years. Some of the group were younger because not all had their first examination in 1961. The researchers examined most of the participants often enough to provide the full range of records through adolescence. They examined about one-third on six or more occasions.

Table 8.1 The distribution of 288 participants with the full range of records by age at first examination and the number of sets of serial records

Age at first examination	Number of serial records										Maximum age
	1	2	3	4	5	6	7	8	9	10	
4	2	2	2	2	2	1	1	1	1	–	13
5	10	9	6	6	5	5	4	4	2	–	14
6	31	28	23	22	20	15	14	14	10	1	15
7	34	30	25	24	20	15	13	9	5	1	16
8	34	32	30	30	27	21	17	16	6	2	17
9	24	23	22	22	17	15	15	8	3	2	18
10	18	16	16	15	15	15	9	6	1	–	19
11	20	18	13	10	8	5	2	–	–	–	20
12	19	17	10	6	4	3	1	1	–	–	21
13	11	9	6	3	3	1	–	–	–	–	22
14	12	6	2	–	–	–	–	–	–	–	23
15	73	8	1	1	–	–	–	–	–	–	>24
Total	288	198	156	141	121	96	76	59	28	6	

Although considerable progress occurred during the 1960s, further research was urgently required. How such large quantities of material could be analysed was a question that dominated thinking for many years. Complex computer programmes were written to cope with the special difficulties in analysing mixed longitudinal growth data. It was essential to acquire and process data faster and also to apply more sophisticated statistical and mathematical approaches to analyses as computer systems became more powerful. Methods of preservation and storage of the collected materials had to be developed so that future researchers would be able to access well-labelled, undamaged material. Valuable genealogical records had accumulated over many years: these awaited the design and application of genetic analyses for the investigation of heritabilities of measurable characters.

Yuendumu was a dynamic, ever-changing environment in the 1970s and one of the natural occurrences that had a profound effect on the project was the inevitable ageing of the participants in the growth study. The longitudinal part of the study was at its most intensive throughout the 1950s for collection of the dental cast records and extending into the 1960s for the other growth recordings. By 1970, many of the participants had reached 17-19 years of age when growth processes had either slowed considerably or stopped. At this stage, Barrett and Brown had to decide whether to continue following these young adults for a few further years, even though there would be only small changes occurring in their dentitions and faces, or whether they should recruit new infants into the study.

There were also changes occurring at Yuendumu at that time. For example, in the later years of the study some older Warlpiri people had left Yuendumu to seek employment elsewhere, or they were otherwise unavailable when the research teams were at the Settlement. Aboriginal communities, generally, were becoming less receptive to research that did not bring more immediate tangible benefits to them. Reflecting the changing mood of Aboriginal people, there were also changes in the prioritisation of research funding, with a move away from supporting research in physical anthropology to a preference for projects that focussed more on social anthropology, including linguistics, ethnology, health, art, song etc.

With respect to the original aims of Barrett and Brown, by the end of the 1971 visit there were adequate data to follow a rigorous approach to the analyses using a mixed-longitudinal model, that is, a model in which researchers examined subjects on a varying number of trips from one to ten. The participants' ages at first examination varied from 4 to 15 years and maximum ages ranged from 13 to over 24 years. The researchers used this model subsequently in a number of published reports on physical growth of the Warlpiri people.

Although the visits to Yuendumu to acquire records for the growth study ceased after the 1971 trip, Barrett and Brown made a few short visits to the Settlement thereafter. Barrett spent his final extended sabbatical leave at Yuendumu shortly before his death in 1975. During this visit he worked with the Flemings to consolidate the genealogical information he had gathered in previous years.

He also made a detailed study of the Warlpiri custom of tooth evulsion (Fig. 8.1) at the invitation of the participants (Barrett *et al.*, 1978). This final paper of Barrett was published posthumously after being edited from his drafts.

Brown made two one-day trips to Yuendumu in the 1980s. The first was at the invitation of the Royal Flying Doctor Service in Alice Springs, when he spent some time at the hospital renewing acquaintances with many of the older Warlpiri people who appeared to welcome Jakamarra (Brown's honorary Warlpiri kinship name). On the second occasion he travelled by road with the Fleming's son Jolyon and was fortunate to spend time with Darby Jampijinpa, a Warlpiri elder, for a recorded interview when Darby recalled his memories of Yuendumu and its settlement.

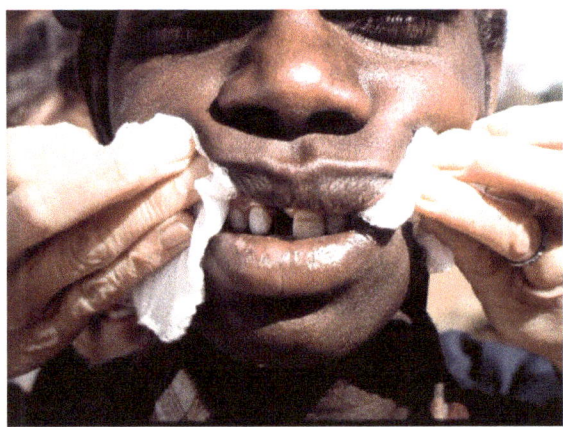

Figure 8.1
Recent evulsion of a central incisor

Ongoing projects and international collaborations

The dental models collected during the Yuendumu Growth Study have provided an invaluable resource for researchers interested in studying dental morphology and development in a population relatively free from dental diseases. The quality of the dental models produced at Yuendumu was excellent and they remain in very good condition, although some damage has occurred over the 40 years since the completion of the study.

Postgraduate students and visiting researchers still access the models, but emphasis is now being placed on indirect methods for obtaining measurements, for example 2D and 3D scanning systems, rather than direct measurements using callipers with sharpened beaks that can scratch the surfaces of the dental stone models. This development highlights the long-term outcomes that can flow from building large collections of permanent records, such as dental models, that can be retained for many years as a resource for study. As new technologies evolve, the same material can be studied with more powerful and precise techniques enabling new research questions to be addressed.

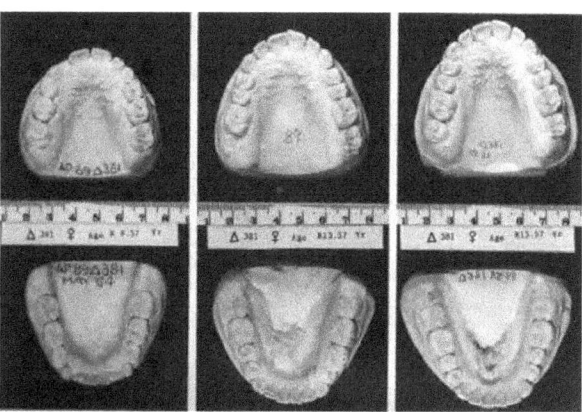

Figure 8.2
Serial dental models of a Warlpiri boy from 8.57-15.57 years

We describe below, with selected references, some of the research themes related to dental and craniofacial morphology and general growth that have grown from the original visits to Yuendumu. A complete bibliography of all of the published papers, theses and films arising directly from the Yuendumu Growth Study up to 2011 appears in Chapter 9.

The Japanese connection

Murray Barrett and Tasman Brown established a long and productive association between the Adelaide research personnel and a number of dental anatomists and anthropologists from Japan during visits to Japan in the 1960s. In 1966, Brown, returning from a period of research in Denmark, visited Professor Kato at the Nihon University in Tokyo. Kato was a distinguished anatomist who had an interest in dental anthropology. He introduced Brown to one of his senior staff, Dr (later Professor) Tadashi Ozaki, who was planning an extended research sabbatical in Adelaide already arranged with Murray Barrett (as discussed in Chapter 7). This was the beginning of a long association between Barrett, Brown and Ozaki that has continued until the present time involving students and colleagues of Ozaki as well as scholars from other Japanese universities who have come to Adelaide to work with Grant Townsend, Lindsay Richards and John Kaidonis in the School of Dentistry.

In May 1969, Tadashi Ozaki became one of the few visiting overseas research personnel to join an Adelaide research team during an annual expedition to Yuendumu. While in Adelaide, Ozaki examined the Yuendumu dental cast collection, helped with somatometry and tutored Adelaide students in dental anatomy. He subsequently visited Adelaide for shorter visits on several occasions, sometimes accompanied by younger colleagues.

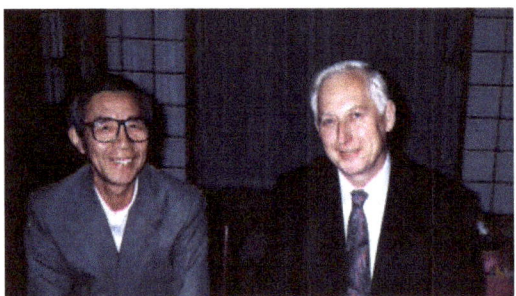

Figure 8.3
Professors Tadashi Ozaki and Tasman Brown

The Adelaide-Japanese connection has been a two-way process, reinforced by research and lecturing visits to Tokyo on separate occasions by Brown, Townsend and Richards and by many visits to Adelaide by Japanese scholars. As Grant Townsend's genetic study of Australian twins and their families has progressed, with the accumulation of extensive dental records, the collaboration has extended to this material with emphasis on tooth morphology and advanced techniques for measuring and describing crown forms. The research associations between Japan and Australia have resulted in many publications dealing with various aspects of dental morphology in the Warlpiri or utilising the Yuendumu data for comparative dental studies with other populations.

The Visitors Register of the Craniofacial Biology Research Group, located in the Murray Barrett Research Laboratory on the 6th Floor of the Adelaide Dental Hospital building, lists the names of all those researchers world-wide who have visited the laboratory since the 1960s (Appendix A). To date, over 30 researchers from Japan alone have spent time in Adelaide studying the Yuendumu collection and associated records.

Research in the 1970s

With the collection of the longitudinal records complete after the June 1971 visit to Yuendumu, attention was now directed to the patterns of dental development, general body growth, skeletal maturation and genetics. Growth curves from childhood through adolescence to young adulthood as well as the secular changes in some body measurements occupied the Adelaide researchers for some time in this decade (Barrett and Brown, 1971; Brown, 1970, 1976, 1979; Brown and Barrett, 1971, 1972, 1973; Brown and Grave, 1976; Grave and Brown, 1976). Barrett and Williamson (1972) and Williamson and Barrett (1972) surveyed oral health and fluorosis in the Warlpiri people. Fanning and Brown (1971) and Brown (1978) investigated tooth formation and emergence.

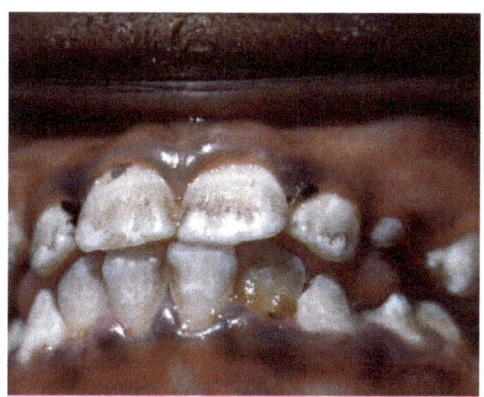
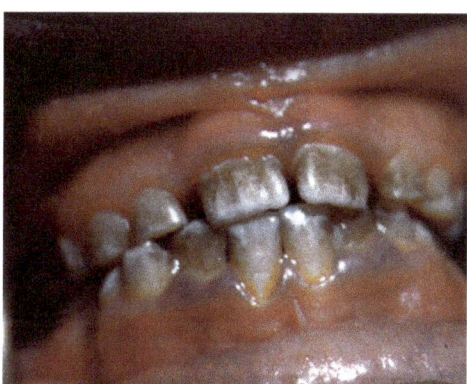

Figure 8.4
Intraoral photographs showing Aboriginal children in the 1950s with considerable staining, oral debris and dental plaque but little evidence of oral disease

Professor Kazuro Hanihara visited Adelaide to examine the cast collection and published several papers between the years 1970–1979 concerning crown size, tooth measurement, sexual dimorphism and dental traits in Australian Aboriginal people (Hanihara, 1970, 1976, 1977, 1978, 1979). He was interested in comparative dental morphology and the genetic distances between human populations and his papers reflect these interests.

Professor William Proffit, an orthodontist from the US, spent a period of sabbatical leave in Adelaide. In May 1972 he visited Yuendumu with Murray Barrett and other Adelaide personnel David Parker and Leslie Reynolds. This was a special visit, separate from the growth study, to investigate lip and tongue pressures and relate them to dental arch morphology. This was accomplished with small intra-oral transducers that registered pressure changes. Several publications soon followed (Proffit,

1975, 1978; Proffit and McGlone, 1975; Proffit *et al.*, 1975). More details of Proffit's connection with Adelaide appears in Chapter 7 and in the Foreword to this book.

With the completion of his PhD studies in 1976, Townsend published a series of papers with Brown on various aspects of the Aboriginal dentition, focusing on inheritance of tooth size, associations between different crown dimensions, and dental asymmetry. These genetic studies relied on the meticulously constructed genealogies of the Yuendumu people by the Flemings and Murray Barrett. They enabled relationships to be studied between full-siblings and also half-siblings with the same father but different mothers, a consequence of the practice of polygyny among the Warlpiri. The studies showed a strong genetic contribution to variation in tooth size, with a lesser influence from environmental factors. The studies also calculated heritability estimates for tooth size, to quantify the amount of genetic influence on observed variation. These estimates can range from zero to one. For the permanent dentition they were 0.72 for mesio-distal diameters and 0.81 for bucco-lingual in the full-siblings and 0.63 and 0.66 respectively for half-siblings. These papers were among the first to report genetic aspects of dental morphology in any population (Townsend, 1978; Townsend and Brown, 1978a,b; 1979a,b).

A significant event in this decade was the publication of Murray Barrett's collected papers as a memorial volume in 1976, achieved through private donations from his friends and colleagues (Barrett, 1976).

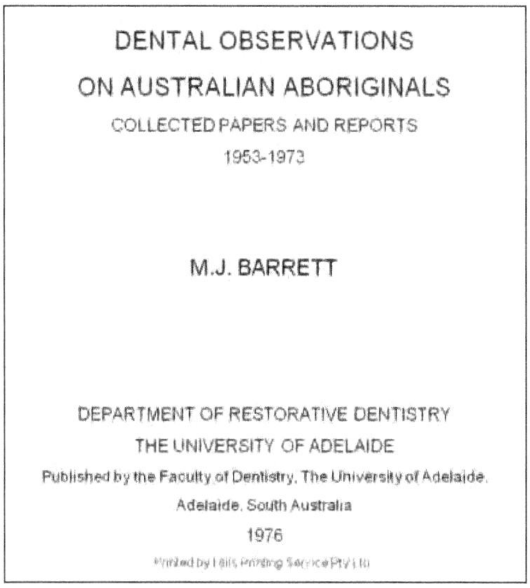
DENTAL OBSERVATIONS
ON AUSTRALIAN ABORIGINALS
COLLECTED PAPERS AND REPORTS
1953-1973

M.J. BARRETT

DEPARTMENT OF RESTORATIVE DENTISTRY
THE UNIVERSITY OF ADELAIDE
Published by the Faculty of Dentistry, The University of Adelaide.
Adelaide, South Australia
1976

Figure 8.5
The title page of the memorial volume of Murray Barrett's collected papers

Research in the 1980s

The analysis of data from the Yuendumu study continued into the 1980s with more frequent visits from overseas researchers as the Adelaide study became widely known through the publications of staff members. Further publications describing crown morphology in the Aboriginal dentition appeared (Townsend and Brown, 1980, 1981a, 1981b; Townsend *et al.*, 1989; Brown *et al.*, 1980a, 1980b; Ozaki *et al.*, 1987; Yamada, 1987a, 1987b; Yamada and Brown, 1988; Sekikawa *et al.*, 1986, 1988, 1989; Richards and Brown, 1986). Townsend also began to study various dental crown features, reporting on their frequency of occurrence and degree of expression, as well as their underlying genetic influence. Patricia Smith from Israel and Hiroyuki Yamada from Japan collaborated in these studies (Townsend *et al.*, 1986).

Several studies of dental arch shape, development and relationships took place in the 1980s. These shed light on the helicoidal plane and alternate intercuspation, two features of the Aboriginal dentition; concepts of dental occlusion were also further refined (Brown *et al.*, 1987a, 1987b; Brown, 1985). The first detailed studies of tooth wear also appeared (Richards and Brown, 1981, 1986; McKee and Molnar, 1988; Molnar *et al.*, 1983; Molnar *et al.*, 1989). A significant study by Björk *et al.*, (1984) used serial cephalograms to compare facial growth in Aboriginal and Danish boys. For the first time, the significant anterior migration of the dentition in Aboriginal people during facial growth and the consequent freeing of dental arch space for later tooth emergence were described by the examination of longitudinal records.

In the early 1980s, after studying the longitudinal material from Yuendumu, Grant Townsend recognised the advantages of studying the dentitions of related individuals to clarify the influences of genetic and environmental factors on dental development. As a result, he commenced a study of Australian twins to further explore genetic influences on dental and facial features. Over subsequent years, he recruited three large cohorts of twins with the focus on the application of sophisticated genetic modelling approaches to dental and facial data. The twin study began to attract a steady stream of established researchers as well as graduate students from Adelaide and abroad. Attention focussed on methods to measure and define the shape of craniofacial hard and soft tissues, including the dentition. New computer-assisted methods for data acquisition were planned, programmed and tested. Powerful desktop computers were becoming available which facilitated these lines of research and freed the investigators from the need to access larger mainframe computers.

Townsend had commenced writing to Professor Lassi Alvesalo in Finland in the early 1980s. Alvesalo's PhD had investigated genetic influences, particularly the roles of the X and Y chromosomes, on tooth size in Finnish families living on the island of Hailuoto off the coast of Finland. Alvesalo's broad aim of clarifying the role of genetic influences on human dental development was very similar to those of Townsend, who had examined the dentitions of Yuendumu Aboriginal people. This led to long-term collaborative studies of dental and facial development in individuals with sex chromosome abnormalities who were enrolled at Alvesalo's Kvantti research project. The 1980s saw the beginning of a steady stream of publications by Townsend with his Adelaide and overseas colleagues dealing with the study of morphological variation in the dentition of South Australian twins and the dental characteristics of subjects with chromosomal aneuploidies (Townsend, 1982, 1983a, 1983b; 1987; Townsend, *et al.*, 1984; Townsend and Alvesalo, 1985a, 1985b; Townsend *et al.*, 1988).

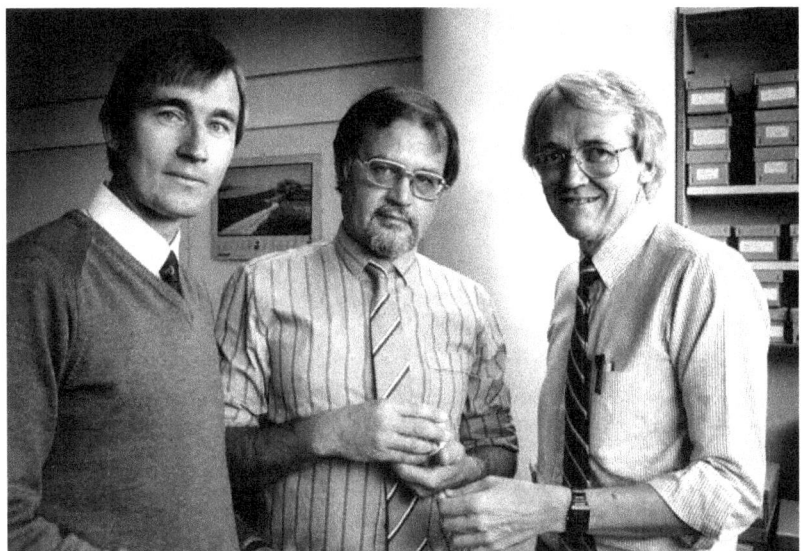

Figure 8.6
Grant Townsend, Lassi Alvesalo and John Mayhall at the University of Turku, Finland, in 1986

Research in the 1990s

Research continued in the 1990s at an accelerated pace with considerable collaborative studies with overseas colleagues and investigations by Adelaide postgraduate students. The research followed three main directions: 1) continuation of the Yuendumu Growth Study with publications on tooth morphology, dental arch shape and occlusion, as well as tooth wear; 2) further genetic research based on the analysis of records from the Grant Townsend's South Australian Twin Study, as well as collaborative studies of subjects with chromosomal aneuploidies; 3) an expansion of the development of two and three dimensional imaging techniques for the diagnosis and treatment of craniofacial abnormalities and trauma.

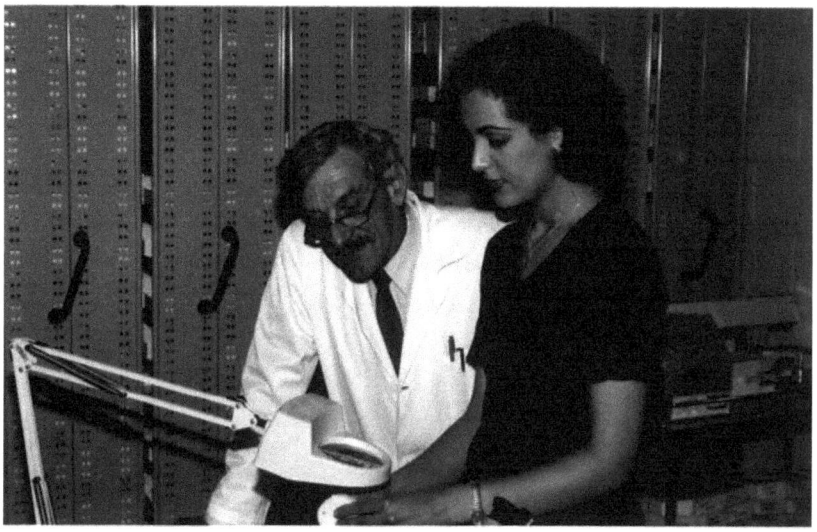

Figure 8.7
James Rogers completed an honours degree based on the twin data housed in the M J Barrett Laboratory, and an increasing number of students began research projects during the 1990s leading to honours or doctorate degrees. One of the students was Sue Taji, shown here discussing with Jim Rogers some dental models of twins

Early in the decade, publications described dental occlusion and the development of occlusion in the Warlpiri people together with the Adelaide team's consolidated views of occlusal function (Brown, 1992, Brown *et al.*, 1990; Corruccini et al., 1990a). In the late 1990s, a team of researchers led by Professor Sen Nakahara from the Nippon Dental University at Niigata, Japan, visited Adelaide and continued the study of development of dental occlusion in the Yuendumu Aboriginal people. This research led to several publications (Nakahara *et al.*, 1997; Nakahara *et al.*, 1998a, 1998b, 1999, 2001). A study based on Moiré photography, led by John Mayhall from Canada and Ikuo Kageyama from Japan, described the three-dimensional occlusal morphology of both the deciduous second molar as well as the three permanent molars in a sample of Yuendumu Aboriginal people (Kageyama, *et al.*, 1999). The emphasis continued to move to using indirect systems of data acquisition from dental models rather than direct measurements using calipers. These methods had the advantages of minimizing damage to the dental models and enabling researchers to make more detailed assessments of crown morphology.

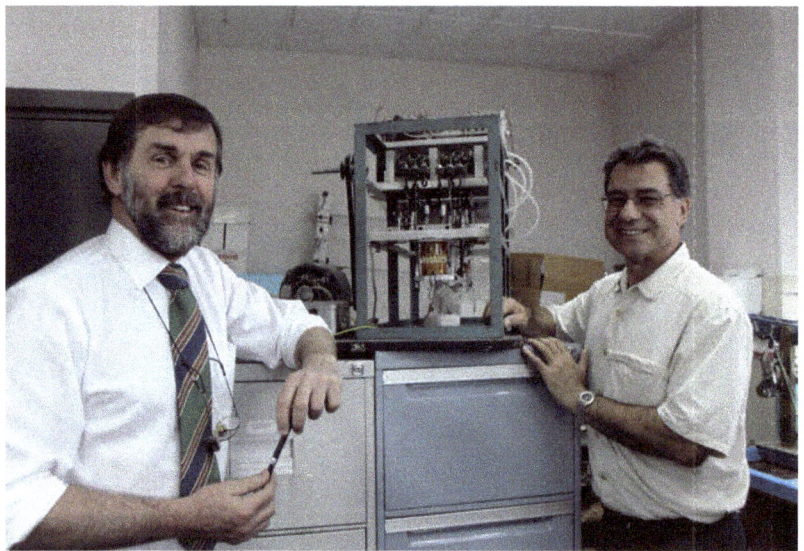

Figure 8.8
Lindsay Richards and John Kaidonis with "Cannibal"

John Kaidonis, who had returned to The University of Adelaide from private dental practice to pursue his interests in tooth wear, began to publish some of his findings with Lindsay Richards and Grant Townsend. Kaidonis was particularly interested in describing the different types of tooth wear that can occur within the dentition, including attrition (caused by tooth-to-tooth contact), abrasion (caused by food and other exogenous factors) and erosion or corrosion (caused by dietary or intrinsic acids). Wear facets, produced by tooth-to-tooth contact during extreme mandibular movements, were evident in nearly all of the dental models of Yuendumu Aboriginal people, supporting the concept that tooth grinding (or bruxism) is a very common activity in all human populations. Following on from his studies of the Aboriginal dentition, Kaidonis extended his investigations of tooth wear to include experimental approaches based on the use of tooth wear machines that allowed dental specimens to be worn at constant loads for a defined number of cycles in the presence of various lubricants (Kaidonis *et al.*, 1992a, b, c, 1993; Kaidonis *et al.*, 1998). It is a matter of some interest that anthropologist Steve Molnar from the

Washington University, St Louis, used his earlier experience as an engineer to develop a motor-driven machine that simulated human masticatory movements. On a visit to Adelaide he presented the machine, affectionately known as "Cannibal", to the Adelaide team for research on tooth wear (Brown, 1994).

Dentofacial studies of Australian twins dominated the direction of genetic research in the 1990s. Dental arch morphology and occlusion were described by Richards *et al.*, (1990), Corruccini *et al.*, (1990b) and Kasai *et al.*, (1995) and aspects of tooth morphology by Townsend and Martin (1992), Townsend *et al.*, (1995) and Dempsey *et al.*, (1995).

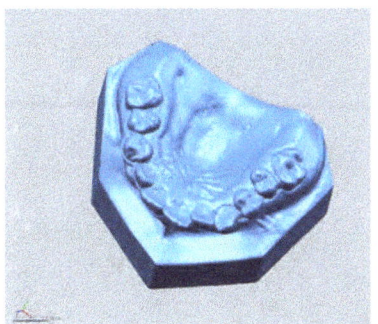 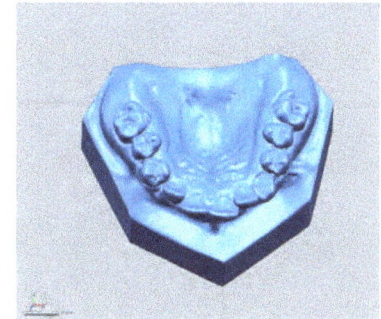

Figure 8.9
Images of the upper dental models of a pair of monozygotic twins generated by a 3D laser scanner and appropriate software available in the Murray Barrett Laboratory at the School of Dentistry, The University of Adelaide (images produced by PhD student, Atika Ashar). This technology now enables "virtual models' to be stored and accurate measurements obtained for research purposes

Mirror imaging of dental and facial morphology is a fascinating characteristic sometimes present in twins. This refers to the tendency for one member of a twin pair to "mirror" the other for one or more features. For example, one twin may have a missing tooth on one side of the mouth, while the co-twin will have the same tooth missing but on the opposite side. Several papers have reported the phenomenon of mirror imaging (Townsend *et al.*, 1992; Brown *et al.*, 1992; Townsend *et al.*, 1994).

Professor Bhim Savara, an orthodontist from Portland, Oregon, came to Adelaide for an extended visit in the 1980s with the support of a Fulbright Scholarship. He was involved in a longitudinal growth study in the US and was one of the first investigators to explore the application of three-dimensional (3D) data acquisition and analysis to assist in the diagnosis and treatment planning of abnormal craniofacial morphology. Under Savara's direction, the Adelaide team designed and built equipment for stereophotography using twin Hasselblad cameras. They then used stereo-pairs to develop facial contour maps by adapting the methods of topographical mapping of land surface contours. George Travan, a member of the Adelaide research team at that time, played a key role in generating facial maps. The stereo-pairs from twins provided information on metric characters of the face and mirror imaging of facial morphology (Brown *et al.*, 1992).

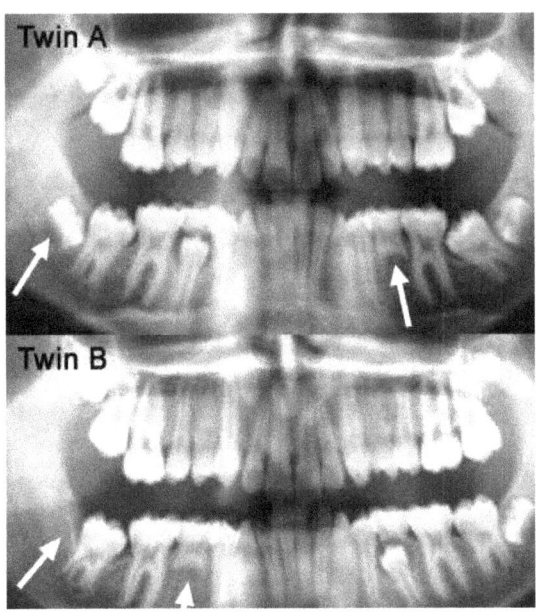

Figure 8.10
Panoral radiographs of a pair of monozygotic (so-called identical) twins showing mirror imaging for congenital absence of a permanent lower second premolar. In Twin A, the arrow shows a missing tooth on the left side whereas the equivalent tooth is missing on the right side in Twin B. The arrows pointing at the lower right third molar region show differences in the stages of dental development between the co-twins, perhaps reflecting epigenetic influences

Dr Amanda Abbott was a PhD student at the time and she and Brown turned their attention to the acquisition of craniofacial landmark data in 3D from bi-planar radiographs, that is, standardised lateral and postero-anterior (or antero-posterior) radiographs of the head, exposed simultaneously. The geometry of the system enables 3D coordinates of key reference points to be determined. Subsequently linear and angular variables can be calculated from the coordinate data. Abbott's PhD thesis dealt with the 3D system and its accuracy. It also explored the application of finite element analysis for mapping one shape onto another.

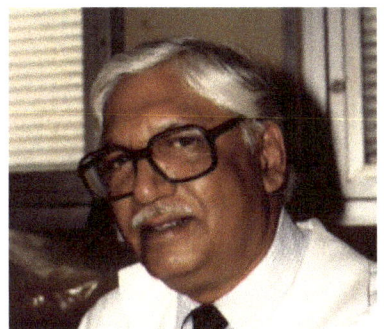 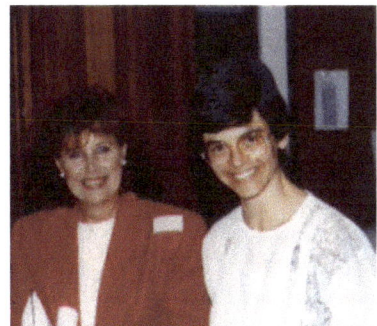

Figure 8.11
Professor Bhim Savara, Sandy Pinkerton and Dr Amanda Abbott

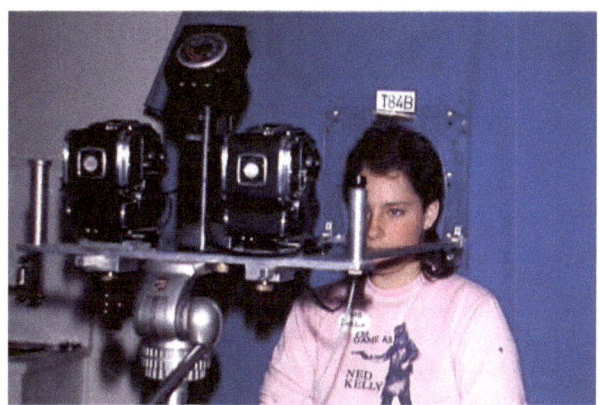

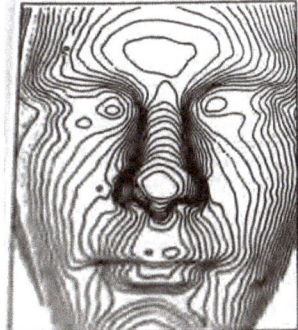 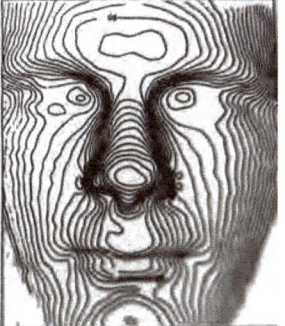

Figure 8.12
Stereo-photography and contour maps of twins

After Brown retired from his position at The University of Adelaide in 1991 he continued working in the field of craniofacial analysis at the Australian Craniofacial Unit of the Women's and Children's Hospital, Adelaide. Dr Abbott and Dr Netherway joined the Unit's research team and together they developed sophisticated computerised systems for rendering 3D images of patients' skulls from computer tomography scans of the head. Data from these scans could be sent to a manufacturing centre to produce accurate 3D models that assisted surgeons prior to craniofacial surgery for congenital malformations or traumatic injuries to the skull. A number of publications dealing with this research and its clinical applications followed (Abbott *et al.*, 1990a, b; Abbott *et al.*, 1994; Abbott and Clarke, 1995). Brown also developed a series of computer-based systems based on his earlier research from Yuendumu. The Unit's orthodontist, Dr John Barker, used these to analyse cephalometric radiographs of patients with dysmorphic conditions requiring surgery and orthodontic treatment (Barker *et al.*, 1991).

Research in the 2000s

In the 2000s, Japanese researchers, including Shintaro Kondo, Eisaku Kanazawa and Hiroyuki Yamada, collaborating with Grant Townsend, undertook further studies of tooth size, now with a focus on the intra-coronal components of teeth rather than overall measures of whole dental crowns (Kondo and Townsend, 2004; 2006; Kondo *et al.*, 2005a; 2005b).

It is possible to calculate from facial photographs of the Yuendumu Aboriginal people, the average faces of the individuals in the collection. Figure 8.13 provides two such examples: the young adult male and female. The male face is calculated from 15 individuals aged between 17 and 20 years at the time of photography (mean = 18 years) while the female face is calculated from 34 individuals aged between 17 and 33 years (mean = 21 years).

These averages were generated by converting the original print photographs to digital format, calibrating them for size (using the in-photo scale), and processing the images in Psychomorph software developed by D Perrett and colleagues (Benson and Perrett, 1992; Rowland and Perrett 1995; Tiddeman *et al.*, 2001). More specifically, the face shape for each individual was delineated using a template of 219 anthropometric landmarks (Stephan *et al.*, 2005), the mean face shape calculated using these templates, and the individual faces warped to the mean shape so that colour and texture information could be averaged (Tiddeman *et al.*, 2001).

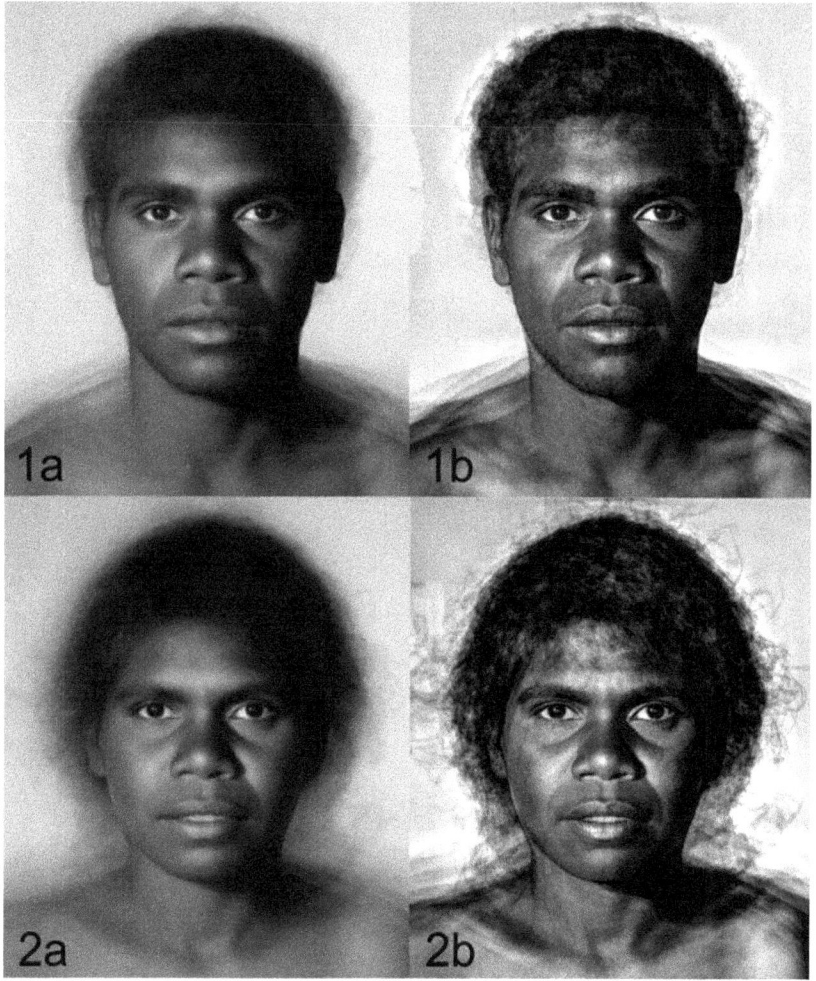

Figure 8.13
Average faces of young adults from the Yuendumu collection.
(1a) The male average. (1b) The same male average as 1a, but with the texture information preserved. (2a) The female average. (2b) The same female average as 2a, but with the texture information preserved
(courtesy of Dr Carl Stephan)

In 2005, Judith Littleton, an anthropologist from New Zealand, published a paper with Townsend that looked at the relationship between linear enamel hypoplasia (LEH) and historical changes in the living conditions of the Aboriginal people at Yuendumu who were born between 1890 and 1960 (Littleton and Townsend, 2005). Linear enamel hypoplasia is a developmental anomaly of teeth that has been often recorded in oral health surveys and in anthropological studies of prehistoric and modern populations to make inferences about the general health of individuals. Although LEH is often recorded directly by clinical examination, the quality of the Yuendumu dental models is good enough to enable the feature to be recorded accurately and reliably by direct examination of the models. Littleton and Townsend made comparisons of the frequency of LEH between different birth cohorts, including those individuals who were born between 1890 and 1929 with those born between 1950 and 1960. They found that the frequency of LEH observed in the permanent dentition increased five times from the 1890-1929 birth cohort of Aboriginal people to the 1950-1960 birth cohort. The changes in LEH frequency corresponded with altered living conditions, with the worst hypoplasia occurring after settlement at Yuendumu. This indicates the effect that resettlement had on the levels of infant morbidity and mortality.

More recently, a further collaboration has been established with Professor Alan Brook in the UK, with the aim of defining new dental phenotypes other than the traditional mesio-distal (length) and bucco-lingual (breadth) crown dimensions and acquiring data with state-of-the-art 2D and 3D scanning systems. An international collaboration has been formally established and the long-term objectives of the International Collaborating Centre in Oro-facial Genetics and Development have been formulated and published recently in the Journal of Dental Research (Townsend *et al.*, 2008). The ultimate aim of these ongoing studies is to identify the genes involved in dental development, a possibility that seemed very remote when the Yuendumu study began but one that is now definitely feasible. The addition of Dr Toby Hughes to the Adelaide research team has provided much-needed expertise in the application of sophisticated genetic modelling approaches to analyse dental data.

The Yuendumu study continues

The research project that commenced at Yuendumu in the 1950s continues to provide an invaluable resource for researchers in Adelaide and from around the world. The findings from the studies of the Yuendumu dentition, particularly the insight into the roles of genetic and environmental influences on observed variation, have provided the stimulus for other long-term studies to be initiated, such as the investigation of Australian twins and their families. Observations of age changes in the dental arches and functional occlusion in the Warlpiri people have led to a better understanding of masticatory physiology and the causes of malocclusions in modern European populations. The research projects concerned with general and craniofacial growth have established base-line data for future studies of the Warlpiri people and also led to applications in the analysis and treatment of craniofacial malformations.

As technologies have improved, more sophisticated approaches have been adopted to address fundamental research questions. However, the value of the Yuendumu material has not diminished in any way. A pressing need is to now scan all of the models and to store their digital images for future use, as has occurred with much of the radiographic material. Over the years since the completion of the record collection phase of the Yuendumu study, corresponding to the major developments in the field of molecular genetics, there has been a gradual change in the focus of the research in Adelaide. Whereas once the emphasis was on describing the nature and causes of phenotypic variation within the human dentition and craniofacial structures, the focus is changing to the application of molecular techniques to locate and identify key genes involved in dental development.

Oral health of Yuendumu Aboriginal people from the 1950s to the present day

As far back as 1953, Murray Barrett had noted that foodstuffs available at the local Yuendumu store were damaging to teeth and did not require the same sort of mastication as a traditional Aboriginal diet (Barrett, 1953). The introduction of refined carbohydrates and high sugar content products that were readily available to the Aboriginal people posed a major threat to the continued good health of their dentitions. Barrett noted the prevalence of dental diseases in the Yuendumu Aboriginal population was low when compared to that in white communities. However, when he compared the Warlpiri people with other typically nomadic native groups in other parts of the world, the prevalence of dental disease was higher (Campbell and Barrett, 1953). This broader comparison made it clear that a Western-imposed diet and culture was already having an adverse influence on Aboriginal teeth, even in the early 1950s.

By 1965, the prevalence of caries had not progressed to any great extent amongst the population, but it was noticeable that there had been a deterioration in the health of the gums, or gingival tissues, leading to chronic gum disease (Barrett, 1965). Researchers attributed the constant tooth decay rate to the naturally occurring high fluoride levels in the bore water at Yuendumu. This had both positive and negative consequences for the population. High levels of fluoride in the drinking water (1.5 parts per million) provided an inhibitory effect on dental caries but there was also an adverse effect on the mineralising tissues of developing teeth in the form of dental fluorosis. Even as far back as 1955, Barrett noted that there was a high prevalence of mottled enamel defects in the teeth of the young Aboriginal children: 30 per cent in children from 6 to 20 years (Barrett, 1956). Barrett suggested that consideration be given to reducing the fluoride levels in the water by the appropriate filtration. The problem was addressed in 1965 when it was found that by using a different bore the fluoride levels could be reduced to between 0.4 and 0.8 parts per million (Barrett and Williamson, 1972).

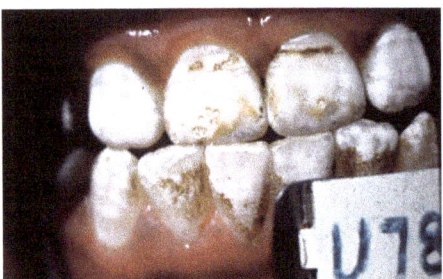 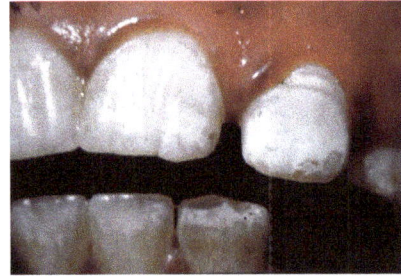

Figure 8.14
Evidence of dental fluorosis

However, with the reduction of fluoride in the water supplies and the increasing consumption of soft sticky foods, the caries rates amongst the population began to rise. Using the dmft index to quantify the number of decayed, missing and filled teeth in 309 individuals at Yuendumu, researchers found that the percentage of those affected ranged from 40 per cent for infants with primary teeth to 66 per cent in adults with one or more third molars. Barrett and Williamson concluded that:

> At the present time it would be difficult for a departmental dentist to provide conservative dental treatment for the people by periodic brief visits to the Settlement. The problem will be much more difficult in the future (Barrett and Williamson, 1972).

Soon after the field trips to Yuendumu ceased, responsibility for the provision of dental treatment for school children came under Government control. Dr Bruce Simmons, long-term General Manager of the Central Australia Oral Health Services in the Northern Territory, notes that from the time of the implementation, development and coordination of the Federal Government-funded School Dental Services Scheme in 1972, it was possible to monitor the oral health status of children enrolled in the School Dental Service in each state and territory of Australia. Over the 36 years from 1975 to 2011 the caries experience of children in remote Aboriginal communities changed from being roughly half that of the Australian population to double the national average.

A 1979 report on Aboriginal health published by the House of Representatives Standing Committee on Aboriginal Affairs expressed concern with the state of Aboriginal dental health:

> The low standard of Aboriginal dental health today is a consequence of numerous factors including a lack of understanding of the relationship between diet and dental health, lack of water for dental hygiene and lack of motivation for maintaining regular brushing and tooth care (House of Representatives Standing Committee on Aboriginal Affairs, 1979).

In 1980, Dr Simmons and his team were promoting the incorporation of oral health education messages within the remote community health services. They provided dental health education and training as well as support training for Aboriginal Health Workers to run school-based toothbrushing programs in all remote communities in the southern region of the Northern Territory. They established a course of clinical training and support for selected Aboriginal Health Workers to provide a mix of preventative and basic conservative care in small dental clinics in the larger communities. The *Northern Territory Dental Act* was also amended to incorporate a schedule of services that could be provided by a registered Aboriginal Dental Health Worker.

Rob Coruccini, an anthropologist from the US, came to Adelaide in the late 1980s to examine the Yuendumu dental cast collection. The purpose of his research was to note any changes that had occurred following adoption of Western food habits, with a decrease in consumption of tough, fibrous foodstuffs requiring vigorous masticatory activity and an increase in the intake of softer, refined foods.

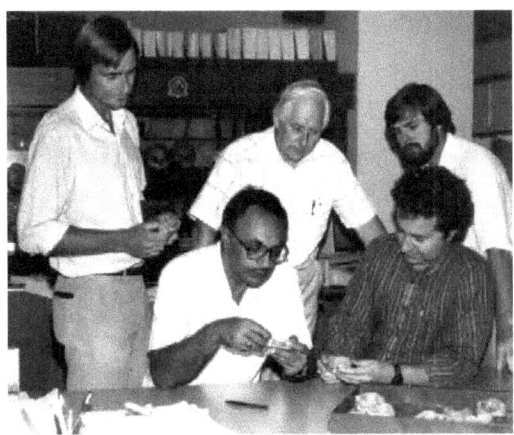

Figure 8.15
Working in the Adelaide laboratory in the early 1990s. Standing are Grant Townsend, Tas Brown and Lindsay Richards with Samvit Kaul and Rob Corruccini seated

Corruccini measured various occlusal features in a sample of older, originally nomadic Aboriginal people and compared the findings with a younger group who had lived at Yuendumu all of their lives. Differences, albeit relatively small ones, were found in the relationships of the incisor teeth, the alignment of teeth, and the relative breadths of the dental arches between the older and younger groups (Corruccini *et al.*, 1990a). The authors of the study offered several reasons to explain the differences, including the possibility that a reduction in vigorous masticatory activity may lead to reduced growth of the maxilla and an increase in dental crowding. In summarising the findings of this study, they state that:

> The present study reinforces the view that concepts of normal occlusion in modern societies need to take note of the changing nature of occlusal relationships in man, not only in individuals during growth but also in populations as a result of the complex interactions between genetic and environmental influences.

Corruccini expanded on these anthropological concepts to explain the causes of malocclusion in modern societies in a book titled *How anthropology informs the orthodontic diagnosis of malocclusion's causes* (Corruccini, 1999).

Another study (Davies *et al.*, 1997) has emphasised the differences in oral health of Aboriginal and non-Aboriginal children in the Northern Territory. This study considered the dental health profiles of Australian children who were of non-Aboriginal descent, those who were born overseas, and those who were of Aboriginal descent. Comparisons of caries experience showed a low level of dental decay for the general population of the Northern Territory, with the aggregate dmft scores (number of decayed, missing and filled permanent teeth) for both Aboriginal and non-Aboriginal children being similar in 1989. Although dmft scores were similar in these two groups, the Aboriginal children had a greater number of untreated decayed teeth. However, by 1997 Aboriginal children had a higher prevalence of caries experience, higher numbers of decayed teeth, and lower numbers of filled or missing teeth. As the authors state, these findings show that:

> Aboriginal children have not benefited to the same extent as non-Aboriginal children from the improvements in dental health in the Northern Territory or the delivery of dental services (Davies *et al.*, 1997).

Table 8.2 presents dmft scores (number of decayed, missing and filled primary teeth) for children living at Yuendumu from the year 2000 as calculated by the Australian Research Centre for Population Oral Health, School of Dentistry, The University of Adelaide. When compared with data published by Williamson and Barrett (1972), these more recent data paint a pessimistic picture of the current trends in oral health of the young children at Yuendumu. For example, the average dmft score for children aged 5-10 years in 2004 was 4.05.

Table 8.2 Mean deciduous dmft scores of Yuendumu children aged 5-10 years

Year	n	Decayed (d)		Missing (m)		Filled (f)		Dmft	
		Mean	95% CI	Mean	95% CI	Mean	95% CI	Mean	95% CI
2000	46	1.52	0.94–2.10	0.02	0.02–0.07	0.07	0.01–0.14	1.61	0.99–2.22
2002	70	2.87	2.18–3.56	0.01	0.01–0.04	0.19	0.01–0.36	3.07	2.39–3.75
2004	56	4.05	3.01–5.10					4.05	3.01–5.10
2005	42	1.93	1.10–2.76			0.17	0.03–0.36	2.10	1.28–2.91

Data courtesy of Professor John Spencer and Dr Diep Ha, Australian Research Centre for Population Oral Health (ARCPOH), School of Dentistry, The University of Adelaide

A 2006 study of the health of Indigenous Australians living in rural and remote regions of the Northern Territory, confirmed that the dental health of indigenous children aged between 4-12 years of age had not shown any real improvement since the beginning of the present millennium (Jamieson *et al.*, 2006a). Using a system of interviews and questionnaires, researchers sought information from carers of children about the use of available community dental services, sources and levels of community dental education, and diet and fluoridation effects in the local water supplies. The results of this study identified the main problems associated with the steady decline in Aboriginal children's dental health as follows:

> Our study showed there were low levels of preventive dental care, irregular use of dentrifices, negligible implementation of alternative fluoride sources, high consumption of sweetened snacks and drinks in the evening ... The findings provide some insights into factors contributing to the poor and declining state of children's dental health, and should aid in the planning and implementation of oral health promotion initiatives (Jamieson *et al.*, 2006a).

Jamieson and her colleagues also considered why oral health disparities should exist between indigenous and non-indigenous children. They outlined the disadvantages of living in a remote location, as over 80 per cent of indigenous children do in the Northern Territory. These authors point out that common factors such as low birth weights, high levels of morbidity, and higher child abuse statistics mean that indigenous children who live in remote communities and who experience poor systemic health in early life are likely to experience equally poor dental health in early childhood and throughout life (Jamieson *et al.*, 2006b).

General health and oral health in Yuendumu Aboriginals at the present time

With the current trend for an increasing prevalence of obesity in both the industrialised and non-industrialised world, there are concerns for the future health of the indigenous population at Yuendumu. Marquisa LaVelle, a biological anthropologist, has highlighted the problems associated with obesity, including Type 2 diabetes, heart disease and obesity-related cancers (LaVelle, 2000). She considers obesity to have reached epidemic proportions associated with diets of packaged and processed foods, sedentary lifestyles and often associated with high unemployment.

These obesity-associated factors are very relevant to the conditions prevailing at Yuendumu. To test her ideas, LaVelle examined the Warlpiri people living at Yuendumu and obtained physical measurements of 270 adults and children (LaVelle and Henneberg, 2002). The data she obtained confirmed that obesity rates were increasing among adolescents and adults, especially in the women (LaVelle, 2000).

A further concern is the possibility of obese mothers giving birth to underweight children. With low birth weight being a concern in isolated Aboriginal communities, LaVelle made the observation that children under the age of 5 years who are underweight are often beset by a myriad of chronic infections, including pneumonia, meningitis, respiratory infection and diarrhoea. She also noted that under-nutrition in early life can serve as a precursor for obesity in later life (LaVelle, 2000).

The combination of welfare payments, (85 per cent of indigenous adults depend upon welfare payments in the Northern Territory), high unemployment, and the effects of community de-institutionalisation introduced in 1970, has created problems in isolated Aboriginal communities, including relatively high levels of anti-social activity (Jamieson *et al.*, 2006a, 2006b). Social anthropologist Yasmine Musharbash has identified "boredom" as a factor associated with anti-social behaviour such as petrol sniffing and smoking marijuana among teenagers, and relatively high levels of adult, domestic and other forms of violence (Musharbash, 2007). She has researched the "boredom" question at Yuendumu, both its definition and its manifestations within the community. Brought about by a loss of cultural values and circumstances of the traditional Warlpiri ways, and an inability to associate fully with modernity, Musharbash believes that the social health of the Yuendumu community is in jeopardy. She argues that if "the oppressive seeming present" does not offer hope of any future change, both "boredom" and its associate evils will prevail in the years ahead.

As time passes, changes continue to occur at Yuendumu. Aboriginal leaders are aware of the problems they face and have developed youth programmes to combat petrol sniffing. They are also attempting to channel the youth into activities that promote traditional Warlpiri ways and, therefore, to reduce juvenile crime. Their future health and happiness would seem to lie in their ability to draw from the past those things that are important to them, and to adapt the merits of their past culture with the demands of the present. It is unlikely that such a solution will be found in the near future, although ultimately time and altered circumstances may provide an answer. In the meantime, Dr Bruce Simmons proposes that accessible, prevention-oriented general dental care integrated into community-controlled primary health care services incorporating oral heath prevention and promotion, seems to be the desirable way forward.

There is now growing scientific evidence that there is a relationship between poor oral health and systemic diseases. A large number of studies have shown links between poor oral health and various medical conditions, including cardiovascular diseases, Type 2 diabetes, adverse pregnancy outcomes, osteoporosis, rheumatoid arthritis and aspiration pneumonia (Cullinan *et al.*, 2009). It is also apparent that this relationship is a two-way process. That is, poor oral health can predispose an individual to various systemic conditions but, conversely, systemic diseases and illnesses can also be associated with significant detrimental effects on oral health. As Cullinan *et al.*, (2009) point out, old sayings such as "The mouth is part of the body" and "You cannot have good general health without good oral health" are now gaining renewed recognition through the evidence being obtained from well-designed scientific studies. These established links between poor oral health and poor general health represent a "double whammy" for indigenous populations.

A recent study of clinical oral health outcomes in young Australian Aboriginal adults showed that the mean number of decayed teeth was eight times higher in Aboriginal people than a representative sample of the Australian population. The prevalence of untreated decayed teeth was 3.1 times higher and Aboriginals showed 10.8 times the prevalence of moderate or severe periodontal disease (Jamieson *et al.*, 2010). These authors stress that: "Any program that includes prevention of chronic oral diseases among Indigenous Australians should start at an early age and continue throughout life." One such educational initiative uses an interactive CD, "The Strong Teeth CD", translated into Arrernte and Warlpiri, to encourage young Aboriginal people to practise good oral health (Roberts-Thomson *et al.*, 2008).

Dr Bruce Simmons' view for the future, based on his extensive experience with Aboriginal people, is that change will come with the taking of responsibility for self-education, for finding work and for good parenting. He goes on to say:

> "Boredom" for which one might exchange "not taking self-responsibility" seems to me to come from a lack of hope, from disempowerment and low self esteem. A critical task for us white fellas seems to be to help individuals, families and community leaders to turn that around. "Education" as in oral health education may well be disempowering. I'd suggest that at least as much emphasis should be put on addressing well being and physical health and I am very confident that most Aboriginal people would agree (personal interview).

Did the Aboriginal people at Yuendumu benefit from the research?

Anthropological research does not always bring immediate tangible benefits to the participants. Indeed, this is not the prime aim of this type of research. However, with respect to the Yuendumu project, it is appropriate to enquire whether the Warlpiri people received any positive outcomes for their 20 years of participation and, if so, what were they?

The Adelaide team members always treated the Yuendumu people with care and respect for their culture. In return, the Warlpiri people displayed friendship to the team and were always willing to teach them about their beliefs and customs. The Warlpiri people appeared to look forward to the annual visits and participated in activities willingly, surely with some humour at the antics of these strange Europeans who wanted to "take" their teeth and measure their heads. On each visit Murray Barrett would carefully explain to the Warlpiri adults and the Settlement staff what the research was about and what would be done. Nevertheless, with little knowledge of Western culture and education, the indigenous population of Yuendumu probably had only a superficial understanding of the reasons why they were involved in the project. They may not have been fully aware that the project's structure, planning, and financing were designed principally to enable the researchers to address research questions in the broad field of dental anthropology. The research was a long-term initiative and was not designed to produce immediate outcomes or improvements in the living conditions of the Aboriginal population at Yuendumu.

Conditions experienced by the indigenous people living at the Settlement during the time of the study were extremely difficult and at times very unhealthy. For example, the mortality and morbidity levels among the Aboriginal children at Yuendumu during the 1950s and 1960s were very high. From 1953-1970 the infant mortality rate was, on average, 16 in every 100 live births (Middleton and Francis, 1976). Unfortunately, there was little the researchers could do to resolve this situation.

Through the knowledge gained by Campbell's and Barrett's examination of Yuendumu's water quality and sources in the past, it has been possible to address problems regarding fluctuating fluoridation levels in present day water supplies. A point of interest concerning the Aboriginal population of Yuendumu, which would have had a bearing on their future dental health, is that Draper Campbell, Murray

Barrett and Tasman Brown were the first visiting researchers with a dental background who many of these Aboriginal people had seen. The research teams routinely carried out dental examinations and charted for all participants and although conservative treatment was not possible, the visitors would carry out emergency extractions, especially for any older people who were in pain from worn or infected teeth. Team members also assisted the nursing sisters at the Yuendumu Hospital with advice on dental matters and they also used their radiographic equipment if the need for X-rays arose in cases of suspected bone fractures.

Perhaps facilitated by the Rev Tom Fleming, members of the Aboriginal community and those leading the research established strong personal relationships. It was essential for the day-to-day running of the research at Yuendumu that everyone was able to participate in an amicable atmosphere. Such circumstances could only have happened if all those involved, including the Aboriginal people, were positive and wanted to make the study work. The team leaders, who visited Yuendumu on many occasions, received Warlpiri names so that their inter-relationships within the community were defined according to Warlpiri culture. Thus, Barrett became a member of the Jungarrayi group while Brown became a Jakamarra. When the visits ended there was certainly sadness on the part of all those Aboriginal elders who had sanctioned the research amongst their people.

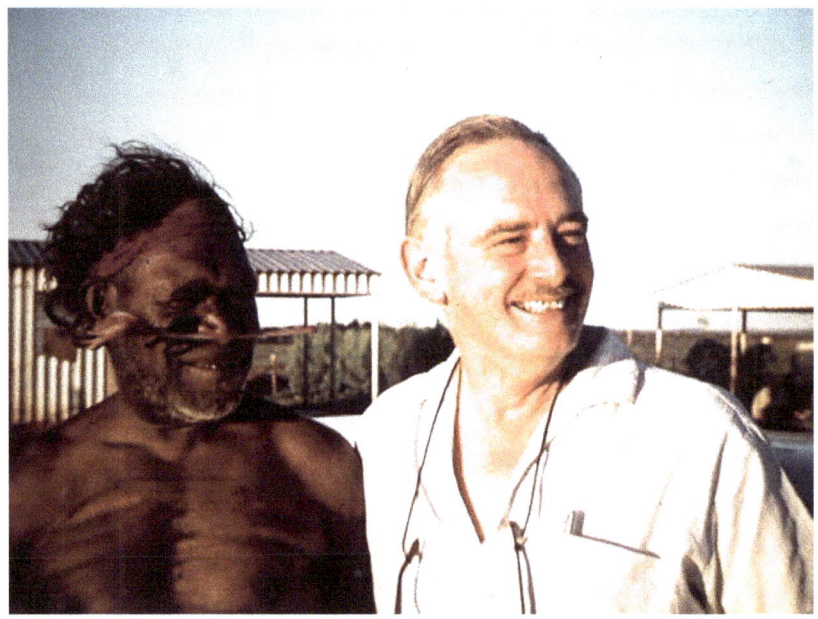

Figure 8.16
Two Jungarrayi, Jimmy and Murray

There were some important tangible outcomes from the research, other than those relating to dentistry and physical anthropology. The construction and documentation of Aboriginal family genealogies by Tom and Pat Fleming and Murray Barrett proved to be important in the seeking of traditional land rights. The success of the application by the Yuendumu people was reflected in the Aboriginal Land Rights Act (NT) 1976, which transformed Yuendumu from a reserve status to a freehold one. This led to the formation of a Community Council with the power to manage all matters concerning the day-to-day activity of the community.

During the planning of the longitudinal project, Barrett and Brown had the foresight to realise that the records and data collected would be an invaluable resource for future studies in the field of dental genetics (Barrett *et al.*, 1965). They acknowledged that this was an area in urgent need of attention and that the investigation of morphological characters and familial trends in tooth formation and eruption would benefit from the Yuendumu genealogies. Barrett recognised that the assistance of a geneticist would be desirable.

In the 1960s, Professor Barry Boettcher, a geneticist who had conducted research previously in the School of Biological Sciences at Flinders University, Adelaide, was on sabbatical leave at The University of Utah in Salt Lake City when he approached Barrett with a view to conducting a new project. Together with three other colleagues, his aim was to collect DNA specimens from the Warlpiri people at Yuendumu to establish genetic markers that would verify the genealogical records already obtained by Barrett.

Firstly, the project had to fulfil the criteria of the National Health and Medical Research Council ethics committee, including being of scientific value, helping the people themselves, respecting the human rights of the Warlpiri people, and not imposing nor interfering with the Settlement routine. Boettcher's research proposal satisfied these criteria and several trips to Yuendumu eventuated. The researchers collated the results and lodged them with the Australian Institute of Aboriginal and Torres Strait Islander Studies in Canberra. The genealogical data compiled by Barrett and the Flemings combined with the DNA contributed solid evidence at the hearings for the land claims by the Warlpiri people in late 1977. These claims were ultimately successful. Professor Nicholas Peterson of the Australian National University, Canberra, used the records of Warlpiri families and relationships to assist his research into tribal boundaries and the legitimacy of land claims.

The longitudinal study produced a series of charts showing growth and growth velocities of a number of body measurements including height and weight (Brown and Barrett, 1971, 1972; Brown and Townsend, 1982). These records form a valuable base-line standard for use in paediatric medicine and for comparison with data from later investigations. Skeletal maturation standards were also derived for the Warlpiri children (Brown and Grave, 1976).

One of the most important and lasting benefits to the people of Yuendumu came from the efforts of Campbell and Barrett to record as much of the Warlpiri culture and customs that the limited time allowed. Campbell scripted and produced several movie films on visits to Yuendumu made for that specific purpose. They recorded the skills and knowledge applied by the men and women in their daily lives. Included in the series were films depicting hunting and gathering food, preparing and cooking food and making the various implements and weapons in common use. Barrett was the photographer for the series and it was his practice to arrange a viewing of the latest film on his visits to Yuendumu. Many of the Warlpiri people would attend and there was great merriment and encouragement when the "star" of the movie appeared, always a well-known Warlpiri identity. The numerous films made by Draper Campbell and Murray Barrett captured many Warlpiri craft skills used in weapon making, hunting techniques and food preparation (*So they did eat*). One film dealt with a young girl growing up under settlement conditions (*Nabarula*). There were also opportunities to record the Warlpiri language and traditional songs. Whenever possible, Barrett would record Warlpiri language and songs that Warlpiri people willingly performed for his tape recorder. All this material is now in the archives of the Australian Institute of Aboriginal and Torres Strait Islander Studies where it forms a permanent record of some aspects of Warlpiri life and customs as they were over 50 years ago.

The future of human longitudinal growth studies

There have been many longitudinal studies of growth carried out in different human populations over the past 60 years or so. The Yuendumu Growth Study was one of several longitudinal studies that were underway during the 1960s. In England, James Tanner and his colleagues in London were involved in the large Harpenden Growth Study. In the US, Lester Sontag and then Alex Roche led the Fels Study (Eveleth and Tanner, 1976). As Barry Bogin points out in his book, *Patterns of Human Growth*, there were several other important studies underway in the US, including the University of Iowa Child Welfare Station Study, the Harvard Growth Study, the University of Colorado Child Research Council Study, the Brush Foundation Study of Western Reserve University (Cleveland, Ohio) and several studies at the University of California (Berkeley). Interestingly, Bogin notes that, except for the Fels Study, all of these studies ended either when the funding dried up, when the collection of data without any specific purpose could not be justified, or when the philosophy of a "whole child" approach to growth research became untenable (Bogin, 1999).

A few other longitudinal studies that focussed more on growth of the dento-facial region also occurred. For example, Coenraad Moorrees was involved in a study of dental and facial development of twins in Boston, US, while Arne Björk in Copenhagen, Denmark, was involved in a study of craniofacial growth using metallic implants. While these two landmark studies were more focussed than many others, they serve to highlight two important problems that still confront researchers wanting to carry out large-scale longitudinal growth studies: the ethical issues associated with studies of healthy individuals and the need for ongoing financial support to carry out these sorts of studies and to also analyse the masses of data that accrue.

Björk's findings have revolutionised the way we think about human craniofacial growth, enabling researchers and clinicians to study craniofacial growth patterns in individuals by superimposing successive radiographic landmarks on relatively stable landmarks. However, these discoveries were based on embedding small metallic implants into the skulls of healthy children, something that would not be approved by ethics committees nowadays. In relation to the Yuendumu Growth Study, researchers obtained all appropriate ethical approvals at the time of the study and the researchers did their best to explain what was involved and what the implications of the study were to the Aboriginal participants. Certainly, there were no invasive procedures performed in the Yuendumu study, such as the use of metallic implants. Record collection involved procedures commonly used by dentists at the time, such as making dental impressions, that carried minimal risk of harm or injury.

The longitudinal twin study of Moorrees that included age-matched siblings was a very ambitious undertaking. It also had the potential to provide fundamentally new insights into the influences of genetic and environmental factors on human craniofacial growth but, unfortunately, very few scientific papers were ever published from the study, apparently due to funding inadequacies (Peck and Will, 2004). As we have mentioned earlier, lack of certainty about ongoing funding was one of the reasons that the record collection phase of the Yuendumu study ended in 1971. However, in contrast to Moorrees' study, analyses of the data from Yuendumu have proceeded up until the present time, resulting in a very large collection of published papers that we list in Chapter 9.

While the Yuendumu project was not the largest of these studies in terms of participants, it had the advantage of involving an isolated group of Aboriginal Australians most of whom belonged to the same tribe and who had only recently moved onto a settlement having formerly lived a traditional lifestyle. It was assumed for the research that nearly all of the Aboriginal people at Yuendumu were of pure Aboriginal ancestry. This homogeneity overcame the difficulty of having to identify participants based on their ethnicity, which is a common problem in similar studies of European populations. Because of the geographical isolation of Yuendumu, and given that many of the Aboriginal people never left the Settlement, the population was not greatly influenced by European customs during the course of the longitudinal study. The homogeneity of the environment also minimised the potential confounding effects that can be introduced into growth studies when there are major differences in living conditions between family groups. The relative stability of the population facilitated the collection of longitudinal growth data, although we have already mentioned that the Aboriginal people became more mobile towards the end of the record collection phase. The custom of polygyny, whereby a male may have more than one wife, provided a rare opportunity to obtain family data from both full-siblings and half-siblings who had the same father but different mothers. This information, recorded in the genealogies produced by the Flemings and Barrett, has been of considerable value for genetic studies. The good condition of the dentitions of the Aboriginal people at Yuendumu enabled researchers to carry out studies of tooth size and morphology of nearly all erupted teeth, with only a very small number of teeth needing to be excluded because of decay or developmental defects. At the time of the visits to Yuendumu, dental caries experience of the young people was amongst the lowest in the world but, as we have noted earlier in this chapter (see Table 8.2), the situation has deteriorated as food habits have changed.

It is highly unlikely that another study like the one led by Barrett and Brown could ever be commenced again at Yuendumu. Physical anthropology, with its sub-discipline dental anthropology, has progressed through many phases starting with descriptions of the physical characteristics of population groups, especially smaller isolated communities. As statistical theory developed, pure descriptive studies gave way to more penetrative analyses of relationships between measurable features. There is little need for more descriptive and analytic studies of physical characteristics. More recently, investigations of growth patterns and genetic studies to explore within group and between group affinities have become more relevant. Documentation of the health and disease status of indigenous populations, particularly those in developing countries, have become very relevant. Research funding tends to be directed towards those fields that are in more urgent need of investigation.

There have been substantial changes at Yuendumu since the termination of the field trips in 1971. The population has more than doubled to almost 1,000. There are now around 100 houses with indigenous occupants and the school has around 30 staff including about 10 teachers of whom several are Aboriginal. The Warlpiri people are less settled than previously and they tend to move away from Yuendumu for extended periods to live and work in other localities including several outstations. In 1971, amenities at Yuendumu were minimal: they included a school, hospital, childcare centre, church and community store. Relatively few Warlpiri families lived in houses. There is now a Community Council structure (Yuendumu being one of several communities that form from the Central Desert Shire Council), supervising facilities such as a media centre, adult education centre, old people's programmes, internet access, a housing officer, police station, youth centre and child care and others. Limited local employment is in mining and traditional paintings through Warlukurlangu Artists. Almost two generations and a different social environment separate the Warlpiri people of 1971 from those of today. It is unlikely that the present generation would be as receptive to the intrusion of anthropologists as their forebears were.

Indeed, the future of long-term longitudinal growth studies worldwide is threatened by the tendency for researchers and funding agencies to seek outcomes in the short term from research initiatives rather than invest in long-term initiatives. By definition, human longitudinal growth studies take a long time to run, requiring great commitment by researchers and participants. With the increasing pressures on researchers to "publish or perish" and the increasing mobility of modern societies, beginning a large-scale longitudinal study can be a risky undertaking, and the chances of completing one are slim.

Nevertheless, we need more well-planned, longitudinal studies of human growth, as these are the only types of studies that provide a realistic picture of the nature and timing of the growth changes that occur in individuals. Cross-sectional studies provide some insights into general trends of growth and development within populations, but the data that arise from them are not representative of any one individual because everyone grows at different rates and at different times.

The last large-scale study of Australian children that produced standards for stature and weight was conducted in the 1960s and published by the NHMRC in the 1970s. Since that time, we know that there have been secular changes occurring, with children of a given age tending to be taller and heavier than previously (Ranjitkar *et al.*, 2006; Lin *et al.*, 2006). We have also noted apparent secular trends in the timing of emergence of primary and permanent teeth of Australian children (Diamanti and Townsend, 2003; Woodroffe *et al.*, 2010). It is very important that up-to-date reference data are available to enable health workers to compare individuals against population standards, so that those who fall outside the normal range can be identified and treatment provided if necessary.

Alex Roche, who led the University of Melbourne Child Growth Study in the 1950s and 60s, as well as the Fels Study in the US from the 1970s, has provided an insightful summary of the issues involved in establishing and maintaining longitudinal growth studies (Roche *et al.*, 1999). Roche and his colleagues note that "exciting possibilities exist if funding can be obtained" and they conclude their discussion of longitudinal studies by stating that "The need exists, the methods exist, and success can be attained with focussed efforts and persistence." Barrett and Brown certainly needed to display "focussed efforts" and "persistence" to ensure the success of the Yuendumu Growth Study.

Bruce Simmons, who Yuendumu Aboriginal people gave the skin name Japangardi, has also noted that he appreciated greatly having the anthropological and epidemiological studies and stories of Campbell and Barrett to draw on when talking with Aboriginal people about how the "old ways" and "new ways" have impacted on oral health: "Their papers have provided me with some ideas on why Aboriginal people haven't readily embraced oral hygiene and other health messages."

Although the Yuendumu Growth Study commenced 60 years ago and the record collection phase ceased 40 years ago, research directly related to the original study, or investigations that have been inspired by it, continue to add to our understanding of human growth and development, particularly of the teeth and facial structures. The foresight of Draper Campbell, Murray Barrett and Tasman Brown has produced a unique collection of records of an Australian Aboriginal population that will continue to draw researchers to the School of Dentistry at The University of Adelaide for years to come.

The study has provided a legacy to dental science and practice in terms of the knowledge gained about dental and facial development and particularly improved our understanding about dental occlusion. It has also provided a legacy to past, present and future researchers in terms of the unique collection of records available for study.

Furthermore, we believe it has provided a legacy for the Aboriginal people from Yuendumu, helping to lead to better health outcomes and improved well-being for them. We hope that the journey described in this book will inspire other researchers to continue the tradition of long-term longitudinal growth studies throughout the world.

References

Abbott AH, Clark B (1995). Protocols for examination of craniomaxillofacial injuries by computed tomography. In: *Cranio-Maxillo-Facial Trauma.* Simpson DA, David DJ, editors. Edinburgh: Churchill Livingstone. Appendix II.

Abbott AH, Netherway DJ, David DJ, and Brown T (1990a). Application and comparison of techniques for three-dimensional analysis for craniofacial anomalies. *J Craniofac Surg* 1:119–134.

Abbott AH, Netherway DJ, David DJ, Brown T (1990b). Craniofacial osseous landmark determination from stereo computer tomography reconstruction *Ann Acad Med Singapore* 19:595–604.

Abbott JR, Netherway DJ, Wingate P, Abbott AH (1994). Craniofacial imaging, models and prostheses. *Aust J Otolaryngol* 6:581–587.

Barker J, Brown T, Nugent MAC, David DJ (1991). The treatment of facial dysharmony and malocclusion by jaw surgery. *Aust Dent J* 36:183–205.

Barrett MJ (1953). Dental observations on Australian Aborigines – Yuendumu, Central Australia, 1951–52. *Aust Dent J* 57:127–138.

Barrett MJ (1956). Dental observations on Australian Aborigines: water supplies and endemic dental fluorosis. *Aust Dent J* 1:87–92.

Barrett MJ (1965). Dental observations on Australian Aborigines. *Mankind* 6:249–254.

Barrett MJ (1976). *Dental Observations on Australian Aborigines: Collected Papers and Reports 1953–1973.* Adelaide: Faculty of Dentistry, The University of Adelaide.

Barrett MJ, Brown T (1971). Increase in average height of Australian Aborigines. *Med J Aust* 2:1169–1172.

Barrett MJ, Brown T, Fanning EA (1965). A long-term study of the dental and craniofacial characteristics of a tribe of Central Australian Aborigines. *Aust Dent J* 10:63–68.

Barrett MJ, Williamson JJ (1972). Oral health of Australian Aborigines: survey methods and prevalence of dental caries. *Aust Dent J* 17:37–50.

Barrett MJ, Fleming TJ, Djagamara NA (1978). *Tooth evulsion in the Walbiri area.* Canberra: Australian Institute of Aboriginal Studies. (Restricted Access Publication.)

Benson P, Perrett D (1992). Face to face with the perfect image. *New Sci* 133:26–29.

Björk A, Brown T, Skieller V (1984). Comparison of craniofacial growth in an Australian Aboriginal and Danes, illustrated by longitudinal cephalometric analysis. *Eur J Orthod* 6:1–14.

Bogin B (1999). *Patterns of Human Growth.* 2nd Edition, Cambridge University Press, Cambridge.

Brown T (1970). Skeletal maturity and facial growth assessment. *Aust Orthod J* 2:80–87.

Brown T (1976). Head size increases in Australian Aborigines. An example of skeletal plasticity. In: *The Origin of the Australians.* Kirk RL, Thorne AG, editors. Canberra: Australian Institute of Aboriginal Studies, pp. 195–209.

Brown T (1978). Tooth emergence in Australian Aboriginals. *Ann Hum Biol* 5:41–54.

Brown T (1979). *Skeletal maturation rates in Aboriginal children.* Occasional Papers in Human Biology. Canberra: Australian Institute of Aboriginal Studies, 1:71–86.

Brown T (1985). Occlusal development and function. In: *Functional Orthopaedics of the Jaw.* Vistas in Neuro-occlusal Rehabilitation. Simões WA, editor. Livraria Editora Santos, Sao Paulo. pp. 1–67. (in Portugese).

Brown T (1992). Developmental, morphological and functional aspects of occlusion in Australian Aboriginals. In: *Culture, Ecology and Dental Anthropology.* Lukacs JR, editor. Delhi: Kamla-Ray Enterprises, pp. 73–85.

Brown T (1994). "Cannibal" moves down under. *Dent Anthrop News* 9:11–12.

Brown T, Barrett MJ (1971). Growth in Central Australian Aborigines: stature. *Med J Aust* 2:29–33.

Brown T, Barrett MJ (1972). Growth in Central Australian Aborigines: weight. *Med J Aust* 2:999–1002.

Brown T, Barrett MJ (1973). Increase in average weight of Australian Aborigines. *Med J Aust* 2:25–28.

Brown T, Grave KC (1976). Skeletal maturation in Australian Aborigines. *Aust Paed J* 12:24–30.

Brown T, Townsend GC (1982). Adolescent growth in height of Australian Aboriginals analysed by the Preece-Baines function: a longitudinal study. *Ann Hum Biol* 9:495–505.

Brown T, Abbott A, Burgess VB (1983). Age changes in dental arch dimensions of Australian Aboriginals. *Am J Phys Anthropol* 62:291–303.

Brown T, Abbott A, Burgess VB (1987). Longitudinal study of dental arch relationships in Australian Aboriginals with reference to alternate intercuspation. *Am J Phys Anthropol* 72:49–57.

Brown T, Margetts B, Townsend GC (1980a). Comparison of mesiodistal crown diameters of the deciduous and permanent teeth in Australian Aboriginals. *Aust Dent J* 25:28–33.

Brown T, Margetts B, Townsend GC (1980b). Correlations between crown diameters of the deciduous and permanent teeth of Australian Aboriginals. *Aust Dent J* 25:219–223.

Brown T, Townsend GC, Richards LC, Burgess, VB (1990). Concepts of occlusion: the Australian evidence. *Am J Phys Anthropol* 82:247–256.

Brown T, Townsend GC, Richards LC, Travan GR, Pinkerton SK (1992). Facial asymmetry and mirror imaging in South Australian Twins. In: *Craniofacial variation in Pacific Populations.* Brown T, Molnar S, editors. Adelaide: Anthropology and Genetics Laboratory, The University of Adelaide, pp. 79–98.

Campbell TD, Barrett MJ (1953). Dental observations on Australian Aborigines – a changing environment and food pattern. *Aust Dent J* 57:1–6.

Corruccini R (1999). *How Anthropology Informs the Orthodontic Diagnosis of Malocclusion's Causes.* Lewiston, New York: The Edwin Mellen Press.

Corruccini RS, Townsend GC, Brown T (1990a). Occlusal variation in Australian Aboriginals. *Am J Phys Anthropol* 82:257–265.

Corruccini RS, Townsend GC, Richards LC, Brown T. (1990b). Genetic and environmental determinants of dental occlusal variation in twins of different nationalities. *Hum Biol* 62: 353–367.

Cullinan MP, Ford PJ, Seymour GJ (2009). Periodontal disease and systematic health: current studies. *Aust Dent J* 54 (1 Suppl):S62–S69.

Davies MJ, Spencer AJ, Westwater A, Simmons B (1997). Dental caries among Australian Aboriginal, non Aboriginal Australian-born, and overseas-born children. *Bull World Health Org* 75:197–203.

Diamanti J, Townsend G (2003). New standards for permanent tooth emergence in Australian children. *Aust Dent J* 48:39–42.

Dempsey PJ, Townsend GC, Martin NG, Neale MC (1995). Genetic covariance structure of incisor crown size in twins. *J Dent Res* 74:1389–1398.

Eveleth PB, Tanner JM (1976) *Worldwide Variation in Human Growth.* Cambridge: University Printing House.

Grave KC, Brown T (1976). Skeletal ossification and the adolescent growth spurt. *Am J Orthod* 69:611–619.

Hanihara K (1970). Preliminary reports on dental anthropology of the Australian Aborigines. (in Japanese) *J Anthrop Soc Nippon* 78:75–76.

Hanihara K (1976). *Statistical and Comparative Studies of the Australian Aboriginal Dentition. Bulletin, No.11.* Tokyo: The University Museum, The University of Tokyo.

Hanihara K (1977). Distance between Australian Aborigines and certain other populations based on dental measurements. *J Hum Evol* 6:403–418.

Hanihara K (1978). Difference in sexual dimorphism in dental morphology among several human populations In: *Development, Function and Evolution of Teeth.* Butler PM, Joysey KA, editors. London: Academic Press, pp. 127–133.

Hanihara K (1979). Dental traits in Ainu, Australian Aborigines, and New World populations. In: *The First Americans: Origins, Affinities and Adaptions.* Laughlin WS, Harper AB, editors. New York: Gustav Fischer, pp. 125–134.

House of Representatives Standing Committee on Aboriginal Affairs (1979). *Aboriginal Health.* The Parliament of the Commonwealth of Australia. Canberra: Australian Government Publishing Service. http://www.aph.gov.au/house/committee/atsia/reports.htm

Jamieson LM, Bailie RS, Beneforti M, Koster CR, Spencer AJ (2006a). Dental self-care and dietary characteristics of remote-living Indigenous children. *Rural Rem Health* (online) 6:503 http://www.rrh.org.au

Jamieson LM, Armfield JM, Roberts-Thomson KF (2006b). Oral health inequalities among indigenous and nonindigenous children in the Northern Territory of Australia. *Community Dent Oral Epidemiol* 34:267–276.

Jamieson LM, Sayers SM, Roberts-Thomson KF (2010). Clinical oral health outcomes in young Australian Aboriginal adults compared with national-level counterparts. *Med J Aust* 192:558–561.

Kageyama I, Mayhall J, Townsend GC (1999). A three-dimensional study of the deciduous and permanent molars in Australian Aborigines. *Persp Hum Biol* 4:103–108.

Kaidonis JA, Townsend GC, Richards LC (1992a). Abrasion: an evolutionary and clinical view. *Aust Pros J* 6:9–16.

Kaidonis JA, Townsend GC, Richards LC (1992b). Interproximal tooth wear – a new observation. *Am J Phys Anthropol* 88:105–107.

Kaidonis JA, Townsend GC, Richards LC (1992c). The morphological features and aetiology of interproximal tooth wear. In: *Craniofacial Variation in Pacific Populations.* Brown T, Molnar S, editors. Adelaide, South Australia: Anthropology and Genetics Laboratory, The University of Adelaide, pp. 121–127.

Kaidonis JA, Townsend GC, Richards LC (1993). Nature and frequency of dental wear facets in an Australian Aboriginal population. *J Oral Rehabil* 20: 333–340.

Kaidonis JA, Townsend GC, Richards LC, Tonsley GD (1998). Wear of human enamel: a quantitative in vitro assessment. *J Dent Res* 77:1983–1990.

Kasai K, Richards LC, Townsend GC, Kanazawa E, Iwasawa T (1995). Fourier analysis of dental arch morphology in South Australian twins. *Anthropol Sci* 103:39–48.

Kondo S, Townsend GC (2004) Sexual dimorphism in crown components of mandibular deciduous and permanent molars in Australian Aborigines. *HOMO J Comp Hum Biol* 55:53–64.

Kondo S, Townsend G (2006). Associations between Carabelli trait and cusp areas in human permanent maxillary first molars. *Am J Phys Anthropol* 129:196–203.

Kondo S, Townsend GC, Yamada H (2005). Sexual dimorphism of cusp dimensions in human maxillary molars. *Am J Phys Anthropol* 128:870–877.

Kondo S, Townsend G, Kanazawa E (2005). Size relationships among permanent mandibular molars in Aboriginal Australians and Papua New Guinea Highlanders. *Am J Hum Biol* 17:622–633.

LaVelle M, Henneberg M (2000). Continuing fifty years of longitudinal observations in Yuendumu, a Warlpiri community in the Central Australian Desert. *Am J Hum Biol* 12:289–290. (Abstract)

LaVelle M (2002). URI scientist: Obesity growing threat to world health. www.uri.edu/news/releases/html/02-0226.html

Lin NH, Ranjitkar S, Macdonald R, Hughes T, Taylor J and Townsend G (2006). New growth references for assessment of stature and skeletal maturation in Australians. *Aust Orthod J* 22:1–10.

Littleton J, Townsend G (2005). Linear enamel hypoplasia and historical change in a central Australian Community. *Aust Dent J* 50:101–107.

McKee JK, Molnar S (1988). Measurement of tooth wear among Australian Aborigines: II Intrapopulational variation in patterns of dental attrition. *Am J Phys Anthropol* 76:125–136.

Middleton MR, and Francis, SH (1976). *Yuendumu and its Children. Life and health on an Aboriginal settlement.* Published for the Department of Aboriginal Affairs. Australian Government Publishing Service, pp. 16–17.

Molnar S, McKee JK, Molnar I (1983). Measurements of tooth wear among Australian Aborigines: I. Serial loss of the enamel crown. *Am J Phys Anthropol* 61:51–65.

Molnar S, Richards LC, McKee JK, Molnar I (1989). Tooth wear in Australian Aboriginal populations from the River Murray Valley. *Am J Phys Anthropol* 79:185–196.

Musharbash Y (2007). Boredom, Time, and Modernity: An example from Aboriginal Australia. *Am Anthropol* 109:307–317.

Nakahara S, Takahashi M, Townsend G (1997). Modes of occlusion in humans: a comparison of traditional Aborigines and modern Japanese. *Shigaku (Odontology)* 85:345–356.

Nakahara S, Takahashi M, Kameda T, Kameda A, Townsend G (1998a). Longitudinal changes in the permanent dentition of traditional Aborigines: movements of the first molar and the anterior dentition. *Shigaku (Odontology)* 86:2–6.

Nakahara S, Takahashi M, Kameda T, Kameda A, Townsend G (1998b). Longitudinal changes in the modes of occlusion of permanent teeth – changes in the teeth and dentition of Australian Aborigines – Part 1: Normalization of malocclusion. *Shigaku (Odontology)* 86:209–230.

Nakahara S, Takahashi M, Kameda T, Kameda A, Townsend GC (1999). Longitudinal changes in the modes of occlusion of permanent teeth – changes in the teeth and dentition of Australian Aborigines – Part 2: Transition of normal incisal occlusion into malocclusions. *Shigaku (Odontology)* 87:8–29.

Nakahara S, Kameda T, Masashi T, Akira K, Townsend GC (2001). Re-examining occlusal changes in the development of the Australian Aboriginal dentition – what we have learned as orthodontists. *Orthod Waves* 60:347–353.

Ozaki T, Kanazawa E, Sekikawa M, Akai J (1987). Three-dimensional measurement of occlusal surface of upper first molars in Australian Aboriginals. *Aust Dent J* 32:263–269.

Peck S, Will L (2004). Obituary: Coenraad F. A. Moorrees 1916–2003. *Angle Orthod* 74:286–288.

Proffit WR (1975). Muscle pressure and tooth position: North American Whites and Australian Aborigines. *Angle Orthod* 45:1–11.

Proffit WR (1978). Equilibrium theory re-examined: To what extent do tongue and lip pressures influence tooth position and thereby occlusion? In: *Oral Physiology and Occlusion*. Proceedings of an International Symposium 1976, Newark, NJ. Perryman JH, editor. London: Pergamon, pp. 55–77.

Proffit WR, McGlone RE (1975). Tongue-lip pressure during speech of Australian Aborigines. *Phonetica* 32:200–220.

Proffit WR, McGlone RE, Barrett MJ (1975). Lip and tongue pressure related to dental arch and oral cavity size in Australian Aborigines. *J Dent Res* 54:1161–1172.

Ranjitkar S, Lin NH, Macdonald R, Taylor J, Townsend G (2006). Stature and skeletal maturation of two cohorts of Australian children and young adults over the past two decades. *Aust Orthod J* 22:47–58.

Richards LC, Brown T (1981). Dental attrition and age relationships in Australian Aboriginals. *Arch Oceania* 16:94–98.

Richards LC, Brown T (1986). Development of the helicoidal plane. *Hum Evol* 1:385–398.

Richards LC, Townsend GC, Brown T, Burgess VB (1990). Dental arch morphology in South Australian twins. *Arch Oral Biol* 35:983–989.

Roberts-Thomson K, Simmons B, Brocklebank C (2008). *The Strong Teeth CD*. Department of Health and Community Services and the Australian Research Centre for Population Oral Health, Adelaide: The University of Adelaide. www.isee-ilearn.com

Roche AF, Guo SS, Towne B (1999). The establishment and maintenance of longitudinal growth studies: experience from Melbourne and Fels. In: *Human Growth in Context*. Johnston FE, Zemel B, Eveleth PB, editors. London: Smith-Gordon, pp. 101–119.

Rowland DA, Perrett DI (1995). Manipulating facial appearance through shape and color. *IEEE Comput Graph* 15:70–76.

Sekikawa M, Akai J, Kanazawa E, Ozaki T (1986). Three-dimensional measurement of the occlusal surfaces of lower first molars of Australian Aboriginals. *Am J Phys Anthropol* 71:25–32.

Sekikawa M, Kanazawa E, Ozaki T, Brown T (1988). Principal component analysis of intercusp distances on the lower first molars of three human populations. *Arch Oral Biol* 33:535–541.

Sekikawa M, Namura T, Kanazawa E, Ozaki T, Richards LC, Townsend GC, Brown T (1989). Three-dimensional measurement of the maxillary first molar in Australian whites. *Nihon Univ J Oral Sci* 15:457–464.

Stephan CN, Penton-Voak I, Perrett D, Tiddeman B, Clement JG, Henneberg M (2005). Two-dimensional computer generated average human face morphology and facial approximation. In: *Computer Graphic Facial Reconstruction*. Clement JG, Marks M, editors. Boston: Academic Press, pp. 105–127.

Tiddeman B, Burt M, Perrett D (2001). Computer graphics in facial perception research. *IEEE Comput Graph* 21:42–50.

Townsend GC (1978). Genetics of tooth size. *Aust Orthod J* 5:142–147.

Townsend GC (1982). Dentition of a 48, XYY, +21 male. *Hum Genet* 61:267–268.

Townsend GC (1983a). Fluctuating dental asymmetry in Down's syndrome. *Aust Dent J* 28:39–44.

Townsend GC (1983b). Tooth size in children and young adults with trisomy 21 (Down) syndrome. *Arch Oral Biol* 28:159–166.

Townsend GC (1987). A correlative analysis of dental crown dimensions in individuals with Down syndrome. *Hum Biol* 59:537–548.

Townsend GC, Brown T (1978a). Inheritance of tooth size in Australian Aboriginals. *Am J Phys Anthropol* 48:305–314.

Townsend GC, Brown T (1978b). Heritability of permanent tooth size. *Am J Phys Anthropol* 49:497–504.

Townsend GC, Brown T (1979a). Family studies of tooth size factors in the permanent dentition. *Am J Phys Anthropol* 50:183–190.

Townsend GC, Brown T (1979b). *Tooth size characteristics of Australian Aborigines*. Occasional papers in Human Biology 1, 17–38. Australian Institute of Aboriginal Studies, Canberra.

Townsend GC, Brown T (1980). Dental asymmetry in Australian Aboriginals. *Hum Biol* 52:661–673.

Townsend GC, Brown T (1981a). Carabelli trait in Australian Aboriginal dentition. *Arch Oral Biol* 26:809–814.

Townsend GC, Brown T (1981b). Morphogenetic fields within the dentition. *Aust Orthod J* 7:3–12.

Townsend GC, Alvesalo L (1985a). The size of permanent teeth in Klinefelter (47, XXY) syndrome in man. *Arch Oral Biol* 30:83–84.

Townsend GC, Alvesalo L (1985b). Tooth size in 47, XYY males – evidence for a direct effect of the Y chromosome on growth. *Aust Dent J* 30:268–272.

Townsend GC, Martin NG (1992). Fitting genetic models to Carabelli trait data in South Australian twins. *J Dent Res* 71:403–409.

Townsend GC, Jensen BL, Alvesalo L (1984). Reduced tooth size in 45,X (Turner syndrome) females. *Am J Phys Anthropol* 65:5–13.

Townsend GC, Yamada H, Smith P (1986). The metaconule in Australian Aboriginals: an accessory tubercule on maxillary molar teeth. *Hum Biol* 58:851–862.

Townsend GC, Richards LC, Brown T (1992). Mirror imaging in the dentitions of twins – what is the biological basis? In: *Craniofacial Variation in Pacific Populations*. Brown T, Molnar S, editors. Adelaide: Anthropology and Genetics Laboratory, The University of Adelaide, pp. 67–78.

Townsend G, Alvesalo L, Brook A (2008). Variation in the human dentition: some past advances and future opportunities. *J Dent Res* 87:802–805.

Townsend GC, Alvesalo L, Jensen B, Kari M (1988). Patterns of tooth size in chromosomal aneuploidies. In: *Teeth Revisited*. Proceedings of the VIIth International Symposium on Dental Morphology, Paris 1986. Russell DE, Santoro J-P, Sigogneau-Russell D, editors. Paris, France: Mémoires Du Muséum National D'Histoire Naturelle, Series C, 53:25–45.

Townsend GC, Brown T, Richards LC, Burgess VB (1989). Dental variation in a group of Australian Aboriginals – genetic and environmental determinants. In: *The Growing Scope of Human Biology*. Schmitt LH, Freedman L, Bruce NW, editors. Perth: Centre for Human Biology, The University of Western Australia, pp. 159–170.

Townsend G, Richards L, Brown T, Pinkerton S (1994). Mirror imaging in twins: some dental examples. *Dent Anthrop* 9:2–5.

Townsend GC, Rogers J, Richards LC, Brown T (1995). Agenesis of permanent maxillary lateral incisors in South Australian twins. *Aust Dent J* 40:186–192.

Williamson JJ, Barrett MJ (1972). Oral health of Australian Aborigines: endemic dental fluorosis. *Aust Dent J* 17:266–268.

Woodroffe S, Mihailidis S, Hughes T, Bockmann M, Seow K, Gotjamanos T, Townsend G (2010). Primary tooth emergence in Australian children: timing, sequence and patterns of asymmetry. *Aust Dent J* 55:245–251.

Yamada H (1987a). Study of the crown contours of maxillary molars in Australian Aboriginals. I. Size and variability. *Jpn J Oral Biol* 29:34–43.

Yamada H (1987b). Study of the crown contours of maxillary molars in Australian Aboriginals. II. Principal component analysis of the crown contours. *Jpn J Oral Biol* 29:428–437.

Yamada H, Brown T (1988). Contours of maxillary molars studied in Australian Aboriginals. *Am J Phys Anthropol* 76:399–407.

9
The Research Legacy: Publications, theses and films directly relating to the Yuendumu Study

Publications

Barbera AL, Sampson WJ, Townsend GC (2009). An evaluation of head position and craniofacial reference line variation. *HOMO J Comp Hum Biol* 60:1–28.

Barrett MJ (1953). Dental observations on Australian Aborigines – Yuendumu, Central Australia, 1951–52. *Aust Dent J* 57:127–138.

Barrett MJ (1953). X-Occlusion. *Dent Mag Oral Top* 70: 279.Report of an exhibit at the Thirteenth Australian Dental Congress, University of Queensland, Brisbane, June 1–5, 1953.

Barrett MJ (1956). Dental observations on Australian Aborigines: water supplies and endemic dental fluorosis. *Aust Dent J* 1:87–92.

Barrett MJ (1957). Serial dental casts of Australian Aboriginal children. *Aust Dent J* 2:74.

Barrett MJ (1957). Dental observations on Australian Aborigines: tooth eruption sequence. *Aust Dent J* 2:217–227.

Barrett MJ (1958). Dental observations on Australian Aborigines: continuously changing functional occlusion. *Aust Dent J* 3:39–52.

Barrett MJ (1960). Parafunctions and tooth attrition. In: *Parafunctions of the Masticatory System (Bruxism)*. Lipke D, Posselt U, editors. Report in: *J West Soc Perio* 8:133–148.

Barrett MJ (1964). Walbiri customs and beliefs concerning teeth. *Mankind* 6:95–100.

Barrett MJ (1965). Dental observations on Australian Aborigines. *Mankind* 6:249–254.

Barrett MJ (1966). Handlist of Field Collections of Recorded Music. 50, 51, 59, 64, 113, 125, 155. Canberra: Australian Institute of Aboriginal Studies.

Barrett MJ (1968). Features of the Australian Aboriginal dentition. *Dent Mag Oral Top* 85:15–18.

Barrett MJ (1969). Functioning occlusion. *Ann Aust Coll Dent Surg* 2:68–80.

Barrett MJ (1972). Tooth wear and culture: a survey of tooth functions among some prehistoric populations. Molnar S, editor. Comment in: *Curr Anthropol* 13:516.

Barrett MJ (1976). Dental Observations on Australian Aborigines: Collected Papers and Reports 1953–1973. Adelaide: Faculty of Dentistry, The University of Adelaide.

Barrett MJ (1977). Masticatory and non-masticatory uses of teeth. In: *Stone Tools as Culture Markers: Change, Evolution and Complexity.* Wright RVS, editor. Canberra: Australian Institute of Aboriginal Studies, pp. 18–23.

Barrett MJ, Brown T (1966). Eruption of deciduous teeth in Australian Aborigines. *Aust Dent J* 11:43–50.

Barrett MJ, Brown T (1968). Relations between the breadth and depth of dental arches in a tribe of Central Australian Aborigines. *Aust Dent J* 13:381–386.

Barrett MJ, Brown T (1971). Increase in average height of Australian Aborigines. *Med J Aust* 2:1169–1172.

Barrett MJ, Brown T (1975). Did La Ferrassie use his teeth as a tool? Wallace J, editor. Comment in: *Curr Anthropol* 16:396.

Barrett MJ, Williamson JJ (1972). Oral health of Australian Aborigines: survey methods and prevalence of dental caries. *Aust Dent J* 17:37–50.

Barrett MJ, Brown T, Arato G, Ozols IV (1964). Dental observations on Australian Aborigines: buccolingual crown diameters of deciduous and permanent teeth. *Aust Dent J* 9:280–285.

Barrett MJ, Brown T, Cellier KM (1964). Tooth eruption sequences in a tribe of Central Australian Aborigines. *Am J Phys Anthropol* 22:79–89.

Barrett MJ, Brown T, Fanning EA (1965). A long-term study of the dental and craniofacial characteristics of a tribe of Central Australian Aborigines. *Aust Dent J* 10:63–68.

Barrett MJ, Brown T, Luke JI (1963). Dental observations on Australian Aborigines – mesiodistal crown diameters of deciduous teeth. *Aust Dent J* 8:299–302.

Barrett MJ, Brown T, Macdonald MR (1963). Dental observations on Australian Aborigines: mesiodistal crown diameters of permanent teeth. *Aust Dent J* 8:150–155.

Barrett MJ, Brown T, Macdonald MR (1963). Dental observations on Australian Aborigines: roentgenographic study of prognathism. *Aust Dent J* 8:418–427.

Barrett MJ, Brown T, Macdonald MR (1965). Size of dental arches in a tribe of Central Australian Aborigines. *J Dent Res* 44:912–920.

Barrett MJ, Brown T, McNulty EC (1968). A computer-based system of dental and craniofacial measurement and analysis. *Aust Dent J* 13:207–212.

Barrett MJ, Brown T, Simmons DW (1966). Computers in dental research. *Aust Dent J* 5:329–335.

Barrett MJ, Fleming TJ, Djagamara NA (1978). *Tooth evulsion in the Walbiri area.* Canberra: Australian Institute of Aboriginal Studies. (Restricted Access Publication.)

Beyron H (1962). Investigation of the occlusion and mastication of Australian Aborigines: Survey of Lecture (Undersuckning Hos Australiska Urinvanare). *Svensk TandläkareTidskrift* 55:43.

Beyron H (1964). Occlusal relations and mastication in Australian Aborigines. *Acta Odontol Scand* 22:597–678.

Björk A, Helm S (1969). Need for orthodontic treatment as reflected in the prevalence of malocclusion in various ethnic groups. *Acta Socio-Med Scand* (1 Suppl):209S–214S.

Björk A, Brown T, Skieller V (1984). Comparison of craniofacial growth in an Australian Aboriginal and Danes, illustrated by longitudinal cephalometric analysis. *Eur Orthod J* 6:1–14.

Brace CL (1979). Krapina, "Classic" Neanderthals, and the Evolution of the European face. *J Hum Evol* 8:527–550.

Brace CL (1980). Australian tooth-size clines and the death of a stereotype. *Curr Anthropol* 21:141–164.

Brace CL, Ryan AS (1980). Sexual dimorphism and human tooth size differences. *J Hum Evol* 9:417–435.

Brace CL, Hinton RJ (1981). Oceanic tooth size variation as a reflection of biological and cultural mixing (see comments). *Curr Anthrop* 22: 549–569. Comment in: *Curr Anthropol* 22:558.

Brook A, Griffin R, Townsend G, Levisianos Y, Russell J, Smith R (2009). Variability and patterning in permanent tooth size of four ethnic groups: genetic and environmental effects. *Arch Oral Biol* 54(1 Suppl):79S–85S.

Brown T (1964). Oral pigmentation in Aborigines of Kalumburu, North-West Australia. *Arch Oral Biol* 9:555–564.

Brown T (1965). *Craniofacial Variations in a Central Australian Tribe: A Radiographic Investigation of Young Adult Males and Females.* Adelaide: Libraries Board of South Australia.

Brown T (1965). Physiology of the mandibular articulation. *Aust Dent J* 10:126–131.

Brown T (1965). Program Factoran: Principal components analysis or complete factor analysis including orthogonal rotation. Canberra: CSIRO, Publication G7 CSIR.

Brown T (1967). *Factor analysis package. Five programs and their subroutines for* various *factoring procedures.* Adelaide: Computing Science, The University of Adelaide, Publication 670216.

Brown T (1969). Facial growth patterns and co-ordination. *Aust Orthod J* 2:5–11.

Brown T (1969). Developmental aspects of occlusion. *Ann Aust Coll Dent Surg* 2:61–67.

Brown T (1970). Skeletal maturity and facial growth assessment. *Aust Orthod J* 2:80–87.

Brown T (1973). *Morphology of the Australian Skull Studied by Multivariate Analysis.* Canberra: Australian Institute of Aboriginal Studies. Australian Aboriginal Studies No. 49.

Brown T (1974). Dental decay in Aborigines. In: *Better Health for Aborigines.* Hetzel BS, Dobbin M, Lippman M, Eggleston E, editors. St. Lucia: The University of Queensland Press, pp. 97–101.

Brown T (1974). Dental research in Australia and its practical applications: the Australian Aborigines. *Int Dent J* 24:299–309.

Brown T (1975). Mandibular movements. In: *The Temporomandibular Joint Syndrome: the Masticatory Apparatus of Man in Normal and Abnormal Function.* Monographs in Oral Science 4. Griffin CJ, Harris R, editors. Basel: Karger, pp. 126–150.

Brown T (1976). Head size increases in Australian Aborigines. An example of skeletal plasticity. In: *The Origin of the Australians.* Kirk RL, Thorne AG, editors. Canberra: Australian Institute of Aboriginal Studies, pp. 195–209.

Brown T (1978). Tooth emergence in Australian Aboriginals. *Ann Hum Biol* 5:41–54.

Brown T (1979). *Skeletal maturation rates in Aboriginal children.* Occasional Papers in Human Biology. Canberra: Australian Institute of Aboriginal Studies, 1:71–86.

Brown T (1981). Oceanic tooth size variation as a reflection of biological and cultural mixing (comment). *Curr Anthropol* 22:558. Comment on: *Curr Anthropol* 22:549–569.

Brown T (1982). *Growth Package Programs.* Adelaide: Department of Dentistry, The University of Adelaide, pp. 1–33.

Brown T (1983). Dental research in Australia – present and future. *J Dent Res* 62:1107–1108.

Brown T (1983). The Preece-Baines growth function demonstrated by personal computer: a teaching and research aid. *Ann Hum Biol* 10:487–489.

Brown T (1985). Occlusal development and function. In: *Functional Orthopaedics of the Jaw.* Vistas in Neuro-occlusal Rehabilitation. Simões WA, editor. Livraria Editora Santos, Sao Paulo. pp. 1–67. (in Portugese).

Brown T (1985). The supraorbital torus: a most remarkable peculiarity" (comment). *Curr Anthropol* 26:350–360. Comment on: *Curr Anthropol* 26:337–350.

Brown T (1991). Physical growth and adaptation in the tropics with special reference to the craniofacial structures. In: *Oral Diseases in the Tropics.* Prabhu SR, Wilson DF, Daftary DK, Johnson NW, editors. Oxford; New York: Oxford University Press, pp. 33–44.

Brown T (1992). Developmental, morphological and functional aspects of occlusion in Australian Aboriginals. In: *Culture, Ecology and Dental Anthropology.* Lukacs JR, editor. Delhi: Kamla-Ray Enterprises, pp. 73–85.

Brown T (1992). Dental Anthropology in South Australia. *Dent Anthropol News* 6:1–3.

Brown T (1994). "Cannibal" moves down under. *Dent Anthropol News* 9:11–12.

Brown T (1998). A century of dental anthropology in South Australia. In: *Human Dental Development, Morphology and Pathology: A Tribute to Albert A Dahlberg.* Lukacs JR, editor. Oregon: University of Anthropological Papers 54, pp. 421–431.

Brown T (2001). Thomas Draper Campbell: pioneer dental anthropologist. In: *Causes and Effects of Human Variation.* Henneberg M, editor. Adelaide: Australasian Society for Human Biology, pp. 1–11.

Brown T, Barrett MJ (1964). A roentgenographic study of facial morphology in a tribe of Central Australian Aborigines. *Am J Phys Anthropol* 22:33–42.

Brown T, Barrett MJ (1969). Tables for decimal age conversion by computer. *Aust Dent J* 14:197–198.

Brown T, Barrett MJ (1971). Growth in Central Australian Aborigines: stature. *Med J Aust* 2:29–33.

Brown T, Barrett MJ (1972). Growth in Central Australian Aborigines: weight. *Med J Aust* 2:999–1002.

Brown T, Barrett MJ (1973). Increase in average weight of Australian Aborigines. *Med J Aust* 2:25–28.

Brown T, Barrett MJ (1973). Dental and craniofacial growth studies of Australian Aborigines. In: *The Human Biology of Aborigines in Cape York.* Kirk RL, editor. Canberra: Australian Institute of Aboriginal Studies, Australian Aboriginal Studies No 44, pp. 69–80.

Brown T, Grave KC (1976). Skeletal maturation in Australian Aborigines. *Aust Paed J* 12:24–30.

Brown T, Molnar S (1990). Interproximal grooving and task activity in Australia. *Am J Phys Anthropol* 81:545–553.

Brown T, Molnar S (1992). *Craniofacial Variation in Pacific Populations.* Adelaide: Anthropology and Genetics Laboratory, Department of Dentistry, The University of Adelaide.

Brown T, Reade PC (1963). Temporomandibular joints. Part 1. Biological factors related to mandibular movements and positions. *Aust Dent J* 8:213–220.

Brown T, Rogers R (1993). *Thomas Draper Campbell.* Australian Dictionary of Biography. Volume 13. Ritchie J, editor. Melbourne: Melbourne University Press, pp. 361–362.

Brown T, Smith P (1988). Craniofacial morphology of two skeletal populations from Israel. *Hum Biol* 60:55–68.

Brown T, Townsend GC (1979). *Sex determination by single and multiple tooth measurements.* Occasional Papers in Human Biology. Canberra: Australian Institute of Aboriginal Studies, 1:1–16.

Brown T, Townsend GC (1980). Australian tooth-size clines and the death of a stereotype (comment). *Curr Anthrop* 21:153–154. Comment on: *Curr Anthropol* 21:141–164.

Brown T, Townsend GC (1982). Adolescent growth in height of Australian Aboriginals analysed by the Preece-Baines function: a longitudinal study. *Ann Hum Biol* 9:495–505.

Brown T, Townsend G (2001). Dentofacial morphology, growth and genetics: a study of Australian Aborigines. In: *Perspectives in Human Growth, Development and Maturation.* Dasgupta P, Hauspie RC, editors. The Netherlands: Kluver Academic Publishers, pp. 109–122.

Brown T, Abbott A, Burgess VB (1983). Age changes in dental arch dimensions of Australian Aboriginals. *Am J Phys Anthropol* 62:291–303.

Brown T, Abbott A, Burgess VB (1987). Longitudinal study of dental arch relationships in Australian Aboriginals with reference to alternate intercuspation. *Am J Phys Anthropol* 72:49–57.

Brown T, Barrett MJ, Clarke HT (1970). Refinement of metric data from cephalometric and other records. *Aust Dent J* 15:482–486.

Brown T, Barrett MJ, Darroch JN (1965). Factor analysis in cephalometric research. *Growth* 29:97–107.

Brown T, Barrett MJ, Darroch JN (1965). Craniofacial factors in two ethnic groups. *Growth* 29:109–123.

Brown T, Barrett MJ, Grave KC (1971). Facial growth and skeletal maturation at adolescence. *Tandlaegebladet* 75:1221–1222.

Brown T, Jenner JD, Barrett MJ, Lees GH (1979). *Exfoliation of deciduous teeth and gingival emergence of permanent teeth in Australian Aborigines.* Occasional Papers in Human Biology Canberra: Australian Institute of Aboriginal Studies, 1:47–70.

Brown T, Lambert W, Pinkerton S (1980). Brachymesophalangia-5 in a group of Australian Aboriginals. *Hum Biol* 52:651–659.

Brown T, Margetts B, Townsend GC (1980). Comparison of mesiodistal crown diameters of the deciduous and permanent teeth in Australian Aboriginals. *Aust Dent J* 25:28–33.

Brown T, Margetts B, Townsend GC (1980). Correlations between crown diameters of the deciduous and permanent teeth of Australian Aboriginals. *Aust Dent J* 25:219–223.

Brown T, Pinkerton S, Lambert W (1979). Thickness of the cranial vault in Australian Aboriginals. *Arch Phys Anthrop Oceania* 14:54–71.

Brown T, Townsend GC, Richards LC (1993). Al Dahlberg: The Australian Connection. *Dent Anthrop News* 8:19–20.

Brown T, Townsend GC, Richards LC, Burgess, VB (1990). Concepts of occlusion: the Australian evidence. *Am J Phys Anthropol* 82:247–256.

Campbell TD (1925). *Dentition and Palate of the Australian Aboriginal.* Adelaide: Hassell Press.

Campbell TD (1956). Comparative human odontology. *Aust Dent J* 1:26–29.

Campbell TD, Barrett MJ (1953). Dental observations on Australian Aborigines – a changing environment and food pattern. *Aust Dent J* 57:1–6.

Cawte JE, Djagamara NA, Barrett MJ (1966). The meaning of subincision of the urethra to Aboriginal Australians. *Br J Med Psychol* 39:245–253.

Chegini-Farahini S, Fuss J, Townsend G (2000). Intra- and inter-population variability in mamelon expression on incisor teeth. *Dent Anthrop* 14:1-6.

Clarke NG (1990). Periodontal defects of pulpal origin: evidence in early man. *Am J Phys Anthropol* 82:371–376.

Clarke NG (1992). Some anatomical factors that influence the pathways followed by dental inflammatory exudates. In: *Craniofacial Variation in Pacific Populations*. Brown T, Molnar S, editors. Adelaide, South Australia: Anthropology and Genetics Laboratory, The University of Adelaide, pp.129–137.

Clarke NG, Carey SE, Srikandi W, Hirsch RS, Leppard PI (1986). Periodontal disease in ancient populations. *Am J Phys Anthropol* 71:173–183.

Clement A, Hillson S, de la Torre I, Townsend G (2009). Tooth use in Aboriginal Australia. *Arch Int* 11:37–40.

Corruccini RS (1990). Australian aboriginal tooth succession, interproximal attrition, and Begg's theory. *Am J Orthod Dentofac Orthop* 97:349–57.

Corruccini RS, Kaul SS (1990). Premature tooth loss in relation to occlusion in Australian aboriginals. *Int J Anthropol* 5:289–294.

Corruccini RS, Townsend GC, Brown T (1990). Occlusal variation in Australian Aboriginals. *Am J Phys Anthropol* 82:257–265.

Cran JA (1955). Notes on the teeth and gingivae of Central Australian Aborigines. *Aust Dent J* 59:356–361.

Cran JA (1957). Notes on the teeth and gingivae of Central Australian Aborigines. *Aust Dent J* 2:227–282.

Cran JA (1959). Relationship of diet to dental caries. *Aust Dent J* 4:182–190.

Cran JA (1960). Histological structure of the teeth of Central Australian Aborigines and the relationship to dental caries incidence. *Aust Dent J* 5:100–104.

Cran JA (1964). Incidence of Lancefield groups in oral streptococci. *Aust Dent J* 9:27–28.

Danenberg PJ, Hirsch RS, Clarke NG, Leppard PI, Richards LC (1991). Continuous tooth eruption in Australian Aboriginal skulls. *Am J Phys Anthropol* 85:305–312.

Eguchi S, Townsend G, Richards L, Hughes T, Kasai K (2004). Genetic and environmental contributions to variation in the inclination of human mandibular molars. *Orthod Waves* 63:95–100.

Fanning EA, Moorrees CFA (1969). A comparison of permanent mandibular molar formation in Australian Aborigines and aucasoids. *Arch Oral Biol* 14:999–1006.

Fanning EA, Brown T (1971). Primary and permanent tooth development. *Aust Dent J* 16:41–43.

Fleming DA, Barrett MJ, Fleming TJ (1971). Family records of an Australian Aboriginal community. *Abor Stud News* 3:15.

Floyd B, Littleton J (2006). Linear enamel hypoplasia and growth in an Australian Aboriginal community: not so small but not so healthy either. *Ann Hum Biol* 33:424–443.

Frayer DW (1980). Sexual dimorphism and cultural evolution in the late Pleistocene and Holocene of Europe. *J Hum Evol* 9:399–415.

Frayer DW, Wolpoff MH (1985). Sex dimorphism. *Annu Rev Anthropol* 14:429–473.

Gagliardi A, Winning T, Kaidonis J, Hughes T, Townsend GC (2004). Association of frontal sinus development with somatic and skeletal maturation in Aboriginal Australians: a longitudinal study. *HOMO J Comp Hum Biol* 55:39–52.

Grave B, Brown T, Townsend G (1999). Comparison of cervicovertebral dimensions in Australian Aborigines and Caucasoids. *Eur J Orthod* 21:127–135.

Grave KC (1973). Timing of facial growth. A study of relations with stature and ossification in the hand around puberty. *Aust Orthod J* 3:117–122.

Grave KC, Brown T (1972). Hand and head roentgenograms on one film. *Aust Dent J* 17:331–332.

Grave KC, Brown T (1976). Skeletal ossification and the adolescent growth spurt. *Am J Orthod* 69:611–619.

Grave KC, Brown T (1979). *Reliability of skeletal age assessments in Aborigines.* Occasional Papers in Human Biology. Canberra: Australian Institute of Aboriginal Studies, 1:87–94.

Grave KC, Brown T (1979). Carpal radiographs in orthodontic treatment. *Am J Orthod* 75:27–45.

Grave K, Townsend G (2003). Cervical vertebral maturation as a predictor of the adolescent growth spurt. *Aust Orthod J* 19:25–32.

Grave K, Townsend G (2003). Hand-wrist and cervical vertebral maturation indicators: how can these events be used to time Class II treatments? *Aust Orthod J* 19:33–45.

Gresham HT, Brown T, Barrett MJ (1965). Skeletal and denture patterns in children from Yuendumu, Central Australia and Melbourne. *Aust Dent J* 10:462–468.

Hanihara K (1970). Preliminary reports on dental anthropology of the Australian Aborigines. (in Japanese) *J Anthrop Soc Nippon* 78:75–76.

Hanihara K (1974). Factors controlling crown size of the deciduous dentition. (in English). *J Anthrop Soc Nippon* 82:128–134.

Hanihara K (1976). *Statistical and comparative studies of the Australian Aboriginal dentition. Bulletin, No.11.* The University Museum, The University of Tokyo, Tokyo.

Hanihara K (1977). Distance between Australian Aborigines and certain other populations based on dental measurements. *J Hum Evol* 6:403–418.

Hanihara K (1978). Difference in sexual dimorphism in dental morphology among several human populations In: *Development, Function and Evolution of Teeth.* Butler PM, Joysey KA, editors. London: Academic Press, pp. 127–133.

Hanihara K (1979). Dental traits in Ainu, Australian Aborigines, and New World populations. In: *The First Americans: Origins, Affinities and Adaptions.* Laughlin WS, Harper AB, editors. New York: Gustav Fischer, pp. 125–134.

Hasegawa Y, Rogers J, Kageyama I, Nakahara S, Townsend G (2007). Comparison of permanent mandibular molar crown dimensions between Mongolians and Caucasians. *Dent Anthrop* 20:1–6.

Hayashi S (1974). Occlusal surface index of the Australian Aboriginal molars. *Nihon Univ Dent J* 48:210–212.

Heithersay GS (1959). A dental survey of the Aborigines at Haast's Bluff, Central Australia. *Med J Aust* 1:721–729.

Heithersay GS (1960). Attritional values for Australian Aborigines, Haast's Bluff. *Aust Dent J* 5:84–88.

Heithersay GS (1961). Further observations on the dentition of the Australian aborigine at Haast's Bluff. *Aust Dent J* 6:18–28.

Helm S (1979). Etiology and treatment need of malocclusion. *J Can Dent Assoc* 45:673–676.

Hughes T, Richards LC, Townsend G (2002). Form, symmetry and asymmetry of the dental arch: orthogonal analysis revisited. *Dent Anthrop* 16:3–8.

Kageyama I, Mayhall J, Townsend GC (1999). A three-dimensional study of the deciduous and permanent molars in Australian Aborigines. *Persp Hum Biol* 4:103–108.

Kaidonis JA, Townsend GC, Richards LC (1992). The morphological features and aetiology of interproximal tooth wear. In: *Craniofacial Variation in Pacific Populations*. Brown T, Molnar S, editors. Adelaide, South Australia: Anthropology and Genetics Laboratory, The University of Adelaide, pp. 121–127.

Kaidonis JA, Townsend GC, Richards LC (1992). Interproximal tooth wear – a new observation. *Am J Phys Anthropol* 88:105–107.

Kaidonis JA, Townsend GC, Richards LC (1992). Abrasion: an evolutionary and clinical view. *Aust Pros J* 6:9–16.

Kaidonis JA, Townsend GC, Richards LC (1993). Nature and frequency of dental wear facets in an Australian Aboriginal population. *J Oral Rehab* 20:333–340.

Kaifu Y, Kasai K, Townsend GC, Richards LC (2003). Tooth wear and the "design" of the human dentition: a perspective from evolutionary medicine. *Yearb Phys Anthropol* 46:47–61.

Kanazawa E, Morris DH, Sekikawa M, Ozaki T (1988). Comparative study of the upper molar occlusal table morphology among seven human populations. *Am J Phys Anthropol* 77:271–278

Kapali S, Townsend G, Richards L, Parish T (1997). Palatal rugae patterns in Australian aborigines and caucasians. *Aust Dent J* 42:129–133.

Kasai K, Kanazawa E, Aboshi H, Richards LC, Matsuno M (1997). Dental arch form in three Pacific populations: a comparison with Japanese and Australian Aboriginal samples. *J Nihon Univ Sch Dent* 39:196–201.

Kasai K, Richards LC, Brown T (1993). Comparative study of craniofacial morphology in Japanese and Australian Aboriginal populations. *Hum Biol* 65:821–834.

Kaul SS, Corruccini RS (1992). Dental arch length reduction through interproximal attrition in modern Australian aborigines. *J Hum Ecol Special Issue* 2:195–199.

Keith, Sir Arthur (1926). Review of *Dentition and Palate of the Australian Aboriginal*. Journal of Anatomy LX, IV.

Kohn L, Osborne R, Townsend GC (1999). Craniofacial and dental morphological integration: III. Comparison of North American and Australian Aboriginal populations. In: *Dental Morphology 1998*. Proceedings of 11th International Symposium on Dental Morphology, August, 1998, Oulu. Mayhall J, Heikkinen T, editors. Oulu, Finland: University of Oulu Press, pp. 425–429.

Kondo S, Townsend GC (2004). Sexual dimorphism in crown units of mandibular deciduous and permanent molars in Australian aborigines. *HOMO J Comp Hum Biol* 55:53–64.

Kondo S, Townsend GC, Kanazawa E (2005). Size relationships among permanent mandibular molars in Aboriginal Australians and Papua New Guinea Highlanders. *Am J Hum Biol* 17:622–633.

Kondo S, Townsend G, Nakajima K, Yamada H, Wakatsuki E (1999). Size of crown components of the mandibular deciduous and permanent molars in Australian Aborigines. In: *Dental Morphology 1998*. Proceedings of 11th International Symposium on Dental Morphology, August, 1998, Oulu. Mayhall J, Heikkinen T, editors. Oulu, Finland: University of Oulu Press, pp. 150–166.

Kondo S, Townsend GC, Yamada H (2005). Sexual dimorphism of cusp dimensions in human maxillary molars. *Am J Phys Anthropol* 128:870–877.

Kuusk S, Barrett MJ (1979). *Rotated maxillary central incisors*. Occasional Papers in Human Biology. Canberra: Australian Institute of Aboriginal Studies, 1:39–46.

Lekkas D, Townsend G (1996). Cervical enamel projections and enamel pearls in a collection of Australian extracted molars. *Dent Anthrop News* 11:2–6.

Linn J, Srikandi W, Clarke NG, Smith T (1987). Radiographic and visual assessment of alveolar pathology of first molars in dry skulls. *Am J Phys Anthropol* 72:515–521.

Lin NH, Ranjitkar S, MacDonald R, Hughes T, Taylor J, Townsend G (2006). New growth references for assessment of stature and skeletal maturation in Australians. *Aust Orthod J* 22:1–10

Littleton J (2005). Invisible impacts but long-term consequences: hypoplasia and contact in Central Australia. *Am J Phys* Anthropol 126:295–304.

Littleton J, Townsend GC (2005). Linear enamel hypoplasia and historical change in a central Australian community. *Aust Dent J* 50:101–107.

Liversidge HM, Townsend GC (2006). Tooth formation in Australian Aborigines. In: *Current Trends in Dental Morphology Research*. 13th International Symposium on Dental Morphology, August 24–27, 2005, Łódź, Poland. Żądzińska E, editor. Łódź: University of Łódź Press, pp. 405–410.

Madsen D, Sampson W, Townsend G (2008). Craniofacial reference plane variation and natural head position. *Eur J Orthod* 30:532–540.

Margetts B, Brown T (1978). Crown diameters of the deciduous teeth in Australian Aboriginals. *Am J Phys Anthropol* 48:493–502.

Mayhall JT, Townsend GC (2006). The changing crown morphology of maxillary first molars and its effect on the efficiency of mastication. In: *Current Trends in Dental Morphology Research*. 13th International Symposium on Dental Morphology, August 24–27, 2005, Łódź, Poland. Żądzińska E, editor. Łódź: University of Łódź Press, pp. 97–104.

McKee JK, Molnar S (1988). Measurement of tooth wear among Australian Aborigines: II Intrapopulational variation in patterns of dental attrition. *Am J Phys Anthropol* 76:125–136.

McKee JK, Molnar S (1988). Mathematical and descriptive classification of variations in dental arch shape in an Australian Aboriginal population. *Arch Oral Biol* 33:901–906.

McNulty EC, Barrett MJ, Brown T (1968). Mesh diagram analysis of facial morphology in young adult Australian Aborigines. *Aust Dent J* 13:440–446.

Molnar S, McKee JK, Molnar I (1983). Measurements of tooth wear among Australian Aborigines: I. Serial loss of the enamel crown. *Am J Phys Anthropol* 61:51–65.

Molnar S, McKee JK, Molnar I, Przybeck TR (1983). Tooth wear rates among contemporary Australian Aborigines. *J Dent Res* 62:562–564.

Molnar S, Molnar IM (1990). Dental arch shape and tooth wear variability. *Am J Phys Anthropol* 82:385–395.

Molnar S, Molnar I (1992). Dental arch shape and tooth wear among the prehistoric populations of the Murray River valley. In: *Craniofacial Variation in Pacific Populations*. Brown T, Molnar S, editors. Adelaide, South Aust: Anthropology and Genetics Laboratory, The University of Adelaide, pp. 99–112.

Molnar S, Richards LC, McKee JK, Molnar I (1989). Tooth wear in Australian Aboriginal populations from the River Murray Valley. *Am J Phys Anthropol* 79:185–196.

Nagashima S (1975). The measurement of relative sizes of the cusp area in human molars Part 2. The Australian Aboriginal teeth. *Nihon Univ J Oral Science* 33–38.

Nakahara S, Takahashi M, Townsend G (1997). Modes of occlusion in humans: a comparison of traditional Aborigines and modern Japanese. *Shigaku (Odontology)* 85:345–356.

Nakahara S, Takahashi M, Kameda T, Kameda A, Townsend GC (1998). Longitudinal changes in the modes of occlusion of permanent teeth: changes in the teeth and dentition of Australian Aborigines – Part 1: Normalization of malocclusion. *Shigaku (Odontology)* 86:209–230.

Nakahara S, Takahashi M, Kameda T, Kameda A, Townsend GC (1999). Longitudinal changes in the modes of occlusion of permanent teeth – changes in the teeth and dentition of Australian Aborigines – Part 2: Transition of normal incisal occlusion into malocclusions. *Shigaku (Odontology)* 87:8–29.

Nakahara S, Takahashi M, Kameda T, Kameda A, Townsend GC (2000). Longitudinal changes in the modes of occlusion of permanent teeth – stabilities in the teeth and dentitions of Australian Aborigines – Part 3: Constant normal occlusion, constant malocclusions and variable types. *Shigaku (Odontology)* 87:545–581.

Ozaki T, Kanazawa E, Sekikawa M, Akai J (1987). Three-dimensional measurement of occlusal surface of upper first molars in Australian Aboriginals. *Aust Dent J* 32:263–269.

Ozaki T, Ohnuki E, Tsuruoka M (1977). Occlusal surface index of the molars in Indians. *J Anthrop Soc Nippon* 85:237–247.

Pretty GL, Brown T, Kricun ME (1992). Extensive compensatory remodelling of craniofacial structures: a case from prehistoric South Australia. In: *Craniofacial Variation in Pacific Populations*. Brown T, Molnar S, editors. Adelaide, South Australia: Anthropology and Genetics Laboratory, The University of Adelaide, pp. 139–146.

Proffit WR (1975). Muscle pressure and tooth position: North American Whites and Australian Aborigines. *Angle Orthod* 45:1–11.

Proffit WR (1978). Equilibrium theory re-examined: To what extent do tongue and lip pressures influence tooth position and thereby occlusion? In: *Oral Physiology and Occlusion*. Proceedings of an International Symposium 1976, Newark, NJ. Perryman JH, editors. London: Pergamon, pp. 55–77.

Proffit WR, McGlone RE (1975). Tongue-lip pressure during speech of Australian Aborigines. *Phonetica* 32:200–220.

Proffit WR, McGlone RE, Barrett MJ (1975). Lip and tongue pressure related to dental arch and oral cavity size in Australian Aborigines. *J Dent Res* 54:1161–1172.

Prokopec M, Brown T, Barrett MJ (1982). The contribution of Dr. A. Hrdlička to Australia's anthropology In: *IInd Anthropological Congress of Aleš Hrdlička*. Novotný VV, editor. Prague: Universitas Carolina Pragensis, pp. 35–39.

Reade PC (1964). Infantile acute oral moniliasis. *Aust Dent J* 9:14–16.

Reade PC (1965). Dental observations on Australian Aborigines, Koonibba, South Australia. *Aust Dent J* 10:361–370.

Richards LC (1984). Principal axis analysis of dental attrition data from two Australian Aboriginal populations. *Am J Phys Anthropol* 65:5–13.

Richards LC (1984). Form and function of the mastication system. In: *Archaelogy at ANZAAS*

Canberra. Ward GK, editor. Canberra: The Australian National University, pp. 96–109.

Richards LC (1985). Dental attrition and craniofacial morphology in two Australian Aboriginal populations. *J Dent Res* 64:1311–1315.

Richards LC (1987). Temporomandibular joint morphology in two Australian Aboriginal populations. *J Dent Res* 66:1602–1607.

Richards LC (1988). Degenerative changes in the temporomandibular joint in two Australian Aboriginal populations. *J Dent Res* 67:1529–1533.

Richards LC (1990). Tooth wear and temporomandibular joint change in Australian Aboriginal populations. *Am J Phys Anthropol* 82:377–384.

Richards LC (1992). Interproximal tooth wear in Australian Aboriginal populations. In: *Craniofacial Variation in Pacific Populations.* Brown T, Molnar S, editors. Adelaide, South Aust: Anthropology and Genetics Laboratory, The University of Adelaide, pp. 113–119.

Richards LC, Brown T (1981). Dental attrition and degenerative arthritis of the temporomandibular joint. *J Oral Rehabil* 8:293–307.

Richards LC, Brown T (1981). Dental attrition and age relationships in Australian Aboriginals. *Arch Oceania* 16:94–98.

Richards LC, Brown T (1986). Development of the helicoidal plane. *Hum Evol* 1:385–398.

Richards LC, Gurner IA (1985). An assessment of radiographic methods for the investigation of temporomandibular joint morphology and pathology. *Aust Dent J* 30:323–332.

Richards LC, Miller SLJ (1991). Relationships between age and dental attrition in Australian Aboriginals. *Am J Phys Anthropol* 84:159–164.

Richards LC, Telfer PJ (1979). The use of dental characters in the assessment of genetic distance in Australia. *Arch Phys Anthrop Oceania* 14:184–194.

Richards LC, Beaumont S, Kaidonis J, Townsend GC (1999). Craniofacial morphology and tooth wear in three Australian populations. *Persp Hum Biol* 4:77–84.

Rogers AH (1973). The occurance of streptococcus mutans in the dental plaque of a group of Central Australian Aborigines. *Aust Dent J* 18:157–159.

Rogers J, Townsend G, Brown T (2009). Murray James Barrett dental anthropologist: Yuendumu and beyond. *HOMO J Comp Hum Biol* 60:295–306.

Russell MA (1985). The supraorbital torus: "a most remarkable peculiarity" (see comments). *Curr Anthrop* 26:337–350. Comment in: *Curr Anthrop* 26:350–360.

Sampson WJ, Richards LC (1985). Prediction of mandibular incisor and canine crowding changes in mixed dentition. *Am J Orthod* 88:47–63.

Sekikawa M, Akai J, Kanazawa E, Ozaki T (1986). Three-dimensional measurement of the occlusal surfaces of lower first molars of Australian Aboriginals. *Am J Phys Anthropol* 71:25–32.

Sekikawa M, Kanazawa E, Ozaki T, Brown T (1988). Principal component analysis of intercusp distances on the lower first molars of three human populations. *Arch Oral Biol* 33:535–541.

Smith P, Brown T, Wood WB (1981). Tooth size and morphology in a recent Australian Aboriginal population from Broadbeach, South East Queensland. *Am J Phys Anthropol* 55:423–432.

Sobhi P, Mihailidis S, Rogers J, Hughes T, Townsend G (2007). Asymmetrical eruption of permanent teeth in Australian Aborigines. *Dent Anthrop* 20:33–40.

Solow B, Barrett MJ, Brown T (1982). Craniocervical morphology and posture in Australian

Aboriginals. *Am J Phys Anthropol* 59:33–45.

Springbett S, Townsend GC, Kaidonis JA, Richards LC (1999). Tooth wear in the deciduous dentition: a cross cultural and longitudinal study. *Persp Hum Biol* 4:93–101.

Takahashi M, Kondo S, Townsend G, Kanazawa E (2007). Variability in cusp size of human maxillary molars, with particular reference to the hypocone. *Arch Oral Biol* 52:1146–1154.

Taylor WB (1971). Shape similarity in bone tracings. In: *A Spectrum of Mathematics.* Butcher JC, editor. Auckland: Auckland University Press and Oxford University Press, pp. 214–224.

Townsend GC (1978). Genetics of tooth size. *Aust Orthod J* 5:142–147.

Townsend GC (1980). Heritability of deciduous tooth size in Australian Aboriginals. *Am J Phys Anthropol* 53:297–300.

Townsend GC (1981). Fluctuating asymmetry in the deciduous dentition of Australian Aboriginals. *J Dent Res* 60:1849–1857.

Townsend GC (1985). Intercuspal distances of maxillary premolar teeth in Australian Aboriginals. *J Dent Res* 64:443–446.

Townsend GC (1988). Anthropological aspects of dental morphology with special reference to tropical populations. In: *Oral Diseases in the Tropics.* Prabhu SR, Wilson DF, Daftary DK and Johnson NW, editors. Oxford; New York: Oxford University Press, pp. 45–58.

Townsend GC (1994). Understanding the nature and causes of variation in the dento-facial structures. *Proc Finn Dent Soc* 12:642–648.

Townsend GC, Brown T (1978). Inheritance of tooth size in Australian Aboriginals. *Am J Phys Anthropol* 48:305–314.

Townsend GC, Brown T (1978). Heritability of permanent tooth size. *Am J Phys Anthropol* 49:497–505.

Townsend GC, Brown T (1979). Family studies of tooth size factors in the permanent dentition. *Am J Phys Anthropol* 50:183–190.

Townsend GC, Brown T (1979). *Tooth size characteristics of Australian Aborigines.* Occasional Papers in Human Biology. Canberra: Australian Institute of Aboriginal Studies, 1:17–38.

Townsend GC, Brown T (1980). Dental asymmetry in Australian Aboriginals. *Hum Biol* 52:661–673.

Townsend GC, Brown T (1981). Morphogenetic fields within the dentition. *Aust Orthod J* 7:3–12.

Townsend GC, Brown T (1981). Carabelli trait in Australian Aboriginal dentition. *Arch Oral Biol* 26:809–814.

Townsend GC, Brown T (1983). Molar size sequence in Australian Aboriginals. *Am J Phys Anthropol* 60:69–74.

Townsend G, Alvesalo L, Brook A (2008). Variation in the human dentition: some past advances and future opportunities. *J Dent Res* 87:802–805.

Townsend GC, Brown T, Richards LC, Burgess VB (1989). Dental variation in a group of Australian Aboriginals – genetic and environmental determinants. In: *The Growing Scope of Human Biology.* Schmitt LH, Freedman L, Bruce NW, editors. Perth: Centre for Human Biology, The University of Western Australia, pp. 159–170.

Townsend G, Harris E, Lesot H, Claus F, Brook A (2009). Morphogenetic fields in the dentition: a new, clinically-relevant synthesis of an old concept. *Arch Oral Biol* 54(1 Suppl):34S–44S.

Townsend GC, Richards LC, Carroll A (1982). Sex determination of Australian Aboriginal skulls by discriminant function analysis. *Aust Dent J* 27:320–326.

Townsend GC, Yamada H, Smith P (1986). The metaconule in Australian Aboriginals: an accessory tubercule on maxillary molar teeth. *Hum Biol* 58:851–862.

Townsend GC, Yamada H, Smith P (1990). Expression of the entoconulid (sixth cusp) on mandibular molar teeth of an Australian Aboriginal population. *Am J Phys Anthropol* 82:267–274.

Williamson JJ, Barrett MJ (1972). Oral health of Australian Aborigines: endemic dental fluorosis. *Aust Dent J* 17:266–268.

Winning TA, Brown T, Townsend GC (1999). Quantifying asymmetry in the human facial skeleton. *Persp Hum Biol* 4:53–60.

Wolpoff MH (1985). Tooth size – body size scaling in a human population: theory and practice of an allometric analysis. In: *Size and Scaling in Primate Biology*. Jungers WL, editor. New York: Plenum, pp. 273–318.

Yamada H (1987). Study of the crown contours of maxillary molars in Australian Aboriginals. I. Size and variability. *Jpn J Oral Biol* 29:34–43.

Yamada H (1987). Study of the crown contours of maxillary molars in Australian Aboriginals. II. Principal component analysis of the crown contours. *Jpn J Oral Biol* 29:428–437.

Yamada H, Brown T (1988). Contours of maxillary molars studied in Australian Aboriginals. *Am J Phys Anthropol* 76:399–407.

Yamada H, Brown T (1990). Shape components of the maxillary molars in Australian Aboriginals. *Am J Phys Anthropol* 82:275–282.

Theses

Campbell TD (1923). *Dentition and Palate of the Australian Aboriginal from Observations on the Skull: A Study in Physical Anthropology and Dental Pathology*. DDSc Thesis, The University of Adelaide.

Campbell TD (1939). *Collection of Published Papers on Original Field Research*. DSc Thesis, The University of Adelaide.

Brown T (1963). *Craniofacial Variations in a Central Australian tribe: A Radiographic Investigation of Young Adult Males and Females*. MDS Thesis, The University of Adelaide.

Brown T (1967). *Skull of the Australian Aboriginal. A Multivariate Analysis of Craniofacial Associations*. DDSc Thesis, The University of Adelaide.

McNulty EC (1968). *Growth Changes in the Face. A Semi-longitudinal Cephalometric Study of the Australian Aboriginal by Means of a Coordinate Analysis*. MDS Thesis, The University of Adelaide.

Grave KC (1971). *Timing of Facial Growth in Australian Aborigines: A Study of Relations with Stature and Ossification in the Hand Around Puberty*. MDS Thesis, The University of Adelaide.

Cheng PCK (1972). *Dental-arch Morphology of Australian Aborigines: A Metric Study of Arch Size and Shape*. MDS Thesis, The University of Adelaide.

Taylor WB (1972). *Some Aspects of Statistical Analysis of Shape Similarity with Applications to Bone Morphology*. PhD Thesis, The University of Adelaide.

Jenner J (1972). *Dental Development and Facial Growth Studied in Australian Aborigines*. MDS Thesis, The University of Adelaide.

Townsend GC (1973). *Curve Fitting Methods to Characterise Human Growth.* BScDent (Hons) Research Report, The University of Adelaide.

Kuusk S (1973). *Deciduous Tooth Crown Morphology in a Tribe of Australian Aborigines. A Study of Twelve Non-metric Traits.* MDS Thesis, The University of Adelaide.

Shultz M (1973). *Body-build and Craniofacial Morphology Studied in Australian Aborigines.* MDS Thesis, The University of Adelaide.

Drummond PW (1974). *Mathematic characterization of dental morphology : a theoretical approach to identification in forensic odontology.* MDS Thesis, The University of Adelaide.

Townsend GC (1976). *Tooth Size Variability in Australian Aboriginals: A Descriptive and Genetic Study.* PhD Thesis, The University of Adelaide.

Richards LC (1978). *Attrition and the Temporomandibular Joint: An Investigation of Interactions and Adaptions in the Masticatory System of the Australian Aboriginal.* BScDent Report, The University of Adelaide.

Telfer PJ (1978). *Comparative Study of Dental Arch Morphology and Occlusion.* MDS Thesis, University of Adelaide.

Richards LC (1983). *Adaptation in the Masticatory System: Descriptive and Correlative Studies of a Pre-Contemporary Australian Population.* PhD Thesis, The University of Adelaide.

Abbott AH (1983) *Shape Analysis Methodology.* BScDent(Hons) Research Report, The University of Adelaide.

Dawson P (1983). *An analysis of craniofacial asymmetry in Australian Aboriginals.* BScDent(Hons) Thesis, The University of Adelaide.

Dawson P (1984). *Craniofacial Asymmetry in Australian Aboriginals.* BScDent (Hons) Report, Department of Oral Biology, The University of Adelaide.

McKee JK (1985). *Patterns of Dental Attrition and Craniofacial Shape Among Australian Aborigines.* PhD Thesis, The Washington University, St. Louis.

Abbott AH (1988). *The Acquisition and Analysis of Craniofacial Data in Three Dimensions.* PhD Thesis, The University of Adelaide.

Burgess VB (1989). *Age Changes in the Dental Arches of Australian Aboriginal Children: A Semi-longitudinal Study from Six to Twenty Years.* MDS Thesis, The University of Adelaide.

Kaidonis J (1989). *Tooth wear: facet frequencies in two human populations including a longitudinal study.* BScDent(Hons) Thesis, The University of Adelaide.

Bachtiar M (1990). *An assessment of Pont's Index to predict dental arch form in human populations.* MDS Thesis, The University of Adelaide.

Grave B (1993). *Relationships between the morphology of cervical vertebrae and craniofacial structures in Australian Aborigines.* BScDent(Hons) Thesis, The University of Adelaide.

Bachtiar M (1990). *An Assessment of Pont's Index to Predict Dental Arch Width in Human populations.* MDS Thesis, The University of Adelaide.

Kaidonis J (1990). *Tooth Wear: Facet Frequencies in Two Human Populations including a Longitudinal Study.* BScDent (Hons) Report, The University of Adelaide.

Townsend GC (1994). *Genetic Studies of Morphological Variation in the Human Dentition. Collection of Papers.* DDSc Thesis, The University of Adelaide.

Springbett S (1998). *Tooth wear in children: a longitudinal and cross-cultural study.* MDS Thesis, The

University of Adelaide.

Beaumont S (1995). *Association between tooth wear and craniofacial morphology.* BScDent(Hons) Thesis, The University of Adelaide.

Cheghini-Farahani A (1999). *Incisor mamelon morphology: how important are genetic factors.* BScDent(Hons) Thesis, The University of Adelaide.

Gagliardi A (2000). *Relationship of frontal sinus development with somatic and skeletal development.* BScDent(Hons) Thesis, The University of Adelaide.

Damhuis S (2005). *Can the sex and age of site occupants be determined by analysing rock art hand stencils?* BScDent(Hons) Thesis, Flinders University, South Australia.

Damhuis SJ (2005). *Hand Stencils (manuscript): a Key to Identifying Gender at Rock Art Sites.* BArchaeol (Hons), Department of Archaeology, Flinders University of South Australia.

Barbera AL (2006). *An evaluation of head balance and craniofacial reference lines.* BScDent(Hons) Report, The University of Adelaide.

Barbera A (2006). *Changes in Head Posture With Age – a Cephalometric Assessment.* DClinDent Thesis, The University of Adelaide.

Sobhi P (2006). *Asymmetrical eruption of permanent teeth in Australian Aborigines.* BScDent(Hons) Thesis, The University of Adelaide.

Madsen DP (2007). *Natural head position: a photographic method and an evaluation of cranial reference planes in cephalometric analysis.* DClinDent Thesis, The University of Adelaide.

Thiyagarajan R (2008). *A Longitudinal Study of Interproximal Attrition and Tooth Wear Rates in Modern Native Australians.* DClinDent Thesis, The University of Adelaide.

Films

Tindale NB, Campbell TD (1930). *Macdonald Downs Expedition.* Adelaide: Board for Anthropological Research, The University of Adelaide. (Members of the Loiaura tribe. Leaf spinning and tjebudja games; tree climbing; stone axe making; Alpalaita or grub totem ceremony; food gathering.)

Campbell TD, Barrett MJ (1954). *So They Did Eat.* Adelaide: Board for Anthropological Research, The University of Adelaide. (Food and food habits, gathering and hunting food supplies, preparation and cooking.)

Campbell TD, Dobbie JC, Cornell JG (1955). *Minjena's Lost Ground.* Adelaide: Board for Anthropological Research, The University of Adelaide. (The effect of white contact on life at Yuendumu.)

Barrett MJ (1956). *Mastication – A Dynamic Process.* Adelaide: University of Adelaide.

Campbell TD, Barrett MJ, Cornell JG (1958). *The Boomerang.* Adelaide: Board for Anthropological Research, The University of Adelaide. (Record of Aboriginal technology showing the making and use of the boomerang by the Walbiri.)

Campbell TD, Barrett MJ, Cornell JG (1958). *The Woomera.* Adelaide: Board for Anthropological Research, The University of Adelaide. (Record of Aboriginal technology showing the making and use of spear throwers by the Walbiri.)

Campbell TD (1958). *Nabarula; the Story of an Aboriginal Girl.* Adelaide: Board for Anthropological Research, The University of Adelaide. (The life of a Walbiri girl from childhood to motherhood.)

Campbell TD, Barrett MJ, Cornell JG (1963). *Palya-Prepared Spinifex Gum*. Adelaide: Board for Anthropological Research, The University of Adelaide. (The collection, cleaning, preparation and heat treatment of the grass resin and some of its uses.)

Campbell TD (1963). *Aboriginal Spears*. Adelaide: Board for Anthropological Research, The University of Adelaide. (Illustrating the manufacture and use of two main types of spear used by the Walbiri.)

Campbell TD, Barrett MJ, Cornell JG (1963). *Aboriginal Hair String*. Adelaide: Board for Anthropological Research, The University of Adelaide. (A record of the manufacture and use of human hair string.)

Campbell TD, Barrett MJ, Cornell JG (1965). *Aboriginal Stone Axes*. Adelaide: Board for Anthropological Research, The University of Adelaide. (Shows quarrying, flaking and mounting of stone axeheads by members of the Walbiri tribe.)

Campbell TD, Cornell JG, Barrett MJ (1965). *Ngoora – A Camping Place*. Adelaide: Board for Anthropological Research, The University of Adelaide. (A story of the movement of a small group of Aboriginal people to a new camping site.)

Appendices

Appendix A:

List of Overseas Visiting Researchers to the Murray Barrett Laboratory

Appendix B:

Growth Tables for Variables on Yuendumu Children with Known Birth Dates (Age Range 5.0–20.0 Years in Half Yearly Intervals)

Details of subject selection and the methodology used to produce the growth tables are given in Chapter 2.

Appendix C:

Photographs of Yuendumu and its people

Appendix A

International visiting researchers include				
Japan		**USA**	**Scandinavia**
Tadashi Ozaki	Takahashi Kameda	Murray Ricketts	Henry Beyron
Kazuro Hanihara	Ryuji Ueno	Bill Proffit	Sven Helm
Tsunehiko Hanihara	Ryuta Kataoka	Harry Sicher	Arne Björk
Hiroyuki Yamada	Shintaro Kondo	Steve Molnar	Vibeke Skieller
Mitsuo Sekikawa	Tadashi Ideguchi	Iva Molnar	Beni Solow
Koh Nakajima	Masutaka Mizutani	Ed McNulty	Lassi Alvesalo
Soichiro Tomo	Masame Takahashi	Rob Coruccini	Juha Varrela
Ikuko Tomo	Yuh Hasegawa	C. Loring Brace	Torstein Sjovold
Ikuo Kajeyama	Hiroshi Takayama	Mary Russell	Tuomo Heikkinen
Kazutaka Kasai	Tsuneo Sekimoto	Ron Presswood	Raija Lähdesmäki
Sen Nakahara	Masashi Takahashi	Christy Turner	Inger Kjaer
Hiro Aboshi	Ken Yoshimura	Bhim Savara	
Eisaku Kanazawa	Satoshi Tanaka		
Shosei Eguchi	Akira Kameda		
Shintaro Kondo	Takashi Kameda		
New Zealand		**England**	
Michael Shultz	Kevin Scally	Graham Lees	Alan Brook
Jules Kieser	Judith Littleton	Helen Liversidge	Anna Clement
Bruce Floyd			
Canada	**Brazil**	**Czech Republic**	**Israel**
John Mayhall	Wilma Simóes	Miroslav Prokopec	Pat Smith
India	**South Africa**		
Samvit S Kaul	Nicky Veres	Peter Owen	

Appendix B
Table B.1 Growth of Yuendumu Aboriginals - Stature (cm)

Age	N	SD	Males centiles			N	SD	Females centiles		
			10th	50th	90th			10th	50th	90th
5.0	1	—	106.7	110.0	113.3	3	—	99.9	105.0	110.1
5.5	3	—	107.9	111.2	114.5	4	3.9	103.4	108.4	113.4
6.0	4	3.2	109.6	113.6	117.6	3	—	106.9	111.8	116.7
6.5	6	3.2	111.9	116.0	120.1	8	3.8	110.4	115.2	120.0
7.0	15	3.4	114.7	119.0	123.3	11	3.8	114.0	118.8	123.6
7.5	18	3.6	117.0	121.6	126.2	18	3.8	117.1	122.0	126.9
8.0	24	3.8	119.1	124.0	128.9	26	4.0	120.1	125.2	130.3
8.5	29	4.2	121.5	126.8	132.1	27	4.2	122.6	128.0	133.4
9.0	38	4.6	122.9	128.8	134.7	31	4.6	125.1	131.0	136.9
9.5	46	5.0	125.2	131.6	138.0	37	5.1	127.3	133.8	140.3
10.0	52	5.4	126.9	133.8	140.7	40	5.5	129.5	136.6	143.7
10.5	54	5.7	127.0	134.2	141.4	43	6.0	131.9	139.6	147.3
11.0	56	5.9	131.2	138.8	146.4	46	6.3	134.3	142.4	150.5
11.5	60	6.2	132.0	140.0	148.0	45	6.4	137.4	145.6	153.8
12.0	63	6.6	135.1	143.6	152.1	48	6.3	140.5	148.6	156.7
12.5	67	7.1	137.1	146.2	155.3	40	6.0	144.0	151.6	159.2
13.0	68	7.7	139.7	149.6	159.5	37	5.6	147.1	154.2	161.3
13.5	63	8.3	142.2	152.8	163.4	38	5.0	149.9	156.4	162.9
14.0	62	8.5	146.1	157.0	167.9	34	4.5	152.6	158.4	164.2
14.5	54	8.6	149.8	160.8	171.8	27	4.2	154.6	160.0	165.4
15.0	48	8.5	152.9	163.8	174.7	30	4.0	155.8	161.0	166.2
15.5	42	8.2	155.6	166.0	176.4	22	3.9	156.6	161.6	166.6
16.0	31	7.7	158.0	167.8	177.6	21	3.9	157.2	162.2	167.2
16.5	33	7.2	160.0	169.2	178.4	27	3.9	157.4	162.4	167.4
17.0	24	6.8	161.2	170.0	178.8	18	4.0	157.3	162.4	167.5
17.5	20	6.6	162.1	170.6	179.1	19	4.1	157.4	162.6	167.8
18.0	14	6.1	163.4	171.2	179.0	15	4.2	157.2	162.6	168.0
18.5	11	6.1	164.1	172.0	179.9	12	4.3	157.2	162.8	168.4
19.0	10	6.2	164.4	172.4	180.4	10	4.5	157.0	162.8	168.6
19.5	9	6.4	164.4	172.6	180.8	5	4.7	156.8	162.8	168.8
20.0	20	6.6	164.3	172.8	181.3	34	4.9	156.5	162.8	169.1

Table B.2 Growth of Yuendumu Aboriginals - Weight (kg)

Age	N	SD	Males centiles			N	SD	Females centiles		
			10th	50th	90th			10th	50th	90th
5.0	1	—	15.8	18.0	20.2	3	—	13.6	15.4	17.2
5.5	3	—	16.1	18.4	20.7	4	1.5	14.2	16.1	18.0
6.0	4	1.8	16.7	19.0	21.3	3	—	14.8	16.9	19.0
6.5	6	1.9	16.8	19.2	21.6	8	1.8	15.7	17.9	20.1
7.0	15	2.1	17.3	20.0	22.7	10	1.9	16.7	19.1	21.5
7.5	18	2.2	18.0	20.8	23.6	17	2.1	17.6	20.3	23.0
8.0	24	2.4	18.9	22.0	25.1	25	2.4	18.5	21.5	24.5
8.5	29	2.6	19.9	23.2	26.5	27	2.6	19.7	23.0	26.3
9.0	39	2.8	20.9	24.4	27.9	31	2.9	20.7	24.4	28.1
9.5	47	3.0	21.6	25.4	29.2	37	3.2	21.7	25.7	29.7
10.0	52	3.3	22.2	26.4	30.6	39	3.7	22.7	27.4	32.1
10.5	54	3.6	22.8	27.4	32.0	42	4.3	23.6	29.0	34.4
11.0	56	3.9	23.4	28.4	33.4	46	5.0	24.4	30.7	37.0
11.5	60	4.3	24.5	30.0	35.5	45	5.7	25.6	32.8	40.0
12.0	63	4.8	25.4	31.6	37.8	48	6.1	26.9	34.7	42.5
12.5	67	5.3	26.6	33.4	40.2	40	6.4	28.8	36.9	45.0
13.0	68	5.9	27.6	35.2	42.8	37	6.5	30.9	39.2	47.5
13.5	63	6.6	29.5	38.0	46.5	38	6.7	33.3	41.8	50.3
14.0	62	7.3	31.0	40.4	49.8	34	6.7	35.3	43.9	52.5
14.5	54	8.0	33.5	43.8	54.1	27	6.7	37.2	45.7	54.2
15.0	48	8.6	36.0	47.0	58.0	30	6.5	38.7	47.0	55.3
15.5	42	8.9	38.6	50.0	61.4	22	6.2	39.8	47.7	55.6
16.0	31	8.8	41.0	52.2	63.4	21	6.0	40.6	48.2	55.8
16.5	33	8.3	43.4	54.0	64.6	27	5.8	40.9	48.3	55.7
17.0	24	7.9	45.3	55.4	65.5	18	5.7	41.1	48.4	55.7
17.5	20	7.9	46.5	56.6	66.7	19	5.6	41.2	48.4	55.6
18.0	14	8.1	47.6	58.0	68.4	15	5.6	41.2	48.4	55.6
18.5	11	8.5	48.1	59.0	69.9	12	5.6	41.2	48.4	55.6
19.0	10	9.2	48.0	59.8	71.6	10	5.6	41.3	48.5	55.7
19.5	9	10.1	47.5	60.4	73.3	5	5.7	41.4	48.6	55.8
20.0	20	11.1	46.6	60.8	75.0	34	5.7	41.3	48.6	55.9

Table B.3 Growth of Yuendumu Aboriginals - Weight/Stature (gm/cm)

Age	N	SD	Males centiles			N	SD	Females centiles		
			10th	50th	90th			10th	50th	90th
5.0	0	—	—	—	—	0	—	—	—	—
5.5	0	—	—	—	—	0	—	—	—	—
6.0	4	9.0	149.5	161.0	172.5	3	—	137.4	151.5	165.6
6.5	6	12.5	147.0	163.0	179.0	8	11.4	141.4	156.0	170.6
7.0	15	15.2	147.3	166.8	186.3	10	12.2	144.9	160.5	176.1
7.5	16	16.8	149.3	170.8	192.3	17	13.2	150.3	167.2	184.1
8.0	24	17.2	153.8	175.9	198.0	25	14.2	154.3	172.5	190.7
8.5	29	17.8	157.7	180.5	203.3	27	15.6	159.0	179.0	199.0
9.0	38	18.0	162.4	185.5	208.6	33	17.0	164.2	186.0	207.8
9.5	44	18.2	167.7	191.0	214.3	39	18.6	168.7	192.5	216.3
10.0	50	19.2	171.9	196.5	221.1	39	20.6	173.1	199.5	225.9
10.5	52	20.3	175.8	201.9	228.0	42	23.1	177.9	207.5	237.1
11.0	56	21.2	179.3	206.5	233.7	46	26.0	181.7	215.0	248.3
11.5	60	22.4	183.6	212.3	241.0	45	28.8	187.8	224.7	261.6
12.0	63	23.8	189.5	220.0	250.5	45	31.4	193.2	233.5	273.8
12.5	67	26.4	194.7	228.5	262.3	40	34.0	200.4	244.0	287.6
13.0	68	29.4	199.8	237.5	275.2	37	35.8	209.1	255.0	300.9
13.5	63	32.0	206.0	247.0	288.0	38	37.2	218.1	265.8	313.5
14.0	60	34.2	214.2	258.0	301.8	34	38.0	227.7	276.4	325.1
14.5	54	36.4	222.3	269.0	315.7	27	37.9	236.7	285.3	333.9
15.0	48	38.4	234.8	284.0	333.2	30	37.4	243.1	291.0	338.9
15.5	42	40.2	248.5	300.0	351.5	22	36.6	247.1	294.0	340.9
16.0	31	42.0	257.7	311.5	365.3	21	35.2	250.7	295.8	340.9
16.5	33	43.2	264.6	320.0	375.4	27	34.8	251.9	296.5	341.1
17.0	22	44.4	269.1	326.0	382.9	18	31.8	256.2	297.0	337.8
17.5	18	45.4	272.3	330.5	388.7	19	29.2	259.8	297.2	334.6
18.0	12	47.2	274.0	334.5	395.0	15	26.4	264.1	297.9	331.7
18.5	11	49.2	275.9	339.0	402.1	12	20.8	271.3	298.0	324.7
19.0	10	52.0	279.3	346.0	412.7	5	14.0	280.6	298.5	316.4
19.5	9	55.1	284.0	354.6	425.2	5	5.0	292.6	299.0	305.4
20.0	20	57.6	288.2	362.0	435.8	34	0.0	299.0	299.0	299.0

Table B.4 Growth of Yuendumu Aboriginals - Radius Length (cm)

Age	N	SD	Males centiles			N	SD	Females centiles		
			10th	50th	90th			10th	50th	90th
5.0	0	—	16.0	16.6	17.2	1	—	14.7	15.8	16.9
5.5	3	—	16.3	17.0	17.7	4	0.9	15.0	16.2	17.4
6.0	4	0.6	16.6	17.4	18.2	3	—	15.5	16.6	17.8
6.5	6	0.7	16.9	17.9	18.8	8	0.9	15.9	17.1	18.2
7.0	15	0.9	17.2	18.3	19.4	10	0.9	16.4	17.6	18.8
7.5	18	1.0	17.5	18.7	19.9	17	1.0	17.0	18.3	19.5
8.0	24	1.0	17.8	19.1	20.4	25	1.0	17.5	18.8	20.1
8.5	29	1.1	18.1	19.5	20.9	27	1.0	18.0	19.3	20.6
9.0	39	1.1	18.4	19.9	21.3	31	1.1	18.4	19.8	21.2
9.5	47	1.1	18.8	20.3	21.7	37	1.2	18.8	20.3	21.8
10.0	52	1.2	19.2	20.7	22.2	40	1.3	19.2	20.8	22.4
10.5	54	1.2	19.7	21.1	22.6	43	1.3	19.7	21.4	23.1
11.0	56	1.2	20.1	21.6	23.1	45	1.4	20.2	22.0	23.7
11.5	60	1.2	20.4	22.0	23.6	44	1.4	20.7	22.5	24.3
12.0	63	1.3	20.9	22.5	24.1	47	1.4	21.1	23.0	24.8
12.5	67	1.4	21.2	22.9	24.6	39	1.4	21.6	23.4	25.2
13.0	68	1.5	21.5	23.4	25.2	36	1.4	21.9	23.7	25.5
13.5	63	1.5	21.8	23.8	25.8	37	1.4	22.2	24.0	25.8
14.0	63	1.6	22.3	24.4	26.4	34	1.3	22.5	24.3	26.0
14.5	55	1.7	22.8	24.9	27.0	27	1.3	22.8	24.4	26.0
15.0	48	1.7	23.3	25.4	27.5	30	1.2	23.0	24.6	26.2
15.5	42	1.6	23.8	25.9	28.0	21	1.2	23.1	24.7	26.3
16.0	31	1.6	24.2	26.3	28.3	20	1.2	23.3	24.8	26.3
16.5	33	1.6	24.5	26.5	28.5	27	1.2	23.4	24.9	26.4
17.0	24	1.5	24.8	26.8	28.7	18	1.2	23.4	25.0	26.5
17.5	20	1.4	25.1	27.0	28.8	20	1.2	23.5	25.0	26.5
18.0	15	1.4	25.4	27.2	28.9	16	1.2	23.4	25.0	26.6
18.5	12	1.3	25.6	27.3	29.0	12	1.2	23.4	25.0	26.6
19.0	10	1.3	25.7	27.3	28.9	10	1.2	23.4	25.0	26.6
19.5	9	1.2	25.8	27.4	28.9	6	1.3	23.4	25.0	26.6
20.0	20	1.2	25.9	27.4	28.9	33	1.3	23.3	25.0	26.7

Table B.5 Growth of Yuendumu Aboriginals - Head Length (cm)

Age	N	SD	Males centiles			N	SD	Females centiles		
			10th	50th	90th			10th	50th	90th
5.0	0	—	17.5	18.2	18.8	1	—	16.4	16.9	17.4
5.5	3	—	17.6	18.2	18.8	4	0.4	16.6	17.1	17.6
6.0	4	0.5	17.6	18.2	18.8	3	—	16.8	17.3	17.8
6.5	6	0.5	17.6	18.2	18.8	8	0.4	16.9	17.5	18.0
7.0	15	0.5	17.6	18.2	18.9	10	0.5	17.0	17.6	18.2
7.5	18	0.6	17.6	18.3	19.0	17	0.5	17.1	17.8	18.4
8.0	24	0.6	17.6	18.3	19.1	25	0.5	17.2	17.9	18.5
8.5	29	0.6	17.6	18.4	19.2	27	0.5	17.3	18.0	18.7
9.0	39	0.7	17.6	18.5	19.3	31	0.6	17.4	18.1	18.8
9.5	47	0.7	17.6	18.6	19.5	37	0.6	17.4	18.2	19.0
10.0	52	0.8	17.7	18.6	19.6	40	0.6	17.5	18.3	19.0
10.5	54	0.8	17.7	18.7	19.7	43	0.6	17.6	18.4	19.2
11.0	56	0.8	17.8	18.8	19.8	46	0.6	17.6	18.4	19.2
11.5	60	0.8	17.9	18.9	19.8	45	0.6	17.7	18.5	19.3
12.0	63	0.8	17.9	18.9	19.9	48	0.6	17.7	18.6	19.4
12.5	67	0.8	18.0	19.0	20.0	40	0.7	17.8	18.6	19.4
13.0	68	0.8	18.1	19.1	20.0	37	0.7	17.8	18.7	19.5
13.5	63	0.7	18.2	19.1	20.1	38	0.6	17.9	18.8	19.6
14.0	63	0.7	18.3	19.2	20.1	34	0.6	18.0	18.8	19.6
14.5	55	0.7	18.4	19.3	20.2	27	0.6	18.1	18.9	19.7
15.0	48	0.7	18.5	19.4	20.3	30	0.6	18.1	18.9	19.7
15.5	42	0.8	18.5	19.5	20.5	22	0.6	18.2	19.0	19.8
16.0	31	0.8	18.6	19.6	20.7	21	0.6	18.2	19.0	19.8
16.5	33	0.8	18.7	19.8	20.8	27	0.6	18.2	19.0	19.8
17.0	24	0.8	18.9	19.9	21.0	18	0.6	18.2	19.0	19.8
17.5	20	0.8	19.0	20.1	21.1	20	0.6	18.3	19.0	19.7
18.0	15	0.8	19.2	20.2	21.2	16	0.6	18.3	19.0	19.7
18.5	12	0.8	19.2	20.1	21.1	12	0.6	18.3	19.0	19.7
19.0	10	0.7	19.4	20.4	21.3	10	0.5	18.3	19.0	19.7
19.5	9	0.7	19.5	20.4	21.3	6	0.5	18.3	19.0	19.7
20.0	20	0.7	19.5	20.4	21.3	34	0.5	18.3	19.0	19.7

Table B.6 Growth of Yuendumu Aboriginals - Head Breadth (cm)

Age	N	SD	Males centiles			N	SD	Females centiles		
			10th	50th	90th			10th	50th	90th
5.0	0	—	12.3	12.8	13.3	1	—	11.9	12.3	12.7
5.5	3	—	12.4	12.8	13.3	4	0.3	12.0	12.4	12.8
6.0	4	0.4	12.4	12.8	13.3	3	—	12.0	12.5	12.9
6.5	6	0.4	12.4	12.9	13.3	8	0.3	12.1	12.5	13.0
7.0	15	0.4	12.4	12.9	13.4	10	0.3	12.2	12.6	13.0
7.5	18	0.4	12.5	13.0	13.4	17	0.4	12.2	12.7	13.1
8.0	24	0.4	12.6	13.0	13.5	25	0.4	12.3	12.7	13.2
8.5	29	0.4	12.6	13.1	13.6	27	0.4	12.3	12.8	13.3
9.0	39	0.4	12.6	13.2	13.7	31	0.4	12.4	12.9	13.3
9.5	47	0.4	12.7	13.2	13.7	37	0.4	12.5	12.9	13.4
10.0	52	0.4	12.7	13.2	13.8	40	0.4	12.5	13.0	13.5
10.5	54	0.4	12.7	13.3	13.8	43	0.4	12.6	13.1	13.6
11.0	56	0.5	12.7	13.3	13.9	46	0.4	12.6	13.1	13.6
11.5	60	0.5	12.7	13.3	13.9	45	0.4	12.6	13.2	13.7
12.0	63	0.5	12.8	13.4	14.0	48	0.4	12.7	13.2	13.8
12.5	67	0.5	12.8	13.5	14.1	40	0.5	12.7	13.3	13.9
13.0	68	0.5	12.9	13.5	14.2	37	0.5	12.8	13.4	13.9
13.5	63	0.5	13.0	13.6	14.2	38	0.5	12.8	13.4	14.0
14.0	63	0.5	13.1	13.7	14.3	34	0.5	12.9	13.5	14.1
14.5	55	0.5	13.2	13.8	14.3	27	0.5	12.9	13.5	14.1
15.0	48	0.5	13.2	13.8	14.4	30	0.5	13.0	13.6	14.2
15.5	42	0.5	13.3	13.9	14.5	22	0.5	13.0	13.6	14.2
16.0	31	0.5	13.4	14.0	14.6	21	0.5	13.0	13.6	14.2
16.5	33	0.5	13.4	14.1	14.7	27	0.5	13.1	13.7	14.2
17.0	24	0.5	13.5	14.1	14.7	18	0.5	13.1	13.7	14.3
17.5	20	0.5	13.5	14.1	14.7	20	0.5	13.1	13.7	14.3
18.0	15	0.5	13.6	14.1	14.7	16	0.4	13.1	13.7	14.3
18.5	12	0.4	13.6	14.1	14.7	12	0.4	13.1	13.7	14.3
19.0	10	0.4	13.6	14.1	14.7	10	0.4	13.2	13.7	14.2
19.5	9	0.4	13.6	14.1	14.7	6	0.4	13.2	13.7	14.2
20.0	20	0.4	13.6	14.1	14.7	34	0.4	13.2	13.7	14.2

Table B.7 Growth of Yuendumu Aboriginals - Head Circumference (cm)

Age	N	SD	Males centiles			N	SD	Females centiles		
			10th	50th	90th			10th	50th	90th
5.0	0	—	49.3	50.7	52.1	1	—	48.2	49.3	50.4
5.5	3	—	49.3	50.8	52.2	4	0.9	48.4	49.5	50.7
6.0	4	1.1	49.4	50.9	52.3	3	—	48.6	49.8	51.0
6.5	6	1.2	49.5	51.0	52.5	8	1.0	48.8	50.1	51.4
7.0	15	1.2	49.6	51.2	52.7	10	1.0	49.0	50.3	51.7
7.5	18	1.3	49.7	51.4	53.0	17	1.1	49.2	50.6	51.9
8.0	24	1.5	49.6	51.5	53.4	25	1.1	50.4	51.8	53.2
8.5	29	1.7	49.6	51.7	53.8	27	1.2	49.5	51.0	52.6
9.0	39	1.7	49.7	51.9	54.1	31	1.2	49.7	51.3	52.9
9.5	47	1.7	49.9	52.0	54.2	37	1.3	49.8	51.5	53.1
10.0	52	1.7	50.1	52.2	54.4	40	1.4	50.0	51.8	53.5
10.5	54	1.6	50.4	52.5	54.6	43	1.4	50.1	52.0	53.8
11.0	56	1.6	50.6	52.7	54.8	46	1.5	50.3	52.2	54.1
11.5	60	1.6	50.9	53.0	55.1	45	1.6	50.4	52.4	54.5
12.0	62	1.7	51.1	53.2	55.3	48	1.6	50.6	52.7	54.7
12.5	66	1.7	51.3	53.5	55.6	40	1.6	50.8	52.9	55.0
13.0	67	1.7	51.5	53.7	56.0	37	1.6	51.1	53.1	55.2
13.5	62	1.8	51.7	54.0	56.3	38	1.6	51.4	53.4	55.4
14.0	63	1.9	51.8	54.2	56.6	34	1.6	51.7	53.7	55.7
14.5	55	1.9	52.0	54.5	57.0	27	1.5	52.1	54.0	56.0
15.0	48	2.0	52.4	54.9	57.5	30	1.5	52.3	54.2	56.1
15.5	42	2.0	52.8	55.4	58.0	22	1.4	52.4	54.2	56.1
16.0	31	2.1	53.1	55.8	58.4	21	1.4	52.5	54.3	56.1
16.5	33	2.1	53.4	56.0	58.7	27	1.3	52.6	54.3	56.0
17.0	24	2.1	53.6	56.2	58.9	18	1.3	52.7	54.4	56.0
17.5	20	2.1	53.7	56.4	59.1	20	1.3	52.8	54.4	56.0
18.0	15	2.0	54.0	56.6	59.2	16	1.2	52.8	54.4	55.9
18.5	12	2.0	54.2	56.8	59.4	12	1.2	52.9	54.4	55.9
19.0	10	2.0	54.6	57.1	59.6	10	1.1	52.9	54.4	55.8
19.5	9	1.9	55.1	57.5	59.9	6	1.1	53.0	54.4	55.8
20.0	20	1.8	55.6	58.0	60.3	33	1.1	53.0	54.4	55.8

Table B.8 Growth of Yuendumu Aboriginals - Cephalic Index (%)

Age	N	SD	Males centiles			N	SD	Females centiles		
			10th	50th	90th			10th	50th	90th
5.0	0	—	69.8	71.7	73.6	1	—	67.8	70.1	72.4
5.5	3	—	69.6	71.6	73.5	4	1.8	67.8	70.2	72.5
6.0	4	1.7	69.3	71.5	73.6	3	—	67.8	70.2	72.7
6.5	6	1.9	68.9	71.4	73.9	8	1.9	67.9	70.4	72.9
7.0	15	2.1	68.6	71.3	74.0	10	2.0	67.9	70.5	73.1
7.5	18	2.3	68.3	71.3	74.2	17	2.1	68.0	70.7	73.4
8.0	24	2.4	68.1	71.2	74.3	25	2.2	68.1	70.9	73.8
8.5	29	2.5	67.9	71.2	74.4	27	2.3	68.3	71.3	74.3
9.0	39	2.6	67.8	71.1	74.4	31	2.4	68.5	71.6	74.7
9.5	47	2.7	67.6	71.1	74.5	37	2.5	68.5	71.7	75.0
10.0	52	2.8	67.5	71.0	74.6	40	2.6	68.3	71.7	75.0
10.5	54	2.8	67.4	71.0	74.6	43	2.7	68.1	71.6	75.0
11.0	56	2.8	67.3	71.0	74.6	46	2.7	67.9	71.4	75.0
11.5	60	2.8	67.3	70.9	74.6	45	2.8	67.8	71.4	74.9
12.0	63	2.8	67.3	70.9	74.5	48	2.8	67.7	71.3	75.0
12.5	67	2.7	67.4	70.9	74.4	40	2.8	67.7	71.4	75.0
13.0	68	2.7	67.5	70.9	74.3	37	2.8	67.8	71.4	75.1
13.5	63	2.6	67.7	71.0	74.3	38	2.8	67.8	71.5	75.1
14.0	63	2.5	68.0	71.2	74.4	34	2.8	67.9	71.5	75.1
14.5	55	2.5	68.0	71.3	74.5	27	2.8	67.9	71.5	75.0
15.0	48	2.6	67.9	71.2	74.6	30	2.7	68.0	71.4	74.8
15.5	42	2.6	67.6	71.0	74.4	22	2.6	68.1	71.4	74.7
16.0	31	2.7	67.2	70.7	74.1	21	2.5	68.2	71.4	74.7
16.5	33	2.7	66.9	70.3	73.8	27	2.5	68.3	71.5	74.7
17.0	24	2.7	66.7	70.1	73.6	18	2.5	68.4	71.7	74.9
17.5	20	2.7	66.5	70.0	73.5	20	2.6	68.4	71.8	75.2
18.0	15	2.7	66.5	69.9	73.4	16	2.7	68.5	72.0	75.4
18.5	12	2.7	66.5	69.9	73.3	12	2.8	68.5	72.1	75.7
19.0	10	2.6	66.5	69.9	73.2	10	2.9	68.6	72.2	75.9
19.5	9	2.6	66.6	69.9	73.1	6	2.9	68.7	72.3	76.0
20.0	20	2.5	66.7	69.9	73.1	34	2.9	68.7	72.4	76.0

Table B.9 Growth of Yuendumu Aboriginals - Bizygomatic Diameter (cm)

Age	N	SD	Males centiles			N	SD	Females centiles		
			10th	50th	90th			10th	50th	90th
5.0	0	—	10.2	10.8	11.4	1	—	10.0	10.4	10.8
5.5	3	—	10.3	10.8	11.4	4	0.3	10.1	10.5	10.9
6.0	4	0.4	10.4	11.0	11.5	3	—	10.3	10.7	11.0
6.5	6	0.4	10.5	11.1	11.6	8	0.3	10.4	10.8	11.2
7.0	15	0.4	10.6	11.2	11.7	10	0.3	10.5	10.9	11.3
7.5	18	0.4	10.7	11.3	11.9	17	0.3	10.7	11.1	11.5
8.0	24	0.4	10.9	11.4	12.0	25	0.4	10.8	11.3	11.7
8.5	29	0.4	11.0	11.5	12.1	27	0.4	10.9	11.4	11.9
9.0	39	0.5	11.1	11.6	12.2	31	0.4	11.0	11.5	12.0
9.5	47	0.5	11.2	11.7	12.3	37	0.4	11.1	11.6	12.2
10.0	52	0.5	11.2	11.8	12.5	40	0.5	11.1	11.7	12.3
10.5	54	0.5	11.3	11.9	12.6	43	0.5	11.2	11.9	12.5
11.0	56	0.5	11.3	12.0	12.7	46	0.5	11.3	11.9	12.6
11.5	60	0.6	11.3	12.0	12.8	45	0.5	11.3	12.0	12.7
12.0	63	0.6	11.3	12.1	12.9	48	0.6	11.4	12.1	12.8
12.5	67	0.6	11.4	12.2	13.0	40	0.5	11.5	12.2	12.9
13.0	68	0.6	11.5	12.3	13.1	37	0.5	11.6	12.3	13.0
13.5	63	0.6	11.6	12.4	13.3	38	0.5	11.8	12.4	13.1
14.0	63	0.6	11.8	12.6	13.4	34	0.5	11.9	12.5	13.2
14.5	55	0.6	12.1	12.8	13.6	27	0.5	12.1	12.6	13.2
15.0	48	0.6	12.3	13.0	13.7	30	0.5	12.1	12.7	13.3
15.5	42	0.6	12.5	13.2	13.9	22	0.4	12.2	12.8	13.4
16.0	31	0.5	12.6	13.3	14.0	21	0.4	12.3	12.9	13.4
16.5	33	0.5	12.8	13.4	14.0	27	0.4	12.4	12.9	13.5
17.0	24	0.5	12.9	13.5	14.1	18	0.4	12.5	13.0	13.5
17.5	20	0.5	12.9	13.5	14.1	20	0.4	12.5	13.0	13.5
18.0	15	0.5	13.0	13.6	14.2	16	0.4	12.5	13.0	13.5
18.5	12	0.5	13.1	13.7	14.3	12	0.4	12.5	13.0	13.5
19.0	10	0.5	13.3	13.9	14.5	10	0.4	12.6	13.0	13.5
19.5	9	0.5	13.4	14.0	14.7	6	0.4	12.6	13.0	13.5
20.0	20	0.5	13.4	14.1	14.8	34	0.4	12.6	13.0	13.5

Table B.10 Growth of Yuendumu Aboriginals - Bigonial Diameter (cm)

Age	N	SD	Males centiles			N	SD	Females centiles		
			10th	50th	90th			10th	50th	90th
5.0	0	—	7.8	8.1	8.5	1	—	7.1	7.5	7.9
5.5	3	—	7.8	8.2	8.5	4	0.3	7.2	7.6	8.0
6.0	4	0.3	7.9	8.3	8.6	3	—	7.3	7.7	8.2
6.5	6	0.3	7.9	8.3	8.7	8	0.4	7.4	7.9	8.4
7.0	15	0.4	8.0	8.4	8.8	10	0.4	7.5	8.0	8.5
7.5	18	0.4	8.0	8.5	9.0	17	0.4	7.6	8.2	8.7
8.0	24	0.4	8.1	8.6	9.1	25	0.4	7.7	8.3	8.8
8.5	29	0.4	8.1	8.7	9.2	27	0.4	7.8	8.4	9.0
9.0	39	0.5	8.2	8.7	9.3	31	0.5	7.9	8.5	9.1
9.5	47	0.5	8.2	8.8	9.4	37	0.5	8.0	8.6	9.2
10.0	52	0.5	8.3	8.9	9.6	40	0.5	8.1	8.7	9.3
10.5	54	0.5	8.3	9.0	9.7	43	0.5	8.2	8.8	9.4
11.0	56	0.6	8.4	9.1	9.8	46	0.5	8.3	8.9	9.6
11.5	60	0.6	8.4	9.2	9.9	45	0.5	8.4	9.0	9.7
12.0	63	0.6	8.5	9.3	10.0	47	0.5	8.4	9.1	9.7
12.5	67	0.6	8.6	9.3	10.1	39	0.5	8.5	9.2	9.8
13.0	68	0.6	8.7	9.4	10.2	36	0.5	8.6	9.3	9.9
13.5	62	0.6	8.8	9.5	10.2	37	0.5	8.6	9.3	10.0
14.0	62	0.5	8.9	9.6	10.3	34	0.5	8.7	9.4	10.1
14.5	54	0.5	9.1	9.7	10.4	27	0.5	8.8	9.5	10.1
15.0	47	0.5	9.2	9.9	10.5	30	0.5	8.9	9.5	10.2
15.5	41	0.5	9.4	10.0	10.6	22	0.5	8.9	9.6	10.2
16.0	30	0.5	9.5	10.1	10.7	21	0.5	9.0	9.6	10.3
16.5	33	0.5	9.6	10.2	10.7	27	0.5	9.1	9.7	10.3
17.0	4	0.5	9.6	10.2	10.8	18	0.5	9.1	9.7	10.3
17.5	20	0.5	9.6	10.3	10.9	20	0.5	9.2	9.8	10.4
18.0	15	0.5	9.6	10.3	10.9	16	0.5	9.2	9.8	10.4
18.5	12	0.5	9.6	10.3	11.0	12	0.4	9.2	9.8	10.4
19.0	10	0.6	9.6	10.3	11.0	10	0.4	9.2	9.8	10.4
19.5	9	0.6	9.5	10.3	11.1	6	0.4	9.3	9.8	10.3
20.0	20	0.7	9.5	10.3	11.2	34	0.4	9.3	9.8	10.3

Table B.11 Growth of Yuendumu Aboriginals - Morphological Face Height (cm)

Age	N	SD	Males centiles			N	SD	Females centiles		
			10th	50th	90th			10th	50th	90th
5.0	0	—	8.9	9.1	9.4	1	—	8.1	8.7	9.3
5.5	3	—	8.9	9.2	9.4	4	0.5	8.2	8.8	9.4
6.0	4	0.3	8.9	9.2	9.5	3	—	8.2	8.9	9.5
6.5	6	0.3	8.9	9.2	9.6	8	0.5	8.3	9.0	9.6
7.0	15	0.3	8.9	9.3	9.7	10	0.5	8.4	9.1	9.7
7.5	18	0.3	9.0	9.4	9.8	17	0.5	8.5	9.2	9.8
8.0	24	0.4	9.0	9.5	9.9	25	0.5	8.6	9.3	9.9
8.5	29	0.4	9.0	9.5	10.0	27	0.5	8.7	9.4	10.0
9.0	39	0.4	9.0	9.5	10.0	31	0.5	8.9	9.5	10.1
9.5	47	0.4	9.0	9.5	10.1	37	0.5	9.0	9.6	10.2
10.0	52	0.4	9.0	9.6	10.1	40	0.5	9.1	9.7	10.3
10.5	54	0.5	9.1	9.6	10.2	43	0.5	9.3	9.8	10.4
11.0	56	0.5	9.1	9.7	10.3	46	0.5	9.3	9.9	10.5
11.5	60	0.5	9.2	9.8	10.4	45	0.5	9.4	10.0	10.6
12.0	63	0.5	9.3	9.9	10.5	48	0.5	9.4	10.1	10.7
12.5	67	0.5	9.4	10.0	10.6	40	0.5	9.5	10.2	10.8
13.0	68	0.5	9.5	10.1	10.7	37	0.5	9.6	10.3	10.9
13.5	63	0.5	9.6	10.2	10.8	38	0.5	9.7	10.4	11.1
14.0	63	0.5	9.7	10.4	11.0	34	0.5	9.8	10.5	11.2
14.5	55	0.5	9.9	10.6	11.2	27	0.5	9.9	10.6	11.3
15.0	48	0.6	10.0	10.7	11.5	30	0.5	10.0	10.7	11.3
15.5	42	0.6	10.1	10.9	11.7	22	0.5	10.1	10.7	11.4
16.0	31	0.7	10.2	11.0	11.9	21	0.5	10.1	10.8	11.4
16.5	33	0.7	10.3	11.1	12.0	27	0.5	10.1	10.8	11.4
17.0	24	0.7	10.3	11.2	12.0	18	0.5	10.2	10.8	11.4
17.5	20	0.6	10.5	11.2	12.0	20	0.5	10.2	10.8	11.4
18.0	15	0.6	10.5	11.3	12.0	16	0.5	10.2	10.8	11.4
18.5	12	0.5	10.7	11.3	12.0	12	0.4	10.2	10.8	11.3
19.0	10	0.5	10.7	11.4	12.1	10	0.4	10.3	10.8	11.3
19.5	9	0.5	10.8	11.5	12.2	6	0.4	10.3	10.8	11.3
20.0	20	0.5	11.1	11.8	12.5	34	0.4	10.3	10.8	11.3

Table B.12 Growth of Yuendumu Aboriginals - Femoral Condyle Diameter (cm)

Age	N	SD	Males centiles			N	SD	Females centiles		
			10th	50th	90th			10th	50th	90th
5.0	0	—	6.5	6.7	6.9	1	—		6.2	6.4
5.5	3	—	6.6	6.8	7.0	4	0.2	6.0	6.2	6.5
6.0	4	0.2	6.6	6.8	7.0	3	—	6.1	6.3	6.6
6.5	6	0.2	6.6	6.9	7.1	7	0.2	6.2	6.5	6.7
7.0	14	0.2	6.7	7.0	7.3	9	0.3	6.2	6.6	6.9
7.5	16	0.3	6.7	7.1	7.4	16	0.3	6.3	6.7	7.0
8.0	23	0.3	6.8	7.2	7.6	25	0.3	6.4	6.8	7.2
8.5	28	0.3	6.9	7.3	7.7	27	0.3	6.5	6.9	7.3
9.0	39	0.4	7.0	7.4	7.9	31	0.3	6.7	7.1	7.4
9.5	47	0.4	7.1	7.5	8.0	37	0.3	6.8	7.2	7.6
10.0	52	0.4	7.2	7.6	8.1	39	0.4	6.9	7.3	7.8
10.5	54	0.4	7.2	7.7	8.2	42	0.4	7.0	7.5	7.9
11.0	56	0.4	7.3	7.8	8.3	45	0.4	7.1	7.6	8.0
11.5	60	0.4	7.4	7.9	8.4	44	0.4	7.2	7.7	8.2
12.0	63	0.4	7.5	8.0	8.6	48	0.4	7.3	7.8	8.3
12.5	67	0.4	7.6	8.2	8.7	40	0.4	7.4	7.9	8.3
13.0	68	0.5	7.7	8.3	8.9	37	0.4	7.5	8.0	8.4
13.5	63	0.5	7.8	8.5	9.1	38	0.3	7.6	8.0	8.4
14.0	63	0.5	8.0	8.6	9.2	34	0.3	7.6	8.1	8.5
14.5	55	0.5	8.2	8.7	9.3	27	0.3	7.7	8.1	8.5
15.0	48	0.4	8.3	8.8	9.4	30	0.3	7.7	8.1	8.5
15.5	42	0.4	8.4	8.9	9.4	22	0.3	7.8	8.1	8.5
16.0	31	0.4	8.4	8.9	9.4	21	0.3	7.8	8.2	8.5
16.5	33	0.4	8.5	9.0	9.4	27	0.3	7.8	8.2	8.5
17.0	24	0.4	8.5	9.0	9.4	18	0.3	7.8	8.2	8.5
17.5	20	0.4	8.5	9.0	9.5	20	0.3	7.8	8.2	8.5
18.0	15	0.4	8.4	9.0	9.6	16	0.3	7.8	8.2	8.5
18.5	12	0.4	8.4	9.0	9.6	12	0.3	7.8	8.2	8.6
19.0	10	0.5	8.4	9.0	9.6	10	0.3	7.8	8.2	8.6
19.5	9	0.5	8.4	9.0	9.6	6	0.3	7.8	8.2	8.6
20.0	20	0.5	8.4	9.0	9.6	34	0.3	7.8	8.2	8.6

Table B.13 Growth of Yuendumu Aboriginals - Wrist Diameter (cm)

Age	N	SD	Males centiles			N	SD	Females centiles		
			10th	50th	90th			10th	50th	90th
5.0	0	—	3.4	3.6	3.8	1	—	3.1	3.4	3.7
5.5	3	—	3.4	3.7	3.9	3	—	3.2	3.5	3.8
6.0	4	0.2	3.5	3.8	4.0	2	—	3.2	3.5	3.8
6.5	6	0.2	3.6	3.8	4.0	5	0.2	3.3	3.6	3.9
7.0	12	0.2	3.6	3.9	4.1	7	0.2	3.4	3.7	4.0
7.5	13	0.2	3.7	3.9	4.2	14	0.3	3.4	3.8	4.1
8.0	20	0.2	3.7	4.0	4.3	22	0.3	3.5	3.8	4.2
8.5	26	0.2	3.8	4.1	4.4	23	0.3	3.6	3.9	4.2
9.0	35	0.2	3.8	4.1	4.4	26	0.3	3.6	4.0	4.3
9.5	43	0.2	3.9	4.2	4.5	31	0.3	3.7	4.1	4.4
10.0	48	0.2	4.0	4.3	4.6	36	0.3	3.8	4.1	4.5
10.5	50	0.2	4.0	4.3	4.6	40	0.3	3.8	4.2	4.6
11.0	53	0.2	4.1	4.4	4.7	44	0.3	3.9	4.3	4.7
11.5	58	0.2	4.2	4.5	4.7	44	0.3	4.0	4.4	4.8
12.0	61	0.2	4.2	4.5	4.8	48	0.3	4.0	4.4	4.8
12.5	66	0.3	4.3	4.6	4.9	40	0.3	4.1	4.5	4.9
13.0	67	0.3	4.3	4.7	5.1	37	0.3	4.2	4.6	4.9
13.5	62	0.3	4.4	4.8	5.2	38	0.3	4.3	4.6	5.0
14.0	62	0.3	4.5	4.9	5.3	34	0.3	4.3	4.7	5.0
14.5	53	0.3	4.6	5.0	5.4	27	0.3	4.4	4.7	5.0
15.0	47	0.3	4.7	5.1	5.5	30	0.2	4.4	4.7	5.0
15.5	40	0.3	4.8	5.2	5.6	22	0.2	4.5	4.8	5.1
16.0	30	0.3	4.9	5.3	5.6	21	0.2	4.5	4.8	5.1
16.5	28	0.3	4.9	5.3	5.6	20	0.2	4.6	4.8	5.1
17.0	24	0.3	5.0	5.3	5.6	18	0.2	4.6	4.8	5.1
17.5	18	0.3	5.0	5.3	5.7	19	0.2	4.6	4.8	5.1
18.0	15	0.3	5.0	5.3	5.7	16	0.2	4.6	4.9	5.1
18.5	11	0.3	5.0	5.4	5.7	10	0.2	4.6	4.9	5.1
19.0	10	0.3	5.0	5.4	5.7	10	0.2	4.6	4.9	5.1
19.5	6	0.3	5.0	5.4	5.7	6	0.2	4.6	4.9	5.1
20.0	7	0.3	5.0	5.4	5.7	23	0.2	4.6	4.9	5.1

Table B.14 Growth of Yuendumu Aboriginals - Stature (cm)

Age	N	SD	Males centiles			N	SD	Females centiles		
			10th	50th	90th			10th	50th	90th
5.0	1	—	106.7	110.0	113.3	3	—	99.9	105.0	110.1
5.5	3	—	107.9	111.2	114.5	4	3.9	103.4	108.4	113.4
6.0	4	3.2	109.6	113.6	117.6	3	—	106.9	111.8	116.7
6.5	6	3.2	111.9	116.0	120.1	8	3.8	110.4	115.2	120.0
7.0	15	3.4	114.7	119.0	123.3	11	3.8	114.0	118.8	123.6
7.5	18	3.6	117.0	121.6	126.2	18	3.8	117.1	122.0	126.9
8.0	24	3.8	119.1	124.0	128.9	26	4.0	120.1	125.2	130.3
8.5	29	4.2	121.5	126.8	132.1	27	4.2	122.6	128.0	133.4
9.0	38	4.6	122.9	128.8	134.7	31	4.6	125.1	131.0	136.9
9.5	46	5.0	125.2	131.6	138.0	37	5.1	127.3	133.8	140.3
10.0	52	5.4	126.9	133.8	140.7	40	5.5	129.5	136.6	143.7
10.5	54	5.7	127.0	134.2	141.4	43	6.0	131.9	139.6	147.3
11.0	56	5.9	131.2	138.8	146.4	46	6.3	134.3	142.4	150.5
11.5	60	6.2	132.0	140.0	148.0	45	6.4	137.4	145.6	153.8
12.0	63	6.6	135.1	143.6	152.1	48	6.3	140.5	148.6	156.7
12.5	67	7.1	137.1	146.2	155.3	40	6.0	144.0	151.6	159.2
13.0	68	7.7	139.7	149.6	159.5	37	5.6	147.1	154.2	161.3
13.5	63	8.3	142.2	152.8	163.4	38	5.0	149.9	156.4	162.9
14.0	62	8.5	146.1	157.0	167.9	34	4.5	152.6	158.4	164.2
14.5	54	8.6	149.8	160.8	171.8	27	4.2	154.6	160.0	165.4
15.0	48	8.5	152.9	163.8	174.7	30	4.0	155.8	161.0	166.2
15.5	42	8.2	155.6	166.0	176.4	22	3.9	156.6	161.6	166.6
16.0	31	7.7	158.0	167.8	177.6	21	3.9	157.2	162.2	167.2
16.5	33	7.2	160.0	169.2	178.4	27	3.9	157.4	162.4	167.4
17.0	24	6.8	161.2	170.0	178.8	18	4.0	157.3	162.4	167.5
17.5	20	6.6	162.1	170.6	179.1	19	4.1	157.4	162.6	167.8
18.0	14	6.1	163.4	171.2	179.0	15	4.2	157.2	162.6	168.0
18.5	11	6.1	164.1	172.0	179.9	12	4.3	157.2	162.8	168.4
19.0	10	6.2	164.4	172.4	180.4	10	4.5	157.0	162.8	168.6
19.5	9	6.4	164.4	172.6	180.8	5	4.7	156.8	162.8	168.8
20.0	20	6.6	164.3	172.8	181.3	34	4.9	156.5	162.8	169.1

Table B.15 Growth of Yuendumu Aboriginals - Weight (kg)

Age	N	SD	Males centiles			N	SD	Females centiles		
			10th	50th	90th			10th	50th	90th
5.0	1	—	15.8	18.0	20.2	3	—	13.6	15.4	17.2
5.5	3	—	16.1	18.4	20.7	4	1.5	14.2	16.1	18.0
6.0	4	1.8	16.7	19.0	21.3	3	—	14.8	16.9	19.0
6.5	6	1.9	16.8	19.2	21.6	8	1.8	15.7	17.9	20.1
7.0	15	2.1	17.3	20.0	22.7	10	1.9	16.7	19.1	21.5
7.5	18	2.2	18.0	20.8	23.6	17	2.1	17.6	20.3	23.0
8.0	24	2.4	18.9	22.0	25.1	25	2.4	18.5	21.5	24.5
8.5	29	2.6	19.9	23.2	26.5	27	2.6	19.7	23.0	26.3
9.0	39	2.8	20.9	24.4	27.9	31	2.9	20.7	24.4	28.1
9.5	47	3.0	21.6	25.4	29.2	37	3.2	21.7	25.7	29.7
10.0	52	3.3	22.2	26.4	30.6	39	3.7	22.7	27.4	32.1
10.5	54	3.6	22.8	27.4	32.0	42	4.3	23.6	29.0	34.4
11.0	56	3.9	23.4	28.4	33.4	46	5.0	24.4	30.7	37.0
11.5	60	4.3	24.5	30.0	35.5	45	5.7	25.6	32.8	40.0
12.0	63	4.8	25.4	31.6	37.8	48	6.1	26.9	34.7	42.5
12.5	67	5.3	26.6	33.4	40.2	40	6.4	28.8	36.9	45.0
13.0	68	5.9	27.6	35.2	42.8	37	6.5	30.9	39.2	47.5
13.5	63	6.6	29.5	38.0	46.5	38	6.7	33.3	41.8	50.3
14.0	62	7.3	31.0	40.4	49.8	34	6.7	35.3	43.9	52.5
14.5	54	8.0	33.5	43.8	54.1	27	6.7	37.2	45.7	54.2
15.0	48	8.6	36.0	47.0	58.0	30	6.5	38.7	47.0	55.3
15.5	42	8.9	38.6	50.0	61.4	22	6.2	39.8	47.7	55.6
16.0	31	8.8	41.0	52.2	63.4	21	6.0	40.6	48.2	55.8
16.5	33	8.3	43.4	54.0	64.6	27	5.8	40.9	48.3	55.7
17.0	24	7.9	45.3	55.4	65.5	18	5.7	41.1	48.4	55.7
17.5	20	7.9	46.5	56.6	66.7	19	5.6	41.2	48.4	55.6
18.0	14	8.1	47.6	58.0	68.4	15	5.6	41.2	48.4	55.6
18.5	11	8.5	48.1	59.0	69.9	12	5.6	41.2	48.4	55.6
19.0	10	9.2	48.0	59.8	71.6	10	5.6	41.3	48.5	55.7
19.5	9	10.1	47.5	60.4	73.3	5	5.7	41.4	48.6	55.8
20.0	20	11.1	46.6	60.8	75.0	34	5.7	41.3	48.6	55.9

Table B.16 Growth of Yuendumu Aboriginals - Weight/Stature (gm/cm)

Age	N	SD	Males centiles			N	SD	Females centiles		
			10th	50th	90th			10th	50th	90th
5.0	0	—	—	—	—	0	—	—	—	—
5.5	0	—	—	—	—	0	—	—	—	—
6.0	4	9.0	149.5	161.0	172.5	3	—	137.4	151.5	165.6
6.5	6	12.5	147.0	163.0	179.0	8	11.4	141.4	156.0	170.6
7.0	15	15.2	147.3	166.8	186.3	10	12.2	144.9	160.5	176.1
7.5	16	16.8	149.3	170.8	192.3	17	13.2	150.3	167.2	184.1
8.0	24	17.2	153.8	175.9	198.0	25	14.2	154.3	172.5	190.7
8.5	29	17.8	157.7	180.5	203.3	27	15.6	159.0	179.0	199.0
9.0	38	18.0	162.4	185.5	208.6	33	17.0	164.2	186.0	207.8
9.5	44	18.2	167.7	191.0	214.3	39	18.6	168.7	192.5	216.3
10.0	50	19.2	171.9	196.5	221.1	39	20.6	173.1	199.5	225.9
10.5	52	20.3	175.8	201.9	228.0	42	23.1	177.9	207.5	237.1
11.0	56	21.2	179.3	206.5	233.7	46	26.0	181.7	215.0	248.3
11.5	60	22.4	183.6	212.3	241.0	45	28.8	187.8	224.7	261.6
12.0	63	23.8	189.5	220.0	250.5	45	31.4	193.2	233.5	273.8
12.5	67	26.4	194.7	228.5	262.3	40	34.0	200.4	244.0	287.6
13.0	68	29.4	199.8	237.5	275.2	37	35.8	209.1	255.0	300.9
13.5	63	32.0	206.0	247.0	288.0	38	37.2	218.1	265.8	313.5
14.0	60	34.2	214.2	258.0	301.8	34	38.0	227.7	276.4	325.1
14.5	54	36.4	222.3	269.0	315.7	27	37.9	236.7	285.3	333.9
15.0	48	38.4	234.8	284.0	333.2	30	37.4	243.1	291.0	338.9
15.5	42	40.2	248.5	300.0	351.5	22	36.6	247.1	294.0	340.9
16.0	31	42.0	257.7	311.5	365.3	21	35.2	250.7	295.8	340.9
16.5	33	43.2	264.6	320.0	375.4	27	34.8	251.9	296.5	341.1
17.0	22	44.4	269.1	326.0	382.9	18	31.8	256.2	297.0	337.8
17.5	18	45.4	272.3	330.5	388.7	19	29.2	259.8	297.2	334.6
18.0	12	47.2	274.0	334.5	395.0	15	26.4	264.1	297.9	331.7
18.5	11	49.2	275.9	339.0	402.1	12	20.8	271.3	298.0	324.7
19.0	10	52.0	279.3	346.0	412.7	5	14.0	280.6	298.5	316.4
19.5	9	55.1	284.0	354.6	425.2	5	5.0	292.6	299.0	305.4
20.0	20	57.6	288.2	362.0	435.8	34	0.0	299.0	299.0	299.0

Table B.17 Growth of Yuendumu Aboriginals - Radius Length (cm)

Age	N	SD	Males centiles			N	SD	Females centiles		
			10th	50th	90th			10th	50th	90th
5.0	0	—	16.0	16.6	17.2	1	—	14.7	15.8	16.9
5.5	3	—	16.3	17.0	17.7	4	0.9	15.0	16.2	17.4
6.0	4	0.6	16.6	17.4	18.2	3	—	15.5	16.6	17.8
6.5	6	0.7	16.9	17.9	18.8	8	0.9	15.9	17.1	18.2
7.0	15	0.9	17.2	18.3	19.4	10	0.9	16.4	17.6	18.8
7.5	18	1.0	17.5	18.7	19.9	17	1.0	17.0	18.3	19.5
8.0	24	1.0	17.8	19.1	20.4	25	1.0	17.5	18.8	20.1
8.5	29	1.1	18.1	19.5	20.9	27	1.0	18.0	19.3	20.6
9.0	39	1.1	18.4	19.9	21.3	31	1.1	18.4	19.8	21.2
9.5	47	1.1	18.8	20.3	21.7	37	1.2	18.8	20.3	21.8
10.0	52	1.2	19.2	20.7	22.2	40	1.3	19.2	20.8	22.4
10.5	54	1.2	19.7	21.1	22.6	43	1.3	19.7	21.4	23.1
11.0	56	1.2	20.1	21.6	23.1	45	1.4	20.2	22.0	23.7
11.5	60	1.2	20.4	22.0	23.6	44	1.4	20.7	22.5	24.3
12.0	63	1.3	20.9	22.5	24.1	47	1.4	21.1	23.0	24.8
12.5	67	1.4	21.2	22.9	24.6	39	1.4	21.6	23.4	25.2
13.0	68	1.5	21.5	23.4	25.2	36	1.4	21.9	23.7	25.5
13.5	63	1.5	21.8	23.8	25.8	37	1.4	22.2	24.0	25.8
14.0	63	1.6	22.3	24.4	26.4	34	1.3	22.5	24.3	26.0
14.5	55	1.7	22.8	24.9	27.0	27	1.3	22.8	24.4	26.0
15.0	48	1.7	23.3	25.4	27.5	30	1.2	23.0	24.6	26.2
15.5	42	1.6	23.8	25.9	28.0	21	1.2	23.1	24.7	26.3
16.0	31	1.6	24.2	26.3	28.3	20	1.2	23.3	24.8	26.3
16.5	33	1.6	24.5	26.5	28.5	27	1.2	23.4	24.9	26.4
17.0	24	1.5	24.8	26.8	28.7	18	1.2	23.4	25.0	26.5
17.5	20	1.4	25.1	27.0	28.8	20	1.2	23.5	25.0	26.5
18.0	15	1.4	25.4	27.2	28.9	16	1.2	23.4	25.0	26.6
18.5	12	1.3	25.6	27.3	29.0	12	1.2	23.4	25.0	26.6
19.0	10	1.3	25.7	27.3	28.9	10	1.2	23.4	25.0	26.6
19.5	9	1.2	25.8	27.4	28.9	6	1.3	23.4	25.0	26.6
20.0	20	1.2	25.9	27.4	28.9	33	1.3	23.3	25.0	26.7

Table B.18 Growth of Yuendumu Aboriginals - Head Length (cm)

Age	N	SD	Males centiles			N	SD	Females centiles		
			10th	50th	90th			10th	50th	90th
5.0	0	—	17.5	18.2	18.8	1	—	16.4	16.9	17.4
5.5	3	—	17.6	18.2	18.8	4	0.4	16.6	17.1	17.6
6.0	4	0.5	17.6	18.2	18.8	3	—	16.8	17.3	17.8
6.5	6	0.5	17.6	18.2	18.8	8	0.4	16.9	17.5	18.0
7.0	15	0.5	17.6	18.2	18.9	10	0.5	17.0	17.6	18.2
7.5	18	0.6	17.6	18.3	19.0	17	0.5	17.1	17.8	18.4
8.0	24	0.6	17.6	18.3	19.1	25	0.5	17.2	17.9	18.5
8.5	29	0.6	17.6	18.4	19.2	27	0.5	17.3	18.0	18.7
9.0	39	0.7	17.6	18.5	19.3	31	0.6	17.4	18.1	18.8
9.5	47	0.7	17.6	18.6	19.5	37	0.6	17.4	18.2	19.0
10.0	52	0.8	17.7	18.6	19.6	40	0.6	17.5	18.3	19.0
10.5	54	0.8	17.7	18.7	19.7	43	0.6	17.6	18.4	19.2
11.0	56	0.8	17.8	18.8	19.8	4	0.6	17.6	18.4	19.2
11.5	60	0.8	17.9	18.9	19.8	45	0.6	17.7	18.5	19.3
12.0	63	0.8	17.9	18.9	19.9	48	0.6	17.7	18.6	19.4
12.5	67	0.8	18.0	19.0	20.0	40	0.7	17.8	18.6	19.4
13.0	68	0.8	18.1	19.1	20.0	37	0.7	17.8	18.7	19.5
13.5	63	0.7	18.2	19.1	20.1	38	0.6	17.9	18.8	19.6
14.0	63	0.7	18.3	19.2	20.1	34	0.6	18.0	18.8	19.6
14.5	55	0.7	18.4	19.3	20.2	27	0.6	18.1	18.9	19.7
15.0	48	0.7	18.5	19.4	20.3	30	0.6	18.1	18.9	19.7
15.5	42	0.8	18.5	19.5	20.5	22	0.6	18.2	19.0	19.8
16.0	31	0.8	18.6	19.6	20.7	21	0.6	18.2	19.0	19.8
16.5	33	0.8	18.7	19.8	20.8	27	0.6	18.2	19.0	19.8
17.0	24	0.8	18.9	19.9	21.0	18	0.6	18.2	19.0	19.8
17.5	20	0.8	19.0	20.1	21.1	20	0.6	18.3	19.0	19.7
18.0	15	0.8	19.2	20.2	21.2	16	0.6	18.3	19.0	19.7
18.5	12	0.8	19.2	20.1	21.1	12	0.6	18.3	19.0	19.7
19.0	10	0.7	19.4	20.4	21.3	10	0.5	18.3	19.0	19.7
19.5	9	0.7	19.5	20.4	21.3	6	0.5	18.3	19.0	19.7
20.0	20	0.7	19.5	20.4	21.3	34	0.5	18.3	19.0	19.7

Table B.19 Growth of Yuendumu Aboriginals - Head Breadth (cm)

Age	N	SD	Males centiles			N	SD	Females centiles		
			10th	50th	90th			10th	50th	90th
5.0	0	—	12.3	12.8	13.3	1	—	11.9	12.3	12.7
5.5	3	—	12.4	12.8	13.3	4	0.3	12.0	12.4	12.8
6.0	4	0.4	12.4	12.8	13.3	3	—	12.0	12.5	12.9
6.5	6	0.4	12.4	12.9	13.3	8	0.3	12.1	12.5	13.0
7.0	15	0.4	12.4	12.9	13.4	10	0.3	12.2	12.6	13.0
7.5	18	0.4	12.5	13.0	13.4	17	0.4	12.2	12.7	13.1
8.0	24	0.4	12.6	13.0	13.5	25	0.4	12.3	12.7	13.2
8.5	29	0.4	12.6	13.1	13.6	27	0.4	12.3	12.8	13.3
9.0	39	0.4	12.6	13.2	13.7	31	0.4	12.4	12.9	13.3
9.5	47	0.4	12.7	13.2	13.7	37	0.4	12.5	12.9	13.4
10.0	52	0.4	12.7	13.2	13.8	40	0.4	12.5	13.0	13.5
10.5	54	0.4	12.7	13.3	13.8	43	0.4	12.6	13.1	13.6
11.0	56	0.5	12.7	13.3	13.9	46	0.4	12.6	13.1	13.6
11.5	60	0.5	12.7	13.3	13.9	45	0.4	12.6	13.2	13.7
12.0	63	0.5	12.8	13.4	14.0	48	0.4	12.7	13.2	13.8
12.5	67	0.5	12.8	13.5	14.1	40	0.5	12.7	13.3	13.9
13.0	68	0.5	12.9	13.5	14.2	37	0.5	12.8	13.4	13.9
13.5	63	0.5	13.0	13.6	14.2	38	0.5	12.8	13.4	14.0
14.0	63	0.5	13.1	13.7	14.3	34	0.5	12.9	13.5	14.1
14.5	55	0.5	13.2	13.8	14.3	27	0.5	12.9	13.5	14.1
15.0	48	0.5	13.2	13.8	14.4	30	0.5	13.0	13.6	14.2
15.5	42	0.5	13.3	13.9	14.5	22	0.5	13.0	13.6	14.2
16.0	31	0.5	13.4	14.0	14.6	21	0.5	13.0	13.6	14.2
16.5	33	0.5	13.4	14.1	14.7	27	0.5	13.1	13.7	14.2
17.0	24	0.5	13.5	14.1	14.7	18	0.5	13.1	13.7	14.3
17.5	20	0.5	13.5	14.1	14.7	20	0.5	13.1	13.7	14.3
18.0	15	0.5	13.6	14.1	14.7	16	0.4	13.1	13.7	14.3
18.5	12	0.4	13.6	14.1	14.7	12	0.4	13.1	13.7	14.3
19.0	10	0.4	13.6	14.1	14.7	10	0.4	13.2	13.7	14.2
19.5	9	0.4	13.6	14.1	14.7	6	0.4	13.2	13.7	14.2
20.0	20	0.4	13.6	14.1	14.7	34	0.4	13.2	13.7	14.2

Table B.20 Growth of Yuendumu Aboriginals - Head Circumference (cm)

Age	N	SD	Males centiles			N	SD	Females centiles		
			10th	50th	90th			10th	50th	90th
5.0	0	—	49.3	50.7	52.1	1	—	48.2	49.3	50.4
5.5	3	—	49.3	50.8	52.2	4	0.9	48.4	49.5	50.7
6.0	4	1.1	49.4	50.9	52.3	3	—	48.6	49.8	51.0
6.5	6	1.2	49.5	51.0	52.5	8	1.0	48.8	50.1	51.4
7.0	15	1.2	49.6	51.2	52.7	10	1.0	49.0	50.3	51.7
7.5	18	1.3	49.7	51.4	53.0	17	1.1	49.2	50.6	51.9
8.0	24	1.5	49.6	51.5	53.4	25	1.1	50.4	51.8	53.2
8.5	29	1.7	49.6	51.7	53.8	27	1.2	49.5	51.0	52.6
9.0	39	1.7	49.7	51.9	54.1	31	1.2	49.7	51.3	52.9
9.5	47	1.7	49.9	52.0	54.2	37	1.3	49.8	51.5	53.1
10.0	52	1.7	50.1	52.2	54.4	40	1.4	50.0	51.8	53.5
10.5	54	1.6	50.4	52.5	54.6	43	1.4	50.1	52.0	53.8
11.0	56	1.6	50.6	52.7	54.8	46	1.5	50.3	52.2	54.1
11.5	60	1.6	50.9	53.0	55.1	45	1.6	50.4	52.4	54.5
12.0	62	1.7	51.1	53.2	55.3	48	1.6	50.6	52.7	54.7
12.5	66	1.7	51.3	53.5	55.6	40	1.6	50.8	52.9	55.0
13.0	67	1.7	51.5	53.7	56.0	37	1.6	51.1	53.1	55.2
13.5	62	1.8	51.7	54.0	56.3	38	1.6	51.4	53.4	55.4
14.0	63	1.9	51.8	54.2	56.6	34	1.6	51.7	53.7	55.7
14.5	55	1.9	52.0	54.5	57.0	27	1.5	52.1	54.0	56.0
15.0	48	2.0	52.4	54.9	57.5	30	1.5	52.3	54.2	56.1
15.5	42	2.0	52.8	55.4	58.0	22	1.4	52.4	54.2	56.1
16.0	31	2.1	53.1	55.8	58.4	21	1.4	52.5	54.3	56.1
16.5	33	2.1	53.4	56.0	58.7	27	1.3	52.6	54.3	56.0
17.0	24	2.1	53.6	56.2	58.9	18	1.3	52.7	54.4	56.0
17.5	20	2.1	53.7	56.4	59.1	20	1.3	52.8	54.4	56.0
18.0	15	2.0	54.0	56.6	59.2	16	1.2	52.8	54.4	55.9
18.5	12	2.0	54.2	56.8	59.4	12	1.2	52.9	54.4	55.9
19.0	10	2.0	54.6	57.1	59.6	10	1.1	52.9	54.4	55.8
19.5	9	1.9	55.1	57.5	59.9	6	1.1	53.0	54.4	55.8
20.0	20	1.8	55.6	58.0	60.3	33	1.1	53.0	54.4	55.8

Table B.21 Growth of Yuendumu Aboriginals - Cephalic Index (%)

Age	N	SD	Males centiles			N	SD	Females centiles		
			10th	50th	90th			10th	50th	90th
5.0	0	—	69.8	71.7	73.6	1	—	67.8	70.1	72.4
5.5	3	—	69.6	71.6	73.5	4	1.8	67.8	70.2	72.5
6.0	4	1.7	69.3	71.5	73.6	3	—	67.8	70.2	72.7
6.5	6	1.9	68.9	71.4	73.9	8	1.9	67.9	70.4	72.9
7.0	15	2.1	68.6	71.3	74.0	10	2.0	67.9	70.5	73.1
7.5	18	2.3	68.3	71.3	74.2	17	2.1	68.0	70.7	73.4
8.0	24	2.4	68.1	71.2	74.3	25	2.2	68.1	70.9	73.8
8.5	29	2.5	67.9	71.2	74.4	27	2.3	68.3	71.3	74.3
9.0	39	2.6	67.8	71.1	74.4	31	2.4	68.5	71.6	74.7
9.5	47	2.7	67.6	71.1	74.5	37	2.5	68.5	71.7	75.0
10.0	52	2.8	67.5	71.0	74.6	40	2.6	68.3	71.7	75.0
10.5	54	2.8	67.4	71.0	74.6	43	2.7	68.1	71.6	75.0
11.0	56	2.8	67.3	71.0	74.6	46	2.7	67.9	71.4	75.0
11.5	60	2.8	67.3	70.9	74.6	45	2.8	67.8	71.4	74.9
12.0	63	2.8	67.3	70.9	74.5	48	2.8	67.7	71.3	75.0
12.5	67	2.7	67.4	70.9	74.4	40	2.8	67.7	71.4	75.0
13.0	68	2.7	67.5	70.9	74.3	37	2.8	67.8	71.4	75.1
13.5	63	2.6	67.7	71.0	74.3	38	2.8	67.8	71.5	75.1
14.0	63	2.5	68.0	71.2	74.4	34	2.8	67.9	71.5	75.1
14.5	55	2.5	68.0	71.3	74.5	27	2.8	67.9	71.5	75.0
15.0	48	2.6	67.9	71.2	74.6	30	2.7	68.0	71.4	74.8
15.5	42	2.6	67.6	71.0	74.4	22	2.6	68.1	71.4	74.7
16.0	31	2.7	67.2	70.7	74.1	21	2.5	68.2	71.4	74.7
16.5	33	2.7	66.9	70.3	73.8	27	2.5	68.3	71.5	74.7
17.0	24	2.7	66.7	70.1	73.6	18	2.5	68.4	71.7	74.9
17.5	20	2.7	66.5	70.0	73.5	20	2.6	68.4	71.8	75.2
18.0	15	2.7	66.5	69.9	73.4	16	2.7	68.5	72.0	75.4
18.5	12	2.7	66.5	69.9	73.3	12	2.8	68.5	72.1	75.7
19.0	10	2.6	66.5	69.9	73.2	10	2.9	68.6	72.2	75.9
19.5	9	2.6	66.6	69.9	73.1	6	2.9	68.7	72.3	76.0
20.0	20	2.5	66.7	69.9	73.1	34	2.9	68.7	72.4	76.0

Table B.22 Growth of Yuendumu Aboriginals - Bizygomatic Diameter (cm)

Age	N	SD	Males centiles			N	SD	Females centiles		
			10th	50th	90th			10th	50th	90th
5.0	0	—	10.2	10.8	11.4	1	—	10.0	10.4	10.8
5.5	3	—	10.3	10.8	11.4	4	0.3	10.1	10.5	10.9
6.0	4	0.4	10.4	11.0	11.5	3	—	10.3	10.7	11.0
6.5	6	0.4	10.5	11.1	11.6	8	0.3	10.4	10.8	11.2
7.0	15	0.4	10.6	11.2	11.7	10	0.3	10.5	10.9	11.3
7.5	18	0.4	10.7	11.3	11.9	17	0.3	10.7	11.1	11.5
8.0	24	0.4	10.9	11.4	12.0	25	0.4	10.8	11.3	11.7
8.5	29	0.4	11.0	11.5	12.1	27	0.4	10.9	11.4	11.9
9.0	39	0.5	11.1	11.6	12.2	31	0.4	11.0	11.5	12.0
9.5	47	0.5	11.2	11.7	12.3	37	0.4	11.1	11.6	12.2
10.0	52	0.5	11.2	11.8	12.5	40	0.5	11.1	11.7	12.3
10.5	54	0.5	11.3	11.9	12.6	43	0.5	11.2	11.9	12.5
11.0	56	0.5	11.3	12.0	12.7	46	0.5	11.3	11.9	12.6
11.5	60	0.6	11.3	12.0	12.8	45	0.5	11.3	12.0	12.7
12.0	63	0.6	11.3	12.1	12.9	48	0.6	11.4	12.1	12.8
12.5	67	0.6	11.4	12.2	13.0	40	0.5	11.5	12.2	12.9
13.0	68	0.6	11.5	12.3	13.1	37	0.5	11.6	12.3	13.0
13.5	63	0.6	11.6	12.4	13.3	38	0.5	11.8	12.4	13.1
14.0	63	0.6	11.8	12.6	13.4	34	0.5	11.9	12.5	13.2
14.5	55	0.6	12.1	12.8	13.6	27	0.5	12.1	12.6	13.2
15.0	48	0.6	12.3	13.0	13.7	30	0.5	12.1	12.7	13.3
15.5	42	0.6	12.5	13.2	13.9	22	0.4	12.2	12.8	13.4
16.0	31	0.5	12.6	13.3	14.0	21	0.4	12.3	12.9	13.4
16.5	33	0.5	12.8	13.4	14.0	27	0.4	12.4	12.9	13.5
17.0	24	0.5	12.9	13.5	14.1	18	0.4	12.5	13.0	13.5
17.5	20	0.5	12.9	13.5	14.1	20	0.4	12.5	13.0	13.5
18.0	15	0.5	13.0	13.6	14.2	16	0.4	12.5	13.0	13.5
18.5	12	0.5	13.1	13.7	14.3	12	0.4	12.5	13.0	13.5
19.0	10	0.5	13.3	13.9	14.5	10	0.4	12.6	13.0	13.5
19.5	9	0.5	13.4	14.0	14.7	6	0.4	12.6	13.0	13.5
20.0	20	0.5	13.4	14.1	14.8	34	0.4	12.6	13.0	13.5

Table B.23 Growth of Yuendumu Aboriginals - Bigonial Diameter (cm)

Age	N	SD	Males centiles			N	SD	Females centiles		
			10th	50th	90th			10th	50th	90th
5.0	0	—	7.8	8.1	8.5	1	—	7.1	7.5	7.9
5.5	3	—	7.8	8.2	8.5	4	0.3	7.2	7.6	8.0
6.0	4	0.3	7.9	8.3	8.6	3	—	7.3	7.7	8.2
6.5	6	0.3	7.9	8.3	8.7	8	0.4	7.4	7.9	8.4
7.0	15	0.4	8.0	8.4	8.8	10	0.4	7.5	8.0	8.5
7.5	18	0.4	8.0	8.5	9.0	17	0.4	7.6	8.2	8.7
8.0	24	0.4	8.1	8.6	9.1	25	0.4	7.7	8.3	8.8
8.5	29	0.4	8.1	8.7	9.2	27	0.4	7.8	8.4	9.0
9.0	39	0.5	8.2	8.7	9.3	31	0.5	7.9	8.5	9.1
9.5	47	0.5	8.2	8.8	9.4	37	0.5	8.0	8.6	9.2
10.0	52	0.5	8.3	8.9	9.6	40	0.5	8.1	8.7	9.3
10.5	54	0.5	8.3	9.0	9.7	43	0.5	8.2	8.8	9.4
11.0	56	0.6	8.4	9.1	9.8	46	0.5	8.3	8.9	9.6
11.5	60	0.6	8.4	9.2	9.9	45	0.5	8.4	9.0	9.7
12.0	63	0.6	8.5	9.3	10.0	47	0.5	8.4	9.1	9.7
12.5	67	0.6	8.6	9.3	10.1	39	0.5	8.5	9.2	9.8
13.0	68	0.6	8.7	9.4	10.2	36	0.5	8.6	9.3	9.9
13.5	62	0.6	8.8	9.5	10.2	37	0.5	8.6	9.3	10.0
14.0	62	0.5	8.9	9.6	10.3	34	0.5	8.7	9.4	10.1
14.5	54	0.5	9.1	9.7	10.4	27	0.5	8.8	9.5	10.1
15.0	47	0.5	9.2	9.9	10.5	30	0.5	8.9	9.5	10.2
15.5	41	0.5	9.4	10.0	10.6	22	0.5	8.9	9.6	10.2
16.0	30	0.5	9.5	10.1	10.7	21	0.5	9.0	9.6	10.3
16.5	33	0.5	9.6	10.2	10.7	27	0.5	9.1	9.7	10.3
17.0	4	0.5	9.6	10.2	10.8	18	0.5	9.1	9.7	10.3
17.5	20	0.5	9.6	10.3	10.9	20	0.5	9.2	9.8	10.4
18.0	15	0.5	9.6	10.3	10.9	16	0.5	9.2	9.8	10.4
18.5	12	0.5	9.6	10.3	11.0	12	0.4	9.2	9.8	10.4
19.0	10	0.6	9.6	10.3	11.0	10	0.4	9.2	9.8	10.4
19.5	9	0.6	9.5	10.3	11.1	6	0.4	9.3	9.8	10.3
20.0	20	0.7	9.5	10.3	11.2	34	0.4	9.3	9.8	10.3

Table B.24 Growth of Yuendumu Aboriginals - Face Height (cm)

Age	N	SD	Males centiles			N	SD	Females centiles		
			10th	50th	90th			10th	50th	90th
5.0	0	—	8.9	9.1	9.4	1	—	8.1	8.7	9.3
5.5	3	—	8.9	9.2	9.4	4	0.5	8.2	8.8	9.4
6.0	4	0.3	8.9	9.2	9.5	3	—	8.2	8.9	9.5
6.5	6	0.3	8.9	9.2	9.6	8	0.5	8.3	9.0	9.6
7.0	15	0.3	8.9	9.3	9.7	10	0.5	8.4	9.1	9.7
7.5	18	0.3	9.0	9.4	9.8	17	0.5	8.5	9.2	9.8
8.0	24	0.4	9.0	9.5	9.9	25	0.5	8.6	9.3	9.9
8.5	29	0.4	9.0	9.5	10.0	27	0.5	8.7	9.4	10.0
9.0	39	0.4	9.0	9.5	10.0	31	0.5	8.9	9.5	10.1
9.5	47	0.4	9.0	9.5	10.1	37	0.5	9.0	9.6	10.2
10.0	52	0.4	9.0	9.6	10.1	40	0.5	9.1	9.7	10.3
10.5	54	0.5	9.1	9.6	10.2	43	0.5	9.3	9.8	10.4
11.0	56	0.5	9.1	9.7	10.3	46	0.5	9.3	9.9	10.5
11.5	60	0.5	9.2	9.8	10.4	45	0.5	9.4	10.0	10.6
12.0	63	0.5	9.3	9.9	10.5	48	0.5	9.4	10.1	10.7
12.5	67	0.5	9.4	10.0	10.6	40	0.5	9.5	10.2	10.8
13.0	68	0.5	9.5	10.1	10.7	37	0.5	9.6	10.3	10.9
13.5	63	0.5	9.6	10.2	10.8	38	0.5	9.7	10.4	11.1
14.0	63	0.5	9.7	10.4	11.0	34	0.5	9.8	10.5	11.2
14.5	55	0.5	9.9	10.6	11.2	27	0.5	9.9	10.6	11.3
15.0	48	0.6	10.0	10.7	11.5	30	0.5	10.0	10.7	11.3
15.5	42	0.6	10.1	10.9	11.7	22	0.5	10.1	10.7	11.4
16.0	31	0.7	10.2	11.0	11.9	21	0.5	10.1	10.8	11.4
16.5	33	0.7	10.3	11.1	12.0	27	0.5	10.1	10.8	11.4
17.0	24	0.7	10.3	11.2	12.0	18	0.5	10.2	10.8	11.4
17.5	20	0.6	10.5	11.2	12.0	20	0.5	10.2	10.8	11.4
18.0	15	0.6	10.5	11.3	12.0	16	0.5	10.2	10.8	11.4
18.5	12	0.5	10.7	11.3	12.0	12	0.4	10.2	10.8	11.3
19.0	10	0.5	10.7	11.4	12.1	10	0.4	10.3	10.8	11.3
19.5	9	0.5	10.8	11.5	12.2	6	0.4	10.3	10.8	11.3
20.0	20	0.5	11.1	11.8	12.5	34	0.4	10.3	10.8	11.3

Appendix C

Photographs of Yuendumu and its People

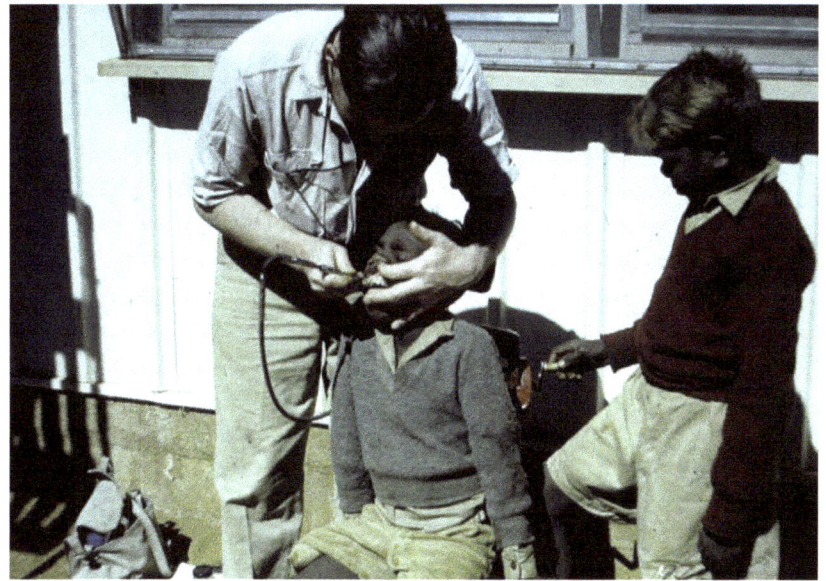

Murray Barrett treating an unidentified Warlpiri boy in the 1950s.

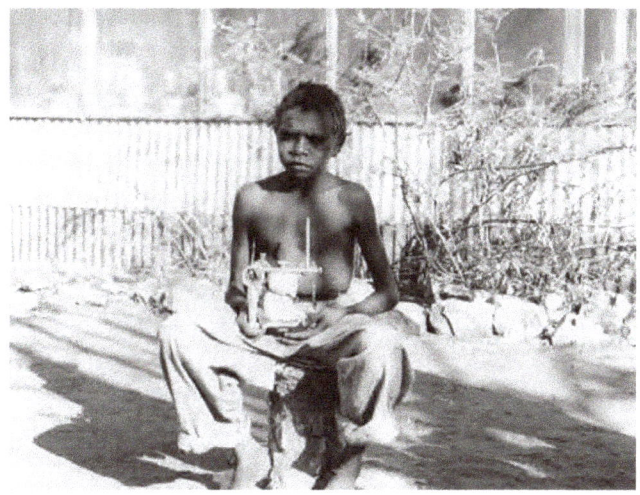

Johnny Wayne Jungarrayi.

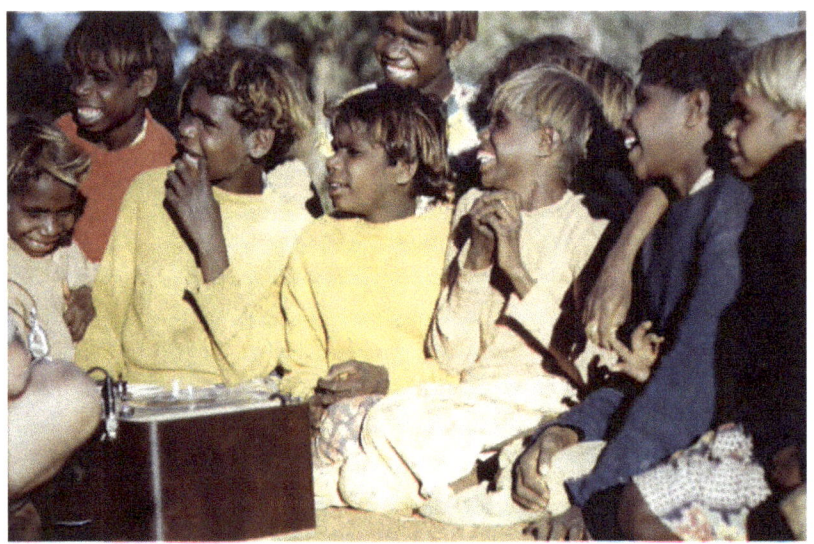
Having fun with a tape recorder.

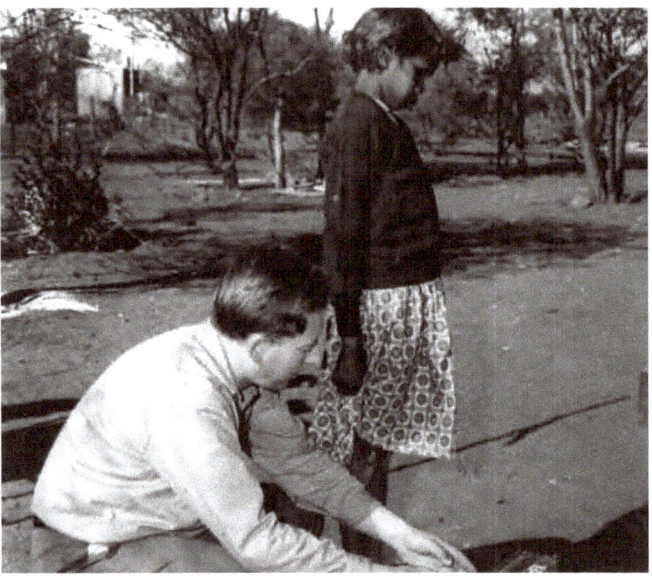
Tasman Brown measuring body weight of an unidentified Aboriginal girl, 1960s.

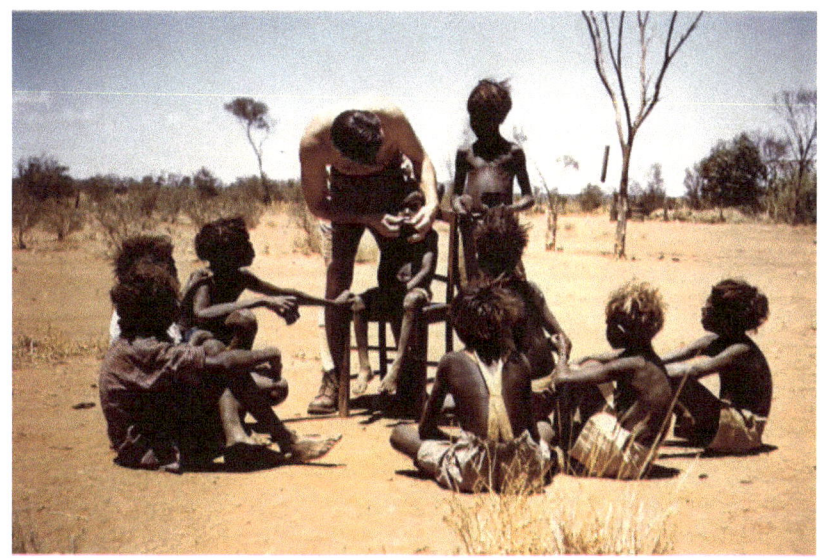
Obtaining a dental impression.

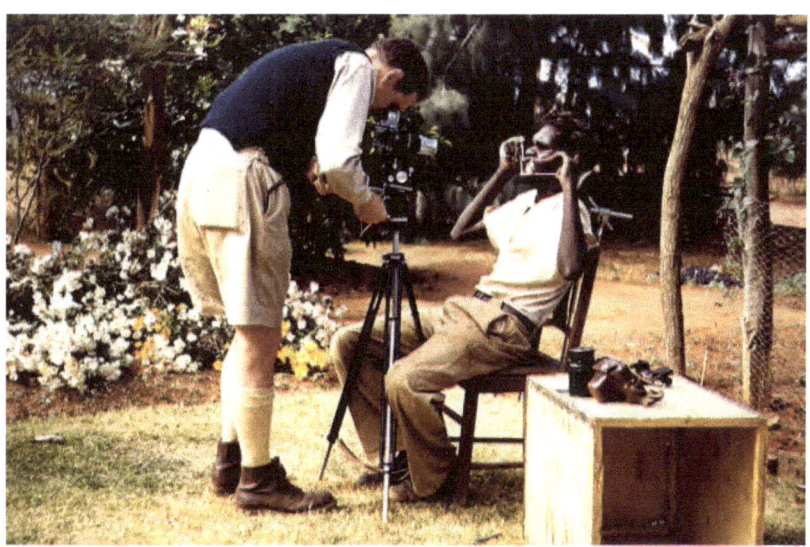
Murray Barrett photographing Harry Jakamarra Nelson's teeth.

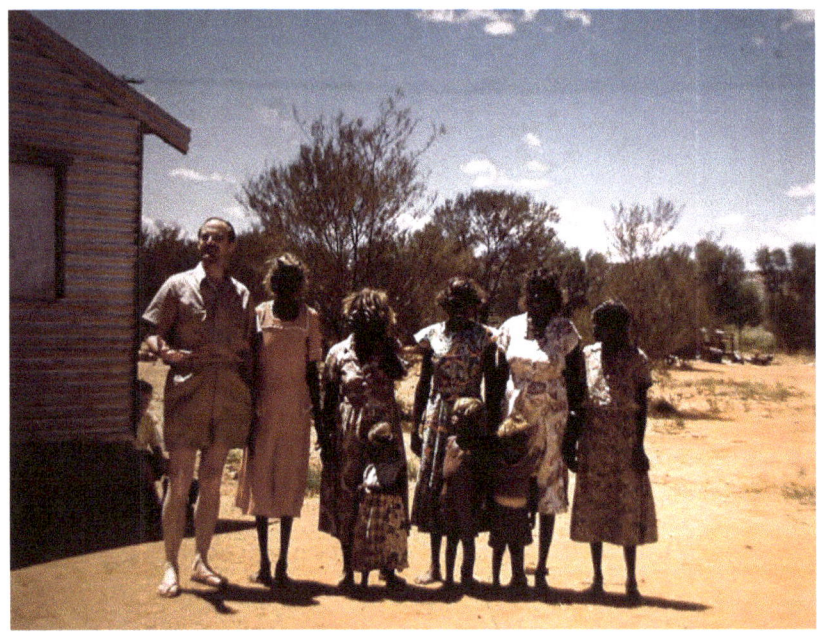
Murray Barrett with mothers and children, Yuendumu 1962.

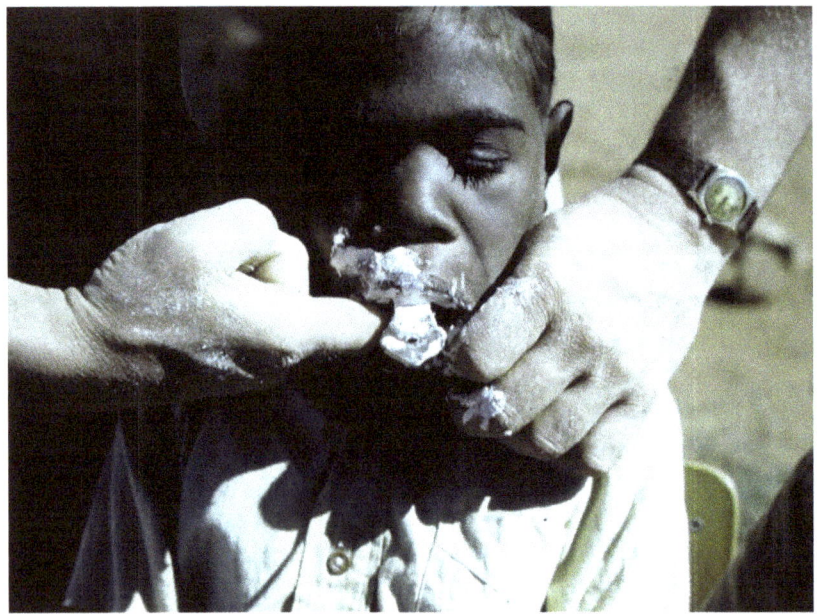
Making some dental impressions.

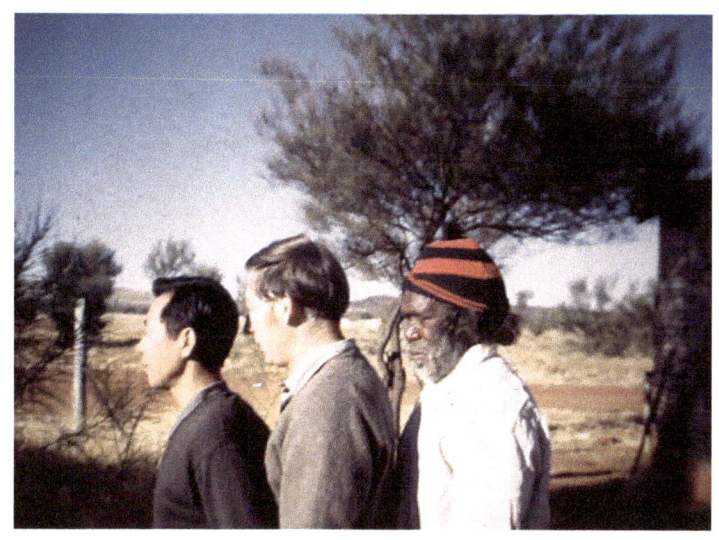

Left to right, Tadashi Ozaki, Tasman Brown and Jimmy Jungarai Spencer, Yuendumu 1962.

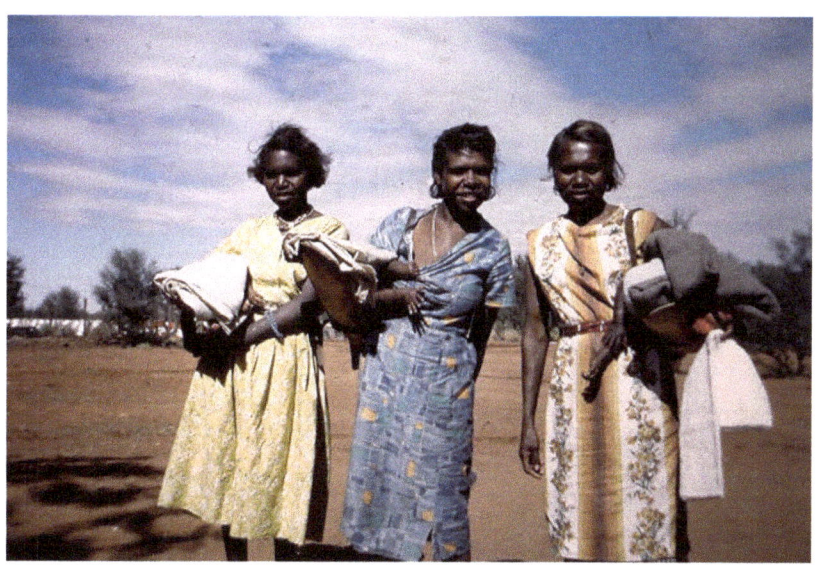

Left to right, Jillie Nakamarra Spencer, Cindy Napaljarri, Judy Nampijinpa Granites 1967.

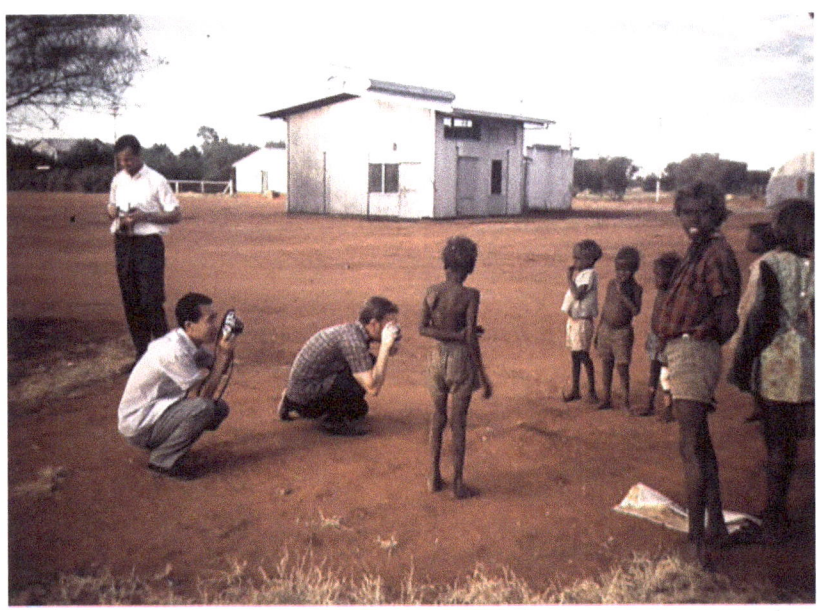
Photographic session at Yuendumu 1969.

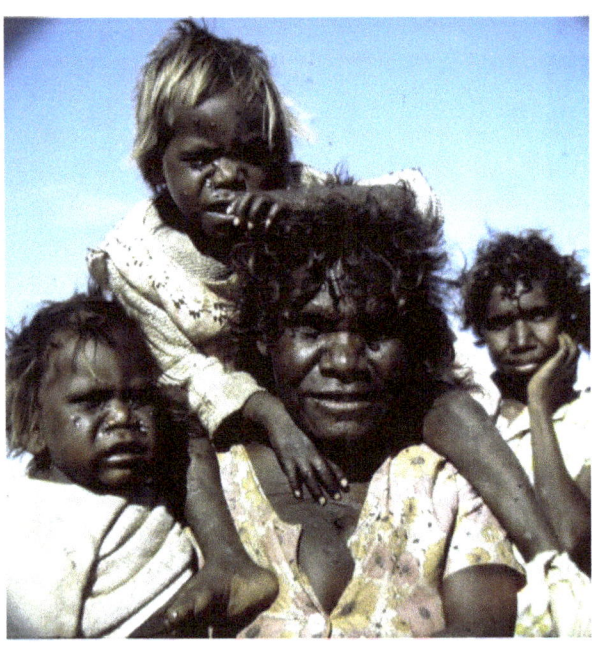
Wikija Nampijinpa (with Portia and Nigel) and Renne Napangardi Marshall.

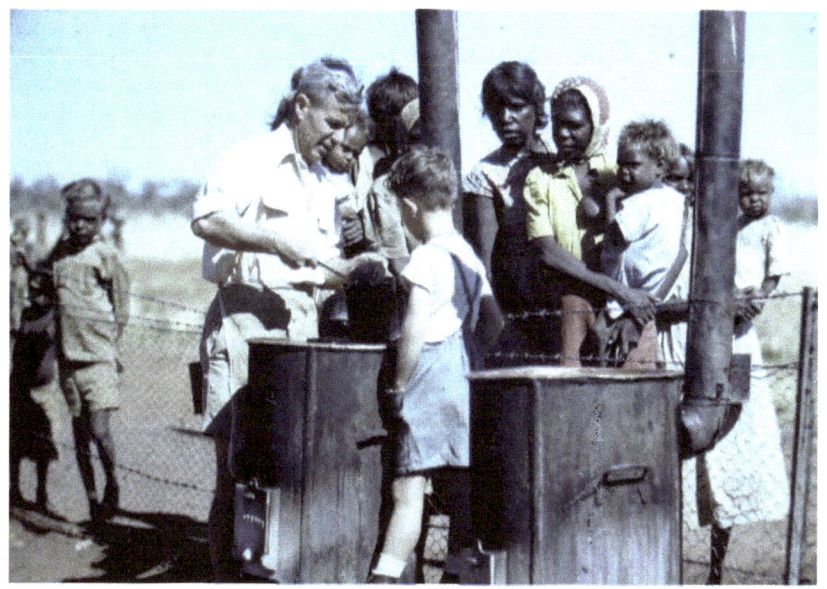
Rev Tom Fleming at the soup kitchen.

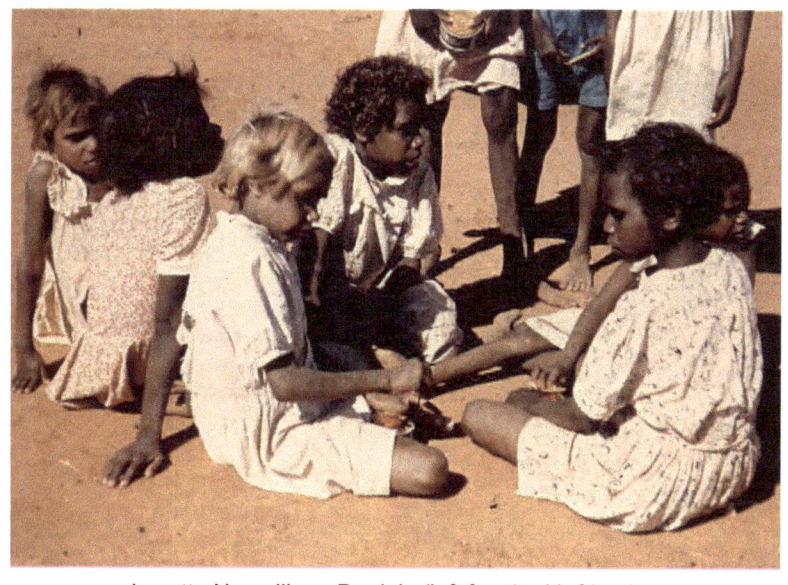
Lynette Nampijinpa Daniels (left front) with friends.

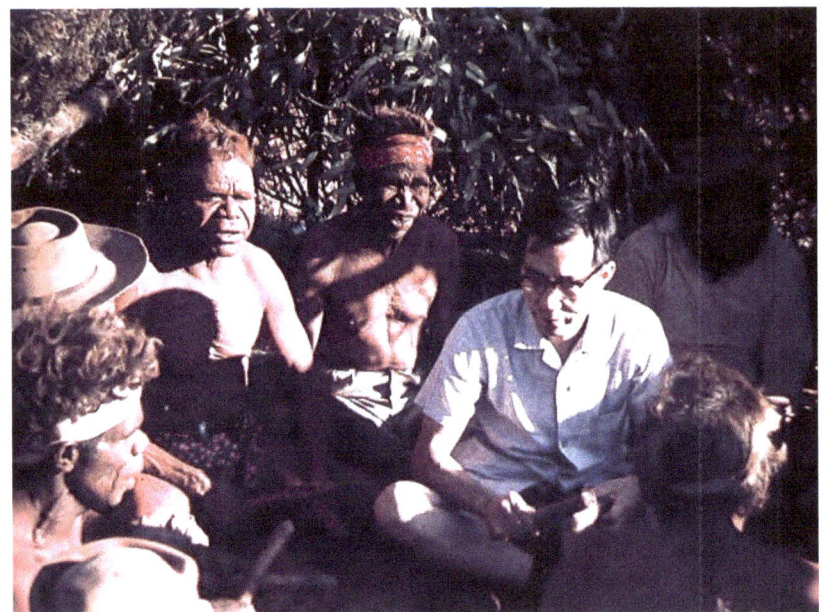
Tadashi Ozaki with Warlpiri men.

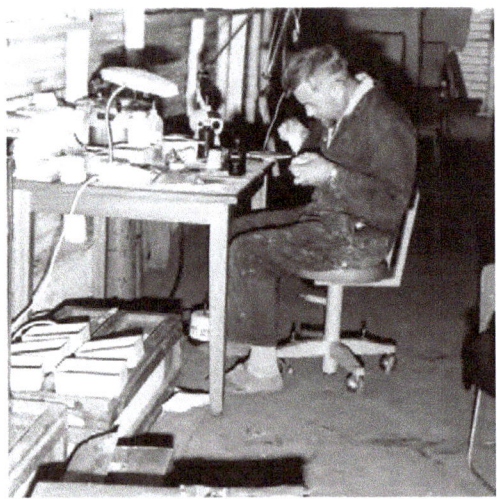
Leslie Reynolds at the technicians' work bench 1972.

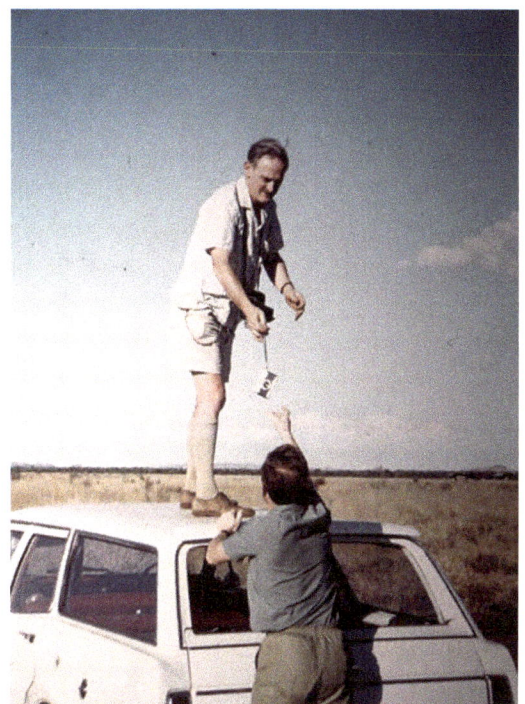
Murray Barrett getting a better view.

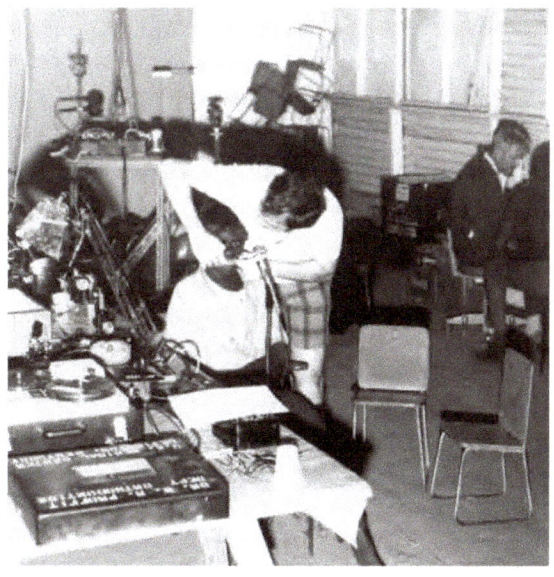
The clinic and laboratory at Yuendumu circa 1972.

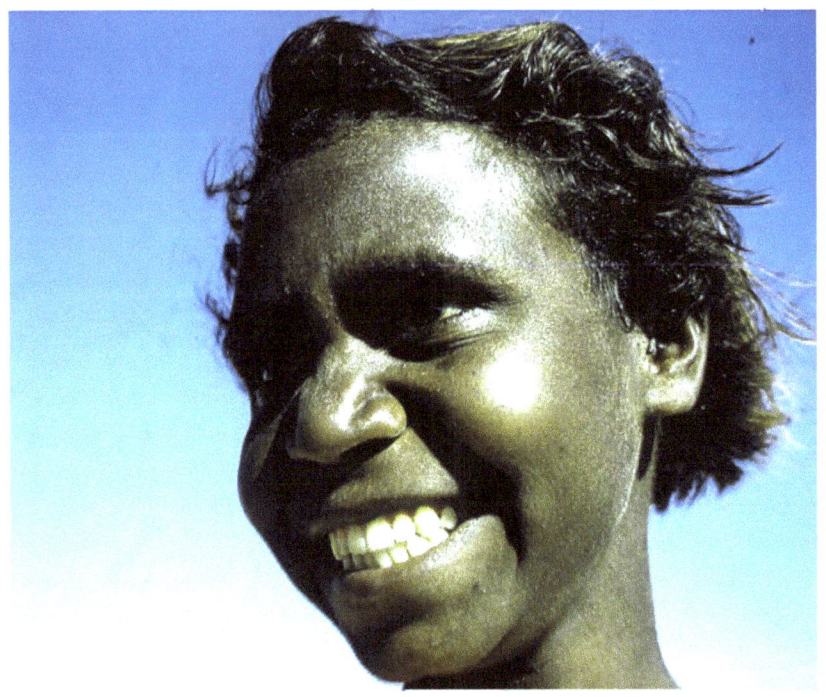

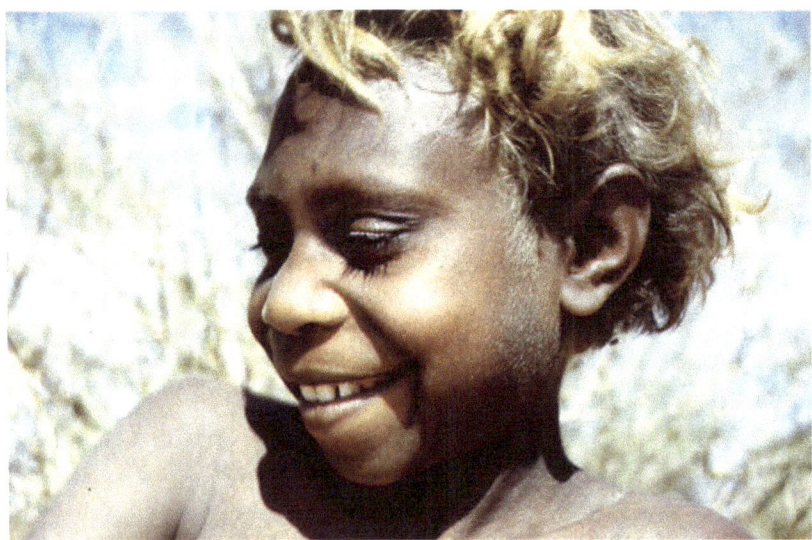

Gracey Napangardi.

Appendices

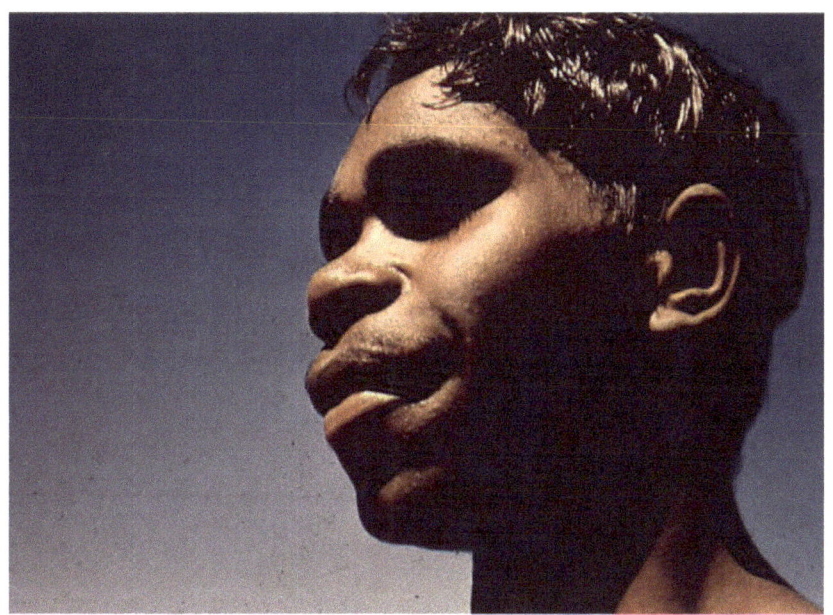

Johnny Wayne Jungarrayi.

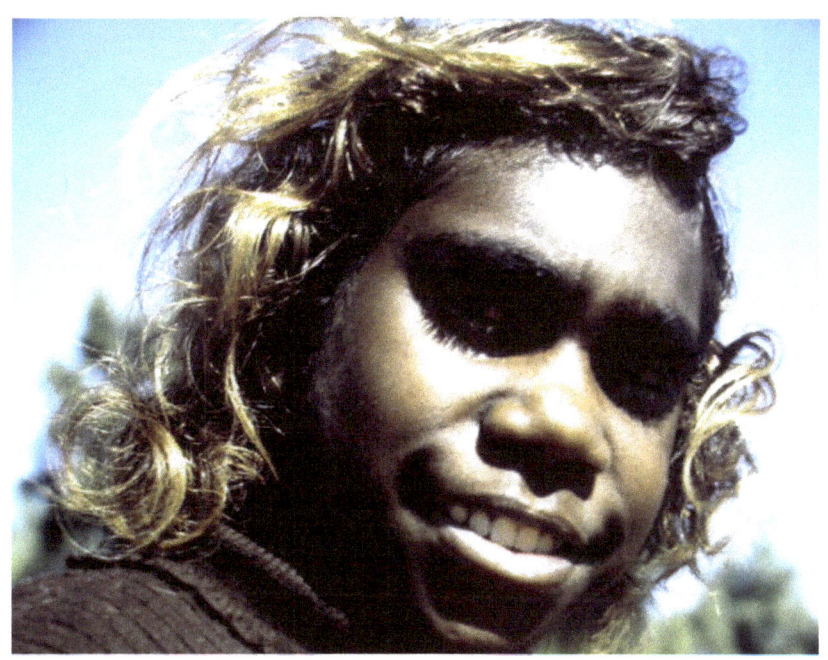

Janey Napanangka Langdon.

A completely searchable PDF edition of this book is available at www.adelaide.edu.au/press

Photographs with fine detail can be viewed in the PDF at up to 400% of their size for readability

www.ingramcontent.com/pod-product-compliance
Lightning Source LLC
Chambersburg PA
CBHW061121010526
44112CB00024B/2943